Living with M.E.

Dr Charles Shepherd qualified in medicine from London's Middlesex Hospital in 1974, where he initially specialised in sexually transmitted diseases. Following this he was appointed to hospital posts in a variety of specialities including psychiatry, paediatrics, infectious diseases and casualty before becoming Resident Medical Officer at Cirencester Hospital in Gloucestershire. He has also worked in both general practice and the pharmaceutical industry. Since becoming ill with M.E. Dr Shepherd has reluctantly had to leave the NHS and now works privately from his home in Gloucestershire. His involvement with the M.E. Association led to him becoming their medical advisor in 1989. In this role he is particularly involved with promoting a better public understanding of the illness through contacts with the media and educating doctors and other health professionals at medical seminars. He has also been personally involved in a number of M.E. research projects, and in 1990 played a major role in bringing together scientists and clinicians from both sides of the Atlantic to the first international symposium on the illness at Cambridge University. Dr Shepherd is also very interested in the area of health fraud, and has helped to bring a number of dubious treatments, including germanium, to the attention of the Department of Health.

Dr CHARLES SHEPHERD

Living
with
M.E.

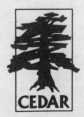

CEDAR

A Mandarin Paperback
LIVING WITH M.E.

First published in Great Britain 1989
by Cedar
This revised edition published 1992 by Cedar
an imprint of Reed Consumer Books Limited
Michelin House, 81 Fulham Road, London SW3 6RB
and Auckland, Melbourne, Singapore and Toronto

Reprinted 1992, 1993

Copyright © 1989, 1992 Charles Shepherd

A CIP catalogue record for this title
is available from the British Library
ISBN 0 7493 1264 5

Printed and bound in Great Britain
by Cox & Wyman Ltd, Reading, Berks

Contents

Part 2: Practical steps towards coping with M.E.

Part 3: Learning to Live with M.E.

Acknowledgement

I should like to acknowledge the help of Dr Melvin Ramsay, who diagnosed my own illness back in 1982.

Dr Ramsay was consultant physician at the Royal Free Hospital in London during the time of an outbreak of an infectious illness that became known as 'the Royal Free disease' and subsequently myalgic encephalomyelitis (M.E.). He did more than anybody else to legitimize this devastating illness, and was prepared to stand up for his patients against a background of controversy and cynicism from the medical establishment. In the end his theories have been shown to be correct.

Sadly, Melvin Ramsay died on 29 March 1990, just a matter of days before he was to be the first speaker at the Cambridge University International Symposium on M.E. where he would have presented the culmination of thirty-five years of painstaking work.

Foreword

There is still a great deal of confusion in the mind of the medical profession regarding the precise clinical identity of myalgic encephalomyelitis and this can, in great measure, be attributed to the current belief that M.E. and the many post-viral fatigue states are synonymous. Far from being synonymous they are distinguishable, in the first place, by the long delay in the restoration of muscle power after even a minor degree of physical effort; secondly, by the extraordinary variability of symptoms even in the course of one day; and finally, by the alarming tendency of the disease to become chronic. On the other hand, the fatigue factor in the post-viral states is merely part of a general fatigue, shows no daily variability and the condition is unlikely to last longer than two years.

The incidence of M.E. among doctors is out of all proportion to their numbers in the general population. Dr Charles Shepherd has now had the disease for close on ten years. His experience of the vagaries of the disease – alternating periods of remission and relapse since the diagnosis was confirmed in 1982 – puts him in an ideal position to help other victims of this distressing complaint.

The chronic M.E. sufferer faces a condition of constant muscle fatigue, often severe muscle pain and discomfort as a result of spasm and twitchings. This is accompanied by cerebral dysfunction in the form of impairment of memory and powers of concentration, emotional lability, disturbed sleep rhythm, vivid dreams, and lack of muscle co-ordination that renders the patient incapable of carrying out simple manoeuvres. This is all too often accompanied by a sense of rejection by friends and relatives as a hopeless neurotic. Dr Shepherd can give these pitiful victims of a disease that is still imperfectly understood, invaluable assistance in the planning of their lives, on a basis that can afford them a sense of purpose in combating what would otherwise be a drab and pointless existence. I thoroughly commend his excellent treatise.

Dr A. Melvin Ramsay
President of the Myalgic Encephalomyelitis Association
Died 29.3.90.

Introduction

It is often said that doctors have no real understanding of a disease unless they contract it themselves. I have now had M.E. for the past twelve years and so have first-hand experience of its debilitating symptoms and of the havoc it can wreak on both career and family life. All thoughts of running my own general practice in the country have had to be abandoned; my wife has become chief breadwinner in addition to shouldering most of the responsibility for running our home and bringing up two young children; M.E. has imposed severe limitations on our lives. Incapacitating though it is, M.E. is only now coming to be recognised by the medical profession as a genuine disease. So, what is it like to have M.E.?

Imagine waking up every single morning for months, even years, with the certain knowledge that for the rest of the day you will be wandering around feeling as though you have flu; that your brain will soon become fogged and completely unable to function correctly, and that after even a short walk to the shops you may be forced to lie down feeling exhausted. Not a very pleasant thought, but that's what it's like having M.E. It not only reduces your day to a few useful hours in which you may be able to function with some degree of normality, it can actually take years out of a whole lifetime.

M.E. is short for myalgic encephalomyelitis, which simply means an illness affecting the muscles (myalgia = muscle pain), the brain (encephalo) and the nervous system (myelitis). The cardinal features of the disease are muscle fatigue induced by exercise and brain malfunction, which follow on in the aftermath of an acute flu-like viral infection, often in a previously fit young adult. These muscle and brain symptoms, although chronic and sometimes lasting for months and even years, will vary in their

1

severity throughout the day, and from day to day – something not seen in any other illness where fatigue is a major feature.

Despite these highly characteristic features, many M.E. patients still visit doctors who don't recognise the disease and regard their symptoms with great scepticism. Patients who complain of being 'tired all the time' (known as 'TATT' in medical shorthand), along with a seemingly endless list of other unrelated symptoms constitute a considerable diagnostic problem. So, unless fully aware of the symptoms of M.E., a doctor may not make the right diagnosis, which means that patients are offered inappropriate advice.

Despite all the recent publicity, M.E. is not a 'new disease'. Outbreaks of the illness have been reported in Europe, America, Australia and New Zealand on a regular basis for the past fifty years, and it is now estimated that there are 100,000 patients in the U.K. alone. In the early days research into M.E. was hampered by the lack of facilities available for identifying 'culprit' viruses; today it is believed that the group of viruses to which polio belongs (the enteroviruses) is likely to be the major cause of the disease. Following the initial infection – which may take the form of flu or gastric enteritis – it seems that a susceptible individual is unable to kill off the virus, which persists in the bowel, then multiplies and passes via the bloodstream to invade the nerve and muscle cells. Why this should be so remains uncertain, but factors such as physical and mental stress during the acute illness are probably quite important.

In addition, the persisting virus could be stimulating excessive production of substances like interferon and interleukin, the body's natural immunising chemicals, which are normally released only in the acute stage of a viral illness. So it could be that both the persisting virus and the immune chemicals are affecting the way muscles, brain and nerves are able to carry out their normal functions.

As yet, there is no drug that will 'cure' M.E., or significantly alter the natural course of the disease. The recent research findings, and the tremendous interest being shown by scientists in other persisting infections (e.g. AIDS) may well open up the way to specific forms of therapy in the near future.

Rest, both physical and mental, is at present the key aspect to recovery from M.E., and this will involve patients and their families in having to make some very significant changes in lifestyle. Patients have to learn to 'listen to their bodies' and to live within their limitations – not very easy advice to take, particularly for previously fit and active young adults.

M.E. patients can and do make a significant – or full – recovery, even after long periods of time, so never give up hope. The aim of my book is to give patients and those caring for them all the information about the disease currently available. Armed with this information I hope you will be better equipped to make the right choices in how to manage your individual case of M.E., and to give your body the optimum conditions for a slow but progressive recovery.

Charles Shepherd

Notes on the second edition

Having been asked to write a second edition of this book has enabled me to completely revise the scientific information and so provide the most up-to-date research findings from neurologists, virologists and immunologists who are studying this complex illness. It has also given me the opportunity to include much more information on the various treatments – both orthodox and unconventional – which are now becoming available.

Charles Shepherd
January 1992

Part 1
WHAT IS M.E.?

1. First Appearances

Introduction

Before looking at some of the numerous outbreaks of M.E. that have hit the headlines over the past sixty years, it is worth noting that this is not a new disease confined to the twentieth century. This baffling syndrome of neurological and muscular symptoms which follow an infective illness has almost certainly been around for very much longer. As early as 1750 Sir Richard Manningham described, in the medical literature, a syndrome of what he termed 'febricula' or the 'little fever' which presented with numerous physical symptoms but few objective clinical findings. There have even been suggestions that both Florence Nightingale and Charles Darwin were early victims of M.E.

However, it wasn't until 1934 (in the U.S.A.) and 1955 (in the U.K.) that the medical profession started to give the subject any serious attention. Following the publicity surrounding these two famous outbreaks, it soon became apparent that M.E. was not just confined to the U.K. and the U.S.A. Similar reports started to emerge from Europe, Australia and South Africa. As a result the illness picked up a large number of different names along the way – Chronic Fatigue and Immune Dysfunction Syndrome/CFIDS (U.S.A.), Icelandic disease (Iceland), Tapanui flu (New Zealand) and Low Natural Killer Cell Syndrome (Japan). Despite this confusing multiplicity of names it now appears that we are all talking about the same illness, even though doctors cannot yet reach a consensus about what to call it!

The Royal Free Disease

In the late spring of 1955 the infectious diseases unit at the Royal Free Hospital in London began admitting patients from all over north London with an infection that had doctors baffled.

Initially the illness was unremarkable, with respiratory symptoms, sore throat, enlarged lymph glands and a slight fever. Some patients also had a gastric upset and a few had marked dizziness (vertigo). Then, instead of getting progressively better, new symptoms started to appear – headaches, blurred or even double vision (diplopia) and abnormal sensations in the skin (paraesthesiae). All the patients had difficulties with brain functioning, particularly with short-term memory and concentration, but the most striking feature of the disease was the severity of muscle fatigue caused by even the most limited exercise. The patients also had cold hands and feet, were troubled by bladder disturbances and were extremely sensitive to any change in external temperatures.

The doctors at the Royal Free were in no doubt: these patients had an infection that the body's front line of defence – the lymphatic glands – seemed unable to filter out, and it was spreading to the nerves and muscles. However, no such illness had been clearly defined in the textbooks.

The degree of muscle weakness the patients complained of initially suggested polio – still a possibility in those days – but there was no muscle wasting taking place, which is one of polio's most characteristic features. Other investigations failed to confirm the presence of polio, so the doctors were left with an infection looking for a cause.

Some patients were given an EEG (electroencephalogram) to measure their brain activity. A few did show abnormalities, and an assumption was made that they were experiencing some form of brain inflammation (encephalitis) and that the cause was a virus, but not the polio virus.

Then the most dramatic events of that year occurred, involving the Royal Free's own medical and nursing staff. The virus broke out at the hospital on 13 July, and over the following twelve days seventy doctors and nurses were taken ill. So many staff became involved that the hospital was forced to close, and it remained closed until 5 October. In all there were 292 cases, but very significantly only twelve of the hospital's patients – who were resting in their beds – fell victim to the disease.

Just like the cases admitted earlier, the hospital staff's illness followed the characteristic pattern of symptoms we now associate with M.E. First came the non-specific flu-like illness with the sort of symptoms that can occur in any viral infection. Following this acute onset some of the staff – now patients themselves – had a short period of remission in which they began to get a little better. Then it became obvious that their defence mechanisms had not limited the spread of the virus after all, and that it had passed through this 'safety net' to reach brain, nerves and muscles. The patients started to feel ill again with the characteristic features of brain malfunction, nervous disturbances and overwhelming muscular fatigue.

Unlike most of the patients we see with M.E. today, many of those involved at the Royal Free had definite abnormalities in their nerves, which could be demonstrated on clinical examination. At the Royal Free nearly 20 per cent of the patients had a paralysis of the facial nerve – the one which controls our facial expressions – and eleven had paralysis of swallowing, and even had to be tube-fed. Clinical examination showed that the nervous system had been affected by the disease in 74 per cent of patients.

Two other important features of the disease that emerged from this outbreak were the pain and sensory changes experienced by some of the staff. Doctors found that the slightest movement of one of the weakened limbs could result in severe pain, and there was often pain too below the ribs which coincided with extreme tenderness in the corresponding muscles. Other patients had significant areas where the skin sensation was lost (hypoaesthesiae); in some cases this involved half the body. Twenty-eight of these cases were investigated with electromyograms (EMG), which show how messages are transmitted from the brain via the nerves to the muscles. The results suggested that there were definite abnormalities in the way these messages were being carried at the level of the spinal cord.

The dramatic way in which this mystery disease paralysed a whole hospital made it headline news, and the papers called it 'the Royal Free disease'. But the inconclusive nature of the tests, which failed to isolate the cause of the epidemic, left many members of the medical profession sceptical, and they lost interest in further research. Some of the patients quickly got better, but others have remained permanently disabled. One person who did not forget their plight was Dr Melvin Ramsay, consultant physician in the infectious diseases unit. He published a report in *The Lancet* on some of the cases at the Royal Free the year after the outbreak, in which a leading article described the disease as 'A New Clinical Entity?', and suggested it be named 'benign myalgic encephalomyelitis'. The term 'benign', implying that M.E. is not a serious or fatal condition, has with hindsight been dropped, but myalgic encephalomyelitis remains the most common name for the disease.

What happened at the Royal Free made the disease briefly famous, but there have been other less spectacular outbreaks – over seventy in fact – reported worldwide, particularly in affluent countries with temperate climates. Outbreaks seem to occur more frequently in closed communities such as schools, hospitals and barracks, where an infectious disease can spread quickly; however, it must be emphasised that though a viral infection can be caught from another person, susceptibility to that infection persisting and turning into M.E. is not something that can be passed on. It should also be noted that M.E. is an endemic disease, meaning that there are individual cases occurring all the time, as well as periodic small outbreaks that present in specific geographic localities.

Other outbreaks of M.E. in Britain

In 1952 an infectious disease, never identified, but which sounds remarkably like M.E., broke out at the Middlesex Hospital in London. In 1955, just before the Royal Free outbreak, there was a cluster of cases with classic M.E. symptoms at a primary school in Cumbria in the north of England. A small outbreak in a teacher training college in Newcastle-upon-Tyne occurred in 1959. The cases here supported the theory that – as with polio

– physical stress during the acute infection was an important co-factor in the development of M.E. The student teachers shared their accommodation with a group of nuns; the students developed M.E., but the nuns, who were naturally leading a very quiet life, did not.

During 1964–6 a large number of cases was reported from the north London practice of Dr Betty Scott, who made the interesting observation that many of her patients had low blood sugars (hypoglycaemia), which may turn out to be important in view of the disordered energy metabolism now being demonstrated in some patients' muscles.

One further outbreak of interest in Britain occurred during 1970–1 at London's Great Ormond Street Children's Hospital. Once again those affected were mainly the nursing staff, and none of the children who were patients on the wards at the time succumbed. There were nearly 150 cases in all. The Great Ormond Street nurses had a list of almost identical symptoms to those experienced at the Royal Free, and again went on to follow the by now familiar pattern of remission followed by relapse or continuing disability.

In 1970 the *British Medical Journal* published a paper by two psychiatrists, Drs McEvedy and Beard (medical reference 71), which concluded that the Royal Free outbreak had all been due to mass hysteria. The effect on U.K. medical opinion was profound – M.E. became a 'dustbin diagnosis', and a subject that few doctors were prepared to take seriously.

One prominent physician who went against the tide of medical opinion was Peter Behan, Professor of Neurology at the Institute of Neurological Sciences in Glasgow. During the late 1970s and early 1980s he started to see a growing number of M.E. patients from all over the country who were being referred to his neurological clinic. Professor Behan became more and more convinced that they did have a genuine organic disorder affecting their brain, muscle and immune system. He also became involved with local general practitioners like Drs Keighley, Calder and Warnock, who had witnessed minor outbreaks in their practices in Balfron and Helensburgh on the Clyde.

In 1985 Professor Behan's first major research paper on the

subject was published in the *Journal of Infection* (medical reference 3) documenting clear abnormalities which were not psychologically based. This was soon followed by steadily increasing publicity for M.E. in both the medical and lay media. In the U.K. the diagnosis once again became 'acceptable', and before long an almost unknown illness became a subject on which all doctors had strong opinions – even if some of them weren't all that complimentary! The link with enteroviruses was pursued, and as you will read in the following chapters, the debate, at last, opened up as to what was really going wrong in M.E.

M.E. in the U.S.A.

In the United States the condition has been variously referred to as epidemic neuromyasthenia, chronic Epstein-Barr virus disease, and 'Yuppie Flu'. Most Americans now call it CFIDS – the Chronic Fatigue and Immune Dysfunction Syndrome.

The first ever recorded outbreak of M.E. in the United States involved doctors and nurses at the Los Angeles County General Hospital in 1934. At first the disease was thought to be polio, but although the patients' muscles remained weak they did not become wasted, so this explanation had to be ruled out. Altogether nearly 200 members of staff were affected, and when they were thoroughly reviewed six months later half were still unwell. Further small outbreaks continued to be reported from various parts of the U.S., but the American public did not really become aware of the condition until 1985, when following an outbreak at Lake Tahoe, Nevada, media attention became overwhelming. There was a general demand that action should be taken, and a proper research programme be initiated.

The shores of Lake Tahoe are a retreat for successful, active, professional 'high achievers' – the last type of person to stay away from work without good reason. Late in 1984 strange things started happening in the area – previously fit adults in their thirties and forties started falling ill with a mysteriously flu-like illness which was then followed by the classic muscular fatigue and intellectual malfunction associated with M.E. So many people were involved that the press got interested and one magazine labelled the area 'Raggedy Ann Town', as the patients said they felt like Raggedy Ann dolls. All the tests were coming back normal, and they began to have doubts as to whether the patients had a physical illness at all. Perhaps, against all the odds, they were just work-shy.

Fortunately, two doctors, Dan Peterson and Paul Cheney, did not share these doubts; they became increasingly convinced that the steady stream of patients arriving at their consulting rooms were genuinely ill. They decided it was time to get to the bottom of the mystery. Their patients had sore throats, glandular swellings and headaches, and they wondered if this might be glandular fever (called in America infectious mono-nucleosis). The problem was that glandular fever is a teenage disease: patients in the age group affected should have developed antibodies and be immune to the virus by now. Nevertheless, the similarity with glandular fever led Peterson and Cheney to research into the Epstein-Barr virus (EBV), which causes it.

The Epstein-Barr virus belongs to the herpes group of viruses, which cause cold sores, genital herpes and chicken-pox. EBV is passed on from person to person by saliva – hence the term 'kissing disease' for glandular fever. Carriers of the disease can pass it on without developing it themselves. By the age of thirty, nearly 90 per cent of all adults will have developed antibodies to EBV, indicating a full degree of immunity, so after this age an attack of glandular fever becomes very rare.

All the viruses in the herpes group have the capacity to stay on in the body after causing an initial infection, so acting as a reservoir of dormant infection. So once a person has been infected by EBV, the virus does not go away, but remains for life, usually without causing any harm, in the salivary glands and the B cells of the immune system, which are responsible for antibody production. The virus is kept in check by other cells of the immune system known as natural killer cells.

What Doctors Peterson and Cheney began to wonder was whether the Epstein-Barr virus, lying dormant in the B cells, had been reactivated and let loose in the body again to produce the American fatigue syndrome that they were witnessing at Lake Tahoe. In other words was something weakening the body's immune system, which up until now had prevented the dormant virus from becoming active? Was the virus now multiplying, and leaving the B cells to start a further episode of glandular fever, from an original infection which the patients had been harbouring since picking it up as children? After all, other members of the herpes group of viruses can be reactivated from their dormant stage, given the right circumstances. Herpes cold sores will reappear at times of stress, during menstruation, in hot sun, or when the patient is feeling run down – exactly the same sort of stimuli now known to cause a relapse or exacerbation of M.E.

Doctors Cheney and Peterson decided to look for evidence of Epstein-Barr virus in the Lake Tahoe patients. They found raised antibodies to EBV in about three-quarters of them, but this still left a quarter with normal levels and a small percentage with no antibodies at all. The hypothesis was further complicated by the fact that EBV antibody tests are difficult to interpret, and that the Lake Tahoe patients produced a fairly similar spread of results that would be expected from a 'normal' group of people of their age. So no conclusions could be drawn to support the EBV theory in Lake Tahoe.

In the meantime the American press and broadcasting media had become extremely interested in the mystery virus, and the outbreak was now receiving extensive publicity throughout the United States. The magazine *Newsweek* referred to it as the 'malaise of the 80s' and other papers used the name 'Yuppie Flu', as so many of them were fit young professionals. Somewhat prematurely, the name chronic Epstein-Barr disease became the accepted term for the illness, and a national CEBV association was founded in Portland, Oregon. They were soon receiving requests for information from all over the U.S. Numerous individual patients started asking their physicians if CEBV could be the cause for their persisting ill health, and pressure came from Congress for researchers to start finding some answers.

Blood samples were then sent to Robert Gallo, the scientist who had been working on the AIDS virus at the National Cancer Institute, and who had recently isolated the first 'new' herpes group virus (human herpes virus type 6/HHV-6) for twenty years. As a result HHV-6 became the next 'culprit' virus to be linked to M.E./CFIDS in the States, but at this point Gallo failed to find any conclusive link.

The Lake Tahoe outbreak eventually subsided, but as in all the other epidemics already described, many of those who were taken ill have still not recovered. It seems that about one-third improved; about one-half followed the familiar pattern of remission alternating with relapse; the rest remain chronically unwell.

New viruses emerge

As the AIDS epidemic quickly gathered pace during the late 1980s, enormous sums of money were spent in trying to identify the virus responsible for this devastating infection. The cause turned out to be HIV (human immunodeficiency virus) which belongs to a group known as the retroviruses. All these viruses contain a unique fingerprint enzyme called reverse transcriptase, hence the name RE-TR-ovirus: RE for 'reverse' and TR for 'transcriptase'. The reverse transcriptase is a vital enzyme which is involved in the way the virus makes copies of itself once inside the cell. In the past these retroviruses had been linked to rare cases of leukaemia in animals, but never to any form of human illness. In the case of HIV infection a picture slowly emerged of a 'new' virus which was capable of attacking key parts of the human immune system – the T helper cells. Two other viruses in the same group, human T-cell leukaemia viruses 1 and 2 (HTLV1 and HTLV2), have also become linked with leukaemia and neurological diseases. Researchers in the States then began to query if there could be a link with CFIDS.

Dr Paul Cheney believed that this was one lead that was well worth following up, and so enlisted the help of Dr Elaine DeFreitas, a virologist, working on HTLV research at the prestigious Wistar Institute in Philadelphia. In March 1988 Dr Cheney sent six blood samples from CFIDS patients to the Wistar – they all turned out to have antibodies to HTLV. During the summer of 1988 he widened the project by enlisting the help of Dr David Bell, a paediatrician from Lyndonville, New York, who had recently become involved in caring for children with CFIDS. The two doctors sent a much larger group of blood samples to Dr DeFreitas, including some from healthy people to act as controls.

Using a new technique for magnifying viral genetic codes (the polymerase chain reaction), Dr DeFreitas set about looking for evidence of retroviral infection. The study took her two years to complete, but the final results suggested that about 80 per cent of the adults and 70 per cent of the children did have evidence of genetic material from HTLV2 (see medical reference 197).

Unfortunately, other research groups, including those at the Centre for Disease Control (CDC) in the States, and Professor Peter Behan in Glasgow have not, so far, been able to replicate these findings. It is possible that the viral DNA sequences found by Dr DeFreitas are very similar to those which can be found in normal cells, and so a big question mark still hangs over any link between M.E./CFIDS and retroviruses.

Further evidence to support a retroviral connection appeared shortly afterwards from Dr John Martin and his colleagues, working at the University of Southern California. Using a similar type of genetic probe, they claimed to have found a spumavirus – a subgroup of the retroviruses – which had not been associated with any specific human disease.

The spumavirus is also known as a foamy virus because of the 'foamy' appearance it can create in infected cells. Dr Martin's claims about finding evidence of a spumavirus in more than 200 patients with M.E./CFIDS were received with considerable scepticism when he presented them to a meeting at the CDC in September 1990. At the time they received considerable media publicity in *Newsweek* and the *New York Times* but not in the mainstream medical journals. Once again, this is a link which requires confirmation by other independent research groups before any firm conclusions can be drawn.

The most recent research findings to come from America are once again implicating HHV-6, but not as a *cause* of M.E./CFIDS. In January 1992, Professor Tony Komaroff's team reported in the *Annals of Internal Medicine* (medical reference 17) that two human herpes viruses were *actively replicating* in a significant number of patients which they had examined – many of whom had first become ill in the communities around Lake Tahoe. The new evidence for an HHV-6 connection came from laboratory experiments in which the patients' white blood cells were placed in a special cell culture. The resulting cellular changes were highly characteristic of HHV-6 damage, and further confirmation of the presence of active HHV-6 came from the use of monoclonal antibodies (see page 33) and polymerase chain reaction analysis.

As with Epstein–Barr virus infection most adults come into contact with HHV-6 during childhood, after which the virus lies dormant in the body. The findings from Professor Komaroff's team suggest that some external factor (infection, stress, toxin) has produced an upset in immune system regulation which, in turn, has led to a *reactivation* of HHV-6 from its dormant state. At the moment we can only speculate as to whether HHV-6 then goes on to affect nerve cells and produce M.E. symptoms, but the possibility is certainly there.

In America the problem of M.E./CFIDS is now being taken very seriously, and the U.S. Congress has granted six million dollars for research projects in 1992. The CDC have also set up a series of surveillance studies in Atlanta, Reno, Grand Rapids and Wichita to try and gather some data on the exact incidence of the disease. And, a growing number of highly respected academic researchers are at last becoming actively involved. Many of these scientists came to Cambridge University in April 1990 to present their findings to the first International Symposium on M.E./CFIDS. Their findings are referred to in later chapters.

As in the U.K. a number of self-help groups have emerged during the past ten years. Undoubtedly the most influential is the CFIDS Association, whose headquarters are in Charlotte, North Carolina. Besides publishing the regular *CFIDS Chronicle* (a highly authoritative and comprehensive review of current medical research and treatment) they have also been responsible for stimulating and financing various research programmes in the United States. The CFIDS Association also organises regular conferences which involve clinicians, researchers and patient participation. Overseas membership is welcomed – see Useful Addresses.

M.E. in other parts of the world

Australia and New Zealand In Australia the history of M.E. dates back to 1949, when a major epidemic occurred in Adelaide. As with many of the other early outbreaks, there was a close and interesting link with poliomyelitis. The polio epidemic had started in May of that year, but it wasn't till August that cases of M.E. started to appear. These continued right through until April 1951 by which time nearly 700 people had been admitted to hospital. No virus was ever isolated, but when material from two of the patients was inoculated into monkeys, damage to the sciatic nerve could clearly be seen under the microscope.

In New Zealand there was a well-publicised outbreak during 1983 in a rural part of Western Otago in the South Island (see medical reference 73). These patients developed extreme fatigue four to six weeks after an initial flu-like illness. Dr Peter Snow, the general practitioner involved in this outbreak, presented his findings to the 1990 Cambridge Symposium. It was quite clear that the Tapanui patients were part of a very hard-working, conscientious community who had obviously succumbed to an illness which was not psychologically based. Not surprisingly, New Zealanders found their own name for M.E. – Tapanui flu.

A number of important research projects are now underway in both Australia and New Zealand. Professor Denis Wakefield and Dr Andrew Lloyd, at the Prince Henry Hospital in Sydney, have assembled an excellent team of neurologists, virologists, immunologists and psychiatrists to look at all aspects of what might be 'going wrong'. The team have now published a series of papers, and they are also looking at specific forms of treatment, especially related to immune system abnormalities. Further information on this research is covered in the next chapter, and the medical reference section gives details of the papers which have been published.

Much of the research taking place in New Zealand centres on the work of Professor Campbell Murdoch and Dr Michael Holmes at the University of Otago Medical School. They, too, have been looking at retroviruses as a possible causative agent, and the development of a computer-assisted profile of white blood cell abnormalities which could turn out to be the basis of a diagnostic test.

Also working at the Otago Medical School is Dr Leslie Simpson, an expert in haematology (the study of the blood). He has published some interesting findings on possible abnormalities in the shape of red blood cells in M.E. (see medical reference 141). Using a high-powered electron microscope, Dr Simpson has found that some of the red cells (which carry oxygen around the body) are not their usual shape. The result, he suggests, is that red blood cells are less able to pass down the smallest blood vessels, the capillaries, which supply vital oxygen and nutrients to tissues such as brain and muscle.

A very active self-help support group (ANZMES) covers both Australia and New Zealand, but there are also locally-based organisations in most of the Australian states. ANZMES publishes a very informative journal called *Meeting Place*. Their address is on page 322, along with the locally based Australian groups.

Canada Recognition of M.E. by both government and the medical profession seems to have seriously lagged behind that in the U.K. and America. This is partly due to the fact that there have not been any major outbreaks in schools or hospitals to stimulate media attention. Nevertheless, the picture does now appear to be changing, and several specialists are taking an active involvement in research projects in Ontario. M.E. Canada is the main self-help support group which is based in Ottawa (address see page 321).

Europe Despite the increasing recognition of M.E. in the U.K. and America, doctors in some parts of Europe still remain sceptical about its very existence. Well-documented outbreaks have, however, occurred in Switzerland – two at military camps in Erstfeld and Degersheim, and the third in a hospital. Smaller outbreaks have also been reported from Denmark, Greece and Iceland.

The outbreak in Iceland during 1948 was of particular interest for a number of reasons. Firstly, it followed several cases of polio around the small northern township of Akureyri. Altogether there were over a thousand cases, mainly in high-school children. Secondly, when an epidemic of polio swept around the coast of Iceland in 1955, the Akureyri township was unaffected. It appeared that the original infective agent (presumably a virus) had produced, just like a vaccination, a degree of immunity to polio. This strongly suggested that both the infections were linked, and belonged to the same group of enteroviruses. And, when these children were eventually given polio vaccination, they responded by producing unusually high levels of polio antibodies, suggesting they had already been exposed to a similar infection. Lastly, when these Akureyri patients were re-examined by a distinguished neurologist in 1955, only 25 per cent of them had made a complete recovery. The remainder still had significant degrees of muscle and brain malfunction. A further assessment, carried out only recently, indicates that many remain permanently disabled, and a few seem to have gone on to develop Parkinson's disease.

Incidentally, on a very positive note, there is apparently no hostility or scepticism from the Icelandic medical profession!

Today, there are active M.E. self-help groups in Belgium, Denmark, Holland and Norway, and I have recently been assisting in the formation of one in Italy. (See addresses on page 321-2). There is also growing interest in Sweden and France – where it is known as Spasmophile – but little in the way of self-help support networks.

South Africa In 1955, a few months earlier than the Royal Free outbreak, an almost mirror image situation occurred 6000 miles away in Durban, South Africa. Once again, as in Iceland and Adelaide, there were close connections with an outbreak of polio. The South African cases occurred at the same time as polio was rife in Durban. In the beginning it was the nursing staff at Addington Hospital who were mainly affected, but as time went on, cases were admitted from the surrounding general population – just as in London. Many of these nurses quickly relapsed when they returned to the wards, and several had to accept permanent retirement from nursing as a result of chronic disablement.

M.E. is steadily being recognised as a significant health problem in South Africa, and their self-help support group is based in Hillcrest (see page 322).

If you would like to follow up any of these previous outbreaks of M.E. in greater detail please refer to the medical references on pages 346-61, and to the magazine articles from *Newsweek*, *In Health* and *Science* which are listed on page 362-3. Dr Melvin Ramsay's book, *Myalgic Encephalomyelitis and Postviral Fatigue States* (see page 362), also gives a comprehensive account of many of these outbreaks with particular reference to the events at London's Royal Free Hospital in 1955.

2. What Triggers M.E.?

Following the outbreak of M.E. at the Royal Free Hospital in 1955, Dr Melvin Ramsay was left with many questions to answer. In all the recorded outbreaks the illness seemed to have been triggered by an infection, presumably a virus, which was impervious to attack by the body's immune system. Which virus or viruses were responsible? Did the virus ever go away, even when a patient apparently got better, or did it remain dormant, with the possibility of being reactivated? A lot of research needed to be done into the way the virus affected the patient's brain, nerves and muscles, and the subsequent response of the immune system.

Dr Ramsay remained utterly convinced that M.E. was a genuine organic disease, but many of his colleagues continued to be sceptical, so it was not easy persuading specialists in the fields of virology, neurology and immunology to become involved in M.E. research. Fifteen years after the Royal Free outbreak two psychiatrists dealt a severe blow to the credibility of M.E. when they published papers concluding that the disease was purely hysterical in origin. This had a devastating effect on the medical establishment, and M.E. became unfashionable and even unmentionable. Even today, with so much concrete evidence that the disease exists, some doctors persist in accusing M.E. patients of malingering and the controversy still rages.

Nevertheless, the search for a cause of M.E. goes on. No single virus has been identified but U.K. scientists now believe that viruses belonging to the enteroviral group are the prime culprits.

The M.E. equation

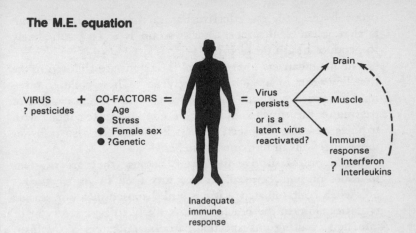

The enteroviruses

These are a group of 72 different viruses which include polio (3 types), Coxsackie and echoviruses (about 30-plus of each), and hepatitis A. It was Hippocrates who first recognised hepatitis (inflammation of the liver), and carvings from the second millennium BC depict cases of polio – these types of infections have been around for a very long time. Today, enteroviruses have a world-wide distribution and are known to cause a variety of illnesses ranging from trivial sore throats through to life-threatening infections involving the brain and heart. Even within the same family an enterovirus may have different effects according to age, sex, occupation and pre-existing immunity. The original outbreaks of M.E. in Australia, Iceland and South Africa all suggested that enteroviruses, particularly the Coxsackie group, were involved.

In underdeveloped tropical countries enteroviral infections occur all the year round, so this population quickly builds up a strong degree of natural immunity from a very early age. This is probably why M.E. is comparatively rare in these countries.

In developed countries with cool temperate climates, enteroviral infections tend to flourish during the warm summer months, often in epidemics that occur every few years. Increased levels of hygiene also mean that fewer enteroviral infections occur leading to less effective natural immunity. The result is that when adults meet a new strain it is far more likely to produce health problems.

The main carriers of enteroviral infections are children in the first few years of life – 'the nappy years'. These children often remain carriers without any ill-effects, whilst being capable of passing on the virus to adults who come into close contact with nappies or excreta. Insects and cockroaches can also transmit these infections in unhygienic kitchens.

Enteroviruses survive in sewage because they are resistant to most of the chemical disinfectants used in its treatment. So, when contaminated waste is still disposed into our seaside estuaries close to the beach, there is likely to be a reservoir of infection awaiting unsuspecting bathers and eaters of shellfish. This is the reason why some people develop M.E. shortly after gastroenteritis contracted during their seaside holiday. It is also possible that the use of sludge as a fertiliser may be infecting fresh fruit and vegetables – a good reason for removing the peel!

Once an enterovirus enters the body via the mouth it may do nothing more than cause a mild sore throat and a few enlarged glands in the neck. This indicates that the body's immune system has responded by producing neutralising antibodies. Important factors which will adversely affect this immune response include physical or mental stress, immunosuppressive drugs, pregnancy, malnutrition, exposure to the cold and recent surgery.

If the primary immune response fails, the virus can then pass down to the lungs or intestines and produce a chest infection or gastroenteritis. Once inside the intestines, enteroviruses remain and multiply to form yet another reservoir of infection. From here they can spread via the blood stream to various other tissues including nerve, muscle and hormone-producing glands. This is how enteroviruses start to cause far more serious problems and why, in some cases, M.E. turns into what is known as a multisystem disease.

A large number of different illnesses are now firmly linked to enteroviral infection. These include summer flu (sore throat, headache, diarrhoea), chest infections (laryngitis, bronchitis), brain infections (meningitis and encephalitis), muscle disease (polymyositis, Bornholm disease), heart inflammation (myocarditis and pericarditis), and glandular inflammation affecting the liver (hepatitis), pancreas, prostate and thyroid glands. Enteroviruses are also being linked with childhood diabetes, and where they persist in the heart muscle to a problem known as cardiomyopathy.

If M.E. really is linked to enteroviral infection, you can appreciate how it can present in a variety of different disguises, and how, as the illness progresses, other parts of the body beside muscle and brain may also become involved. An excellent review of enteroviruses has been written by Dr Elizabeth Dowsett in the *Journal of Hospital Infection* (see medical reference 186); other references to enteroviral research are contained in the same section.

Tests for enteroviruses

During the early 1980s Dr Eleanor Bell, a world authority on enteroviral infection, and her colleagues in Scotland, started to examine the link between M.E. and Coxsackie viruses. Using blood samples from M.E. patients, they looked for increased levels of two different types of antibody – the proteins made by the immune system which attack viruses. The first are known as neutralising antibodies, which tend to persist at high levels after the initial infection. The second are called IgM antibodies, and these usually fade away quite quickly – any persistence would suggest a continuing active infection. Although many of the patients did have raised levels of these antibodies, the results were difficult to interpret because quite a few perfectly healthy people also had exactly the same antibodies from previous infections. Professor Peter Behan has recently reviewed the value of looking for such antibodies and concluded that they cannot be used as a diagnostic test for M.E. (see medical reference 193).

In 1988 Professor James Mowbray and Dr Galal Yousef, both working at St Mary's Hospital in London, published the results of a new sophisticated blood test (the VP1 test) in *The Lancet* (medical reference 194). This test picks up a specific protein called viral protein one (VP1), which helps to form a protective wrapper around the virus. VP1 is common to all the different 72 enteroviruses and the results turned out to be positive in about 60 per cent of cases. Although helpful as a research investigation, VP1 has not turned out to be a useful diagnostic test for M.E. (see also page 115).

At the same time the doctors at St Mary's developed a method of separating and then culturing (growing) enteroviruses in stool specimens. The results, also published in *The Lancet*, showed that about 22 per cent of the patients had a persisting reservoir of enteroviral infection in their intestines. This complicated test is not available from other hospitals.

During the past few years molecular biologists have discovered new techniques which are capable of demonstrating the presence of specific genetic codes (DNA or RNA) which are rather like viral fingerprints. Using one such technique, known as in situ hybridisation, Dr Len Archard, from London's Charing Cross Hospital, has been looking for the presence of both Coxsackie and Epstein-Barr virus particles in biopsies of muscle taken from M.E. patients. His results indicate that enteroviral RNA is present in about 25 per cent of cases and DNA from Epstein-Barr in about 10 per cent (see medical reference 181). The most recent research findings indicate that this enterovirus is 'poorly replicating', meaning that during the process of multiplication it has turned itself into a mutant form, rather like the way that flu viruses change shape from year to year (see medical reference 185). One implication of this may be that the body's immune system is less able to recognise and challenge a virus with which it is not familiar.

Professor Peter Behan's team in Glasgow have been using the same technique as Dr Elaine DeFreitas in America – the polymerase chain reaction (PCR). This enzyme-based investigation allows a massive multiplication of tiny amounts of genetic material. It's the virologists' equivalent of being able to find a needle in a haystack!

Professor Behan's findings, now published in the *British Medical Journal* (medical reference 187), show that about 55 per cent of patients have enterovirus RNA in their muscle. Incidentally, in the hospital patients used as controls, the only other group with enterovirus present were patients with carcinoma of the breast or colon. None of the healthy volunteers had any virus present in the muscle. PCR is a very sensitive way of detecting viral genetic codes, but one problem is that any small amount of contamination can also produce false positive results. So, like all the other viral research, these findings now need to be repeated in other groups of M.E. patients.

A follow-up to these important findings was recently published in the prestigious *British Medical Bulletin* which devoted the entire October 1991 issue to M.E. (see further reading). Here, Professor Behan stated that there may also be abnormalities associated with an intracellular protein known as calsequestrin – a substance with a very similar structure to polio virus. Calsequestrin is stored within the cell in particles known as calcicomes, and acts as an important calcium-carrying protein within the nerve and muscle. When a nerve impulse reaches the cell, the calsequestrin is responsible for distributing calcium, without which the muscle would be unable to contract and function effectively. This new work will be submitted for publication in due course.

Having discovered the fact that enterovirus is persisting in the muscle, the next question that needs answering is what, if anything, is it doing there? Is it just acting as a marker, indicating that the virus is also present in the brain and other body tissues? Or, is it actually interfering with the muscle cell's own genetic codes, and somehow 'switching off' their normal functions and causing a disturbance in energy production? These are questions which I shall address in the next chapter.

Other viruses which may be involved

Although enteroviruses remain the most consistent group of viruses associated with M.E., there are plenty of well-documented cases where the illness has followed other infections, particularly herpes zoster (shingles), chicken-pox, cytomegalovirus and rubella. In Australia the Ross River virus has been implicated and, as described in the previous chapter, researchers in America are currently looking at a possible link with retroviruses. I am also aware of a few cases where vaccination appears to have been the principal trigger factor.

Those cases which have been initiated by chicken-pox seem to be particularly severe and protracted, possibly because this is a virus which is capable of causing chemical problems in both the liver and brain (Reye's syndrome), as well as persisting within the central nervous system to cause various other neurological problems. It has also been suggested that the temporary immune suppression resulting from any viral infection may allow a secondary enteroviral infection to take hold. Yet another possible explanation is that the main action of any of these 'triggering' viruses is to reactivate another virus, such as HHV-6 or measles, which has remained harmless and dormant in the body since childhood (see also page 15).

One last virus to be linked to M.E. is the Epstein-Barr virus – the cause of glandular fever/infectious mononucleosis. Doctors have always recognised that a small minority of teenagers who develop glandular fever go on to develop a protracted illness, which may last for up to two years, consisting of fatigue, low grade fever and enlarged lymph glands. Whether or not reactivation of a dormant (latent) Epstein-Barr virus can result in M.E. remains the subject of debate. However, about 20 per cent of patients with M.E. do seem to have raised levels of specific antibodies (IgG antibodies to what are known as viral capsid antigens and early antigen) which indicate an active production of Epstein-Barr virus. For the moment though it is probably not helpful to be spending a great deal of time and money looking for such antibodies in individual patients as the findings cannot be considered diagnostic. Further details on the role of other viruses, including Epstein-Barr and the antibody tests available, can be followed up by referring to medical references 195–204.

The fight against viruses

All viruses are made up of two parts. On the outside is a protein-coated capsule, called the capsid, which contains the antigens against which human antibodies are mobilised. Inside there is a core of nucleic acid (the genome) which is the genetic material of the virus. Viruses are classified according to the type of nucleic acid within this core. Some, like the herpes viruses (Epstein–Barr virus, chicken–pox), contain DNA (deoxyribonucleic acid). Others, like the enteroviruses, contain RNA (ribonucleic acid).

How viruses invade cells and replicate

1 The virus meets the host cell and becomes attached to its outer surface. This is just like a key fitting into a lock, as the virus has to find specific receptors on the surface to fit into. If antiviral antibodies are being made, part of their function is to block these receptor sites (1(b)).

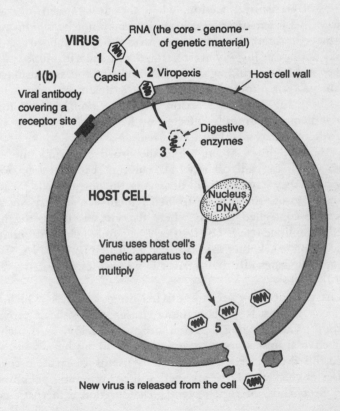

2 The successful virus penetrates the cell wall: this is called viropexis.

3 The capsule or capsid of the virus is stripped off by intra-cellular enzymes, so that its genetic information is freed.
4 The viral nucleic acid (RNA or DNA) then takes over the host cell's own genetic apparatus, using it to manufacture new viral particles. This very complicated process is again controlled by the host cell's own enzymes.
5 The new virus, which has been assembled and recoated by the host cell, then passes out through the cell membrane.

During this process the host cell may end up being so damaged that it ceases functioning normally and dies. However, in some cases of persisting infection, where the virus remains dormant (as with Epstein-Barr virus), the cell may not be significantly damaged. Another possibility is that although the virus itself may not be causing any great harm, the patient's immune system may still be reacting against it, and in the process causing cell damage – an autoimmune process. It is this mechanism which has been suggested as a reason for the continual liver damage in someone chronically infected by hepatitis B, and this type of response may just have some relevance in M.E.

Antiviral drugs are not like the broad spectrum antibiotics, which can kill off a whole range of bacterial infections. Because they have to avoid damaging the normal cells invaded by the virus, the aim is to make them act at very specific enzyme-controlled stages, where the virus is using the host cell to replicate itself. The host cell's enzymes behave differently according to whether the invader contains DNA or RNA. Consequently drugs effective against DNA viruses do not work on RNA viruses.

At present there are no antiviral drugs available which are effective against RNA-containing viruses such as the enteroviral group. There is one antiviral drug – Acyclovir – which is effective against some of the DNA-containing herpes viruses, and this drug is proving particularly useful for treating severe cases of chicken-pox where there is life-threatening pneumonia or encephalitis, or for shortening the duration of herpetic cold sores.

Acyclovir interferes with the replication of the DNA and has no adverse effect on the host cell. It is only effective in cells containing a herpes virus and once inside acts like a magic bullet in its specificity. The problem is that it only works when the virus is actively multiplying, so although it will help to reduce the severity of an acute attack of cold sores it will not prevent a recurrence once the virus becomes latent within the cell. The possible role of Acyclovir in the management of chronic Epstein-Barr virus infection is still being assessed in America, but there appear to be no clear benefits at present.

Antiviral drugs directed at other specific viruses are now in the research stage. No doubt in time antiviral drugs for RNA viruses will become available, but their future use in M.E. remains uncertain. The possible use of antiviral drugs in the treatment of M.E. is considered in further detail on page 124.

Pesticides

I have also come to the conclusion that agricultural and farm pesticides – especially the organophosphorous compounds used in some sheep dips – can no longer be ignored as possible trigger factors in the development of M.E.

Living in a rural part of the country, I have become increasingly aware of the fact that farmers who are in close and regular contact with sheep dips are prone to developing an acute flu-like illness, which is then followed by excessive fatigue, sore throats and limb pains, all of which may be accompanied by a severe depressive illness – a clinical syndrome which is almost equivalent to M.E. Similar cases were also reported at the end of 1991 in the medical journal, *Pulse*, by general practitioners working in farming communities in North Devon.

The Ministry of Agriculture's veterinary medicines directorate is currently reviewing the safety of all sheep dips, and the Health and Safety Executive is developing a test which will detect breakdown products from these particular chemicals in the urine.

In the past the medical profession has always been fairly sceptical about the possibility of these type of chemicals causing long-term damage to the central nervous system. However, a recent paper in *The Lancet* (medical reference 22) seems to provide good evidence from both EEG and psychological studies that such damage does occur.

Clearly, this is now another area which warrants further research, especially to find out if these patients have similar abnormalities in brain and hypothalamic function which are being demonstrated in purely post-viral M.E.

How the body's immune system responds

The Body's Immune Response to Viruses

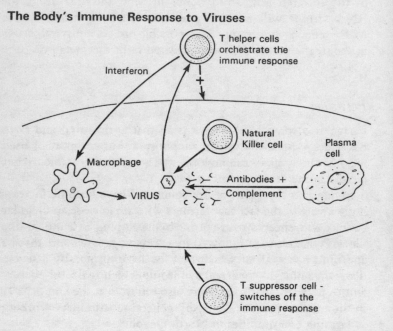

The second part of this 'M.E. Equation' involves the role of the body's immune system, and how it reacts not only to an initial viral infection, but also how it might respond to a persisting or reactivated virus.

The immune system is made up of a number of different components which are 'switched on', rather like a cascade, as soon as the body recognises a foreign invader be it virus, bacteria or fungus. Then, rather like an orchestra, these components should all act in unison to neutralise and remove the invader. Unfortunately, if one part is missing or defective, then the immune response may fail.

As I will discuss in the last part of this chapter, there are several important co-factors which seem to inhibit the body making an effective immune response, and these seem to be particularly important in M.E.

The main players in the immune orchestra are antibodies, immune chemicals like interferon, and cells called lymphocytes which all have their own individual functions. The response is 'switched on' by special white blood cells – the T helper lymphocytes – which recognise the virus, and then 'switched off' again by another group called T suppressor lymphocytes.

The full membership of the immune orchestra is made up of:

Antibodies These are a group of proteins called immuno-globulins, which recognise and lock on to invading organisms. They are produced by plasma cells which originate in the bone marrow where most of the blood cells are produced. This is why bone marrow transplants are sometimes carried out in people whose immune systems have been seriously damaged by leukaemia cells infiltrating the bone marrow. Antibodies make the virus more susceptible to attack by cells called macrophages, and they also activate an immune chemical called complement.

Following any viral infection, antibody production quickly gathers pace. IgA antibodies are the first line of defence, and they act rather like an 'antiseptic paint' to protect the delicate lining membranes of the throat and intestines, and so prevent further spread of the virus via the blood stream. IgA antibodies are produced by the regional lymph glands which is why those in the neck quickly swell up during a throat infection.

IgG and IgM antibodies are the next to be produced, and their role is to prevent blood spread of the virus to tissues like the heart and brain. These type of antibodies often remain long after the initial infection has gone (or after vaccination) and so prevent any further attack by that particular virus.

IgE antibodies are commonly produced during allergic reactions, and a raised level of IgE may indicate a co-existent problem with allergies.

Autoantibodies form a special group of antibodies, whereby the body's immune system 'turns on itself' and starts to attack its own tissues. Some researchers have speculated that this could be happening in M.E. where autoantibodies to the thyroid gland and muscle are occasionally found.

Complement is the name given to a group of about twenty different proteins which circulate in the blood. Along with antibodies, this substance helps to neutralise any invading virus.

Immune complexes are, as the name suggests, combinations of antibody and antigen which also circulate round in the blood. These immune complexes are found in up to 50 per cent of patients with M.E. and their presence has been linked to inflammation in the joints, kidneys and skin.

Lymphokines is the name given to a group of immune chemicals which are mainly produced by the T helper cells. These substances act as messengers within the immune system, and help to co-ordinate the attack on a virus. They also have direct effects on the brain and produce some of the common 'normal' reactions to any type of infection. It now seems that changes in sleep pattern, body temperature control, energy levels and mood which are associated with most infections are largely due to changes in the level of lymphokines called interleukins acting on a particular part of the brain known as the hypothalamus. These lymphokines are also responsible for the general aches and pains in muscles and joints which accompany flu-like infections.

Lymphocytes are a vital group of white blood cells which are also made in the bone marrow. One group, the B cells, turn into short-lived plasma cells and produce the antibodies already described. Another group migrates via the blood to a small gland in the neck called the thymus gland (hence T cells) where they mature into various subgroups, each with a particular number (e.g. T4, T8) according to their specific function. T cells are responsible for general immune surveillance against viruses and bacteria. The T4 (helper) cells have been likened to the conductor of the immune orchestra because of their role in 'switching on' and maintaining the response. These are the cells that become severely depleted in patients with AIDS. The T8 (suppressor) cells send out messages which instruct the immune system to slow down or cease its activities once the infection is under control.

Macrophages and phagocytic cells are another important group of cells which act rather like scavengers, and are literally capable of 'mopping up' all the infected cells and immune complexes. They are one of the first group of cells to recognise an invading organism, and envelop it under their membrane. The macrophage then goes on to present the 'captured virus' to the rest of the immune system, but principally to the T4 helper cells and the antibody-producing B cells.

Monoclonal antibodies are custom-designed antibodies which can be synthetically produced. They are then used to identify all kinds of chosen targets inside the body for both investigative and treatment purposes. In the case of M.E. monoclonal antibodies have been used to detect the presence of enteroviral protein in the blood – Professor Mowbray's VP1 test.

Natural Killer cells (NK cells) are part of our primitive immune system. They are always ready to attack anything that the body recognises as 'foreign', and this ranges from infections through to cancerous cells. The way they do this is to produce proteins which can damage the outer coating of virus-infected cells. These NK cells also help to regulate the production of antibody from the B cells.

Immune system abnormalities in M.E.

To date a large number of subtle immune system abnormalities have been reported by different research groups in the U.K., U.S.A. and Australia. Unfortunately, these results have often been conflicting, and some of the research has not always met high scientific standards. These inconsistencies may well stem from the fact that researchers have been looking at patients who are in different stages of their illness as far as severity and duration are concerned. Equally, the patients' sex, age, level of physical activity and degree of psychiatric involvement will all have an effect on their immune profile, as can the time of day when the blood sample is taken. These variables must be taken into account in the design of any future research if such findings are to be taken seriously.

As far as antibodies are concerned, minor deficiencies in the amounts of IgG1 and IgG3 (which is responsible for virus neutralization) have been reported by Dr Andrew Lloyd and Professor Denis Wakefield's team in Australia (see medical references 92 and 96). Professors Hobbs and Mowbray in the U.K. have found increased levels of IgE in some patients, suggesting a connection with allergies (see medical reference 85). And, Professor Peter Behan has described occasional increases in the level of IgM and decreased amounts of IgA. However, none of these abnormalities can be considered as being specific to M.E., and they are certainly not diagnostic of the illness.

Researchers on both sides of the Atlantic have continued to speculate as to whether raised levels of immune chemicals such as interferons and interleukins could be adversely affecting the brain and muscle. This would fit in nicely with the hypothesis that a continuing viral infection was causing a permanent upregulation of the immune system, and it has already been shown that when patients with severe liver disease are treated with alpha interferon, they commonly develop a set of flu-like symptoms and lethargy along with muscle pains in the shoulders and neck (see medical reference 94). Unfortunately, there is still no consistent evidence that levels of these immune chemicals are raised in the body, although the Australians have reported finding increased amounts of alpha interferon in the spinal fluid (see medical reference 93). Dr Paul Cheney, in America, has reported increased levels of interleukin 2 (medical reference 82), but others have not been able to replicate this observation. Neither is it yet possible to prove or disprove the theory that there might be a *localized* overproduction of interleukins in certain key parts of the brain which only occurs intermittently and fails to show up in blood samples.

All manner of conflicting abnormalities have also been described in both number and function of T4 (helper) and T8 (suppressor) lymphocytes. Probably the most significant observation here comes from both Dr Andrew Lloyd and Professor Peter Behan, who have found that the T4 cells do not function as effectively as normal when they are stimulated with a substance known as phytohaemagglutinin (PHA). Even so, there is no evidence that the virus has infected these key cells of the immune system in the way that the AIDS virus does where it progressively reduces their numbers. Other research groups have noted changes in the T8 (suppressor) lymphocyte subsets which are consistent with a continuing immune response to a viral infection.

Dr Andrew Lloyd's team has also found T cell function to be abnormal in over 80 per cent of patients when their skin sensitivity responses are measured by a technique known as delayed type hypersensitivity skin testing. Many were found to be either hypoergic (a decreased response) or anergic (no response). Details of this work can be found in medical reference 91.

Although routine measurement of the white blood count by your own general practitioner may show slight abnormalities in the numbers of cells, it cannot pick up the changes I've described in these specialist type of lymphocytes – these investigations have to be carried out in research laboratories. Many of these abnormalities probably represent a normal immune response to a persisting infection, and they cannot be considered as diagnostic tests for M.E.

The final immune system abnormality, which has been found by both Professor Behan (medical reference 95) and Dr Nancy Klimas in the States (medical reference 87), is an abnormality in the function of Natural Killer cells, which act as an important front-line defence against viral infections.

So, in conclusion, a number of immune system abnormalities can be demonstrated in M.E. which are more indicative of a normal response to a persisting virus rather than an actual immune-deficiency as seen in conditions like AIDS. In practice, it seems that although the virus has been recognised, the immune system is unable to eliminate it for prolonged periods of time.

With the newly published findings on abnormalities in the

way that hormones controlled by the hypothalamus are affected in M.E. (see pages 67–71) an alternative explanation for some of these immune changes also needs to be seriously considered. So, instead of a persisting viral infection stimulating the immune response, it may be due to a lack of restraint resulting from changes in the levels of the stress hormone cortisol.

If, in due course, a truly consistent and significant abnormality can be identified in the vast majority of patients, it could well form the basis of a diagnostic test, as well as providing a lead into some form of specific immune therapy. The various types of immune system therapy which have already been tried are described on pages 30–33.

Full details of all the recent medical papers giving further information on immune system abnormalities can be found on pages 351–3.

So, why did I develop M.E.?

'Why me?' is a question that everyone suffering from a chronic disability wants an answer to. In the case of M.E., why is it that such a large number of previously fit, active and economically vital members of the community should be struck down with such a devastating illness in the prime of their lives?

The reasons are extremely complex and not yet fully understood, but from looking at the 'M.E. Equation' on page 21 it is clear that two important components have to combine to produce M.E. In essence this means coming into contact with the right virus at the wrong time in your life!

In the first part of the M.E. Equation the different viruses that seem to trigger the illness have already been discussed earlier on in this chapter. The second part also concerns what are known as 'host factors' – a number of reasons why your immune response was not as effective as it should have been.

The most important host factor is obviously the degree to which you'd managed to acquire natural immunity from previous exposure to infections. On top of this are several other co-factors, all of which may combine to reduce the body's immune response. In the case of M.E. it now appears that stress, as well as age, sex and hormones may all have a role to play when it comes to fighting off a viral infection.

Genetic factors

There is also a suggestion that people with M.E. may have an inherited defect in their ability to respond to viral infections, in a similar way that men sometimes develop the severe rheumatic disease, ankylosing spondylitis, following a gastrointestinal bacterial infection. Time and again it is noticed that M.E. affects different members of the same family, with first degree relatives living in different parts of the country developing the illness on separate dates. This strongly suggests that there is some form of inherited predisposition, and is the reason why researchers are now looking for evidence of common genetic markers called HLA antigens. To date Professor Behan has found that the frequencies of HLA-A, HLA-B and DR antigen markers are all fairly normal. However, he has found that when the lymphocytes which carry these markers are cultured for a long period of time, they fail to express certain HLA markers, and that their expression on B cells is also abnormal. These observations on the genetics of M.E. are not easy to interpret, but they may have important implications regarding the exact type of viruses which can infect cells, and the way in which they persist and alter cell functions (see also medical reference 135).

Age

Age is an important factor in determining susceptibility to both enteroviruses and the Epstein-Barr virus, so far considered the likely culprits in M.E. Children who come into contact with EBV usually develop no illness at all, just protective antibodies. When infected with enteroviruses, they likewise tend to suffer only minor self-limiting illnesses with no after-effects.

However, the body's immune system reacts in different ways to a variety of infections according to age, and as it matures it does not necessarily increase its protective role. 'Childhood illnesses' like rubella, mumps and measles often affect adults far more severely and for longer than they do the young. Teenagers who have not developed immunity to EBV get glandular fever, which may leave them debilitated for months; it is now suggested that a reactivation of dormant EBV may be responsible for M.E. in some adults. Enteroviral infections can also cause serious diseases in adults, including inflammation of the brain and heart, and may even prove fatal.

In Drs Dowsett and Ramsay's survey of 420 chronically affected patients the average age at *onset* was 32 years. It is probably significant that women of this age are frequently in contact with young children and babies: the prime sources of enteroviral infections. Altogether about 75 per cent of people with M.E. first develop their illness at some time between their late teens and mid-forties, but there are also plenty of well-documented cases in children as young as seven, as well as more elderly people occasionally being affected.

Table: Age at onset of ME

Age group	Males	Females	Total
‹ 10 years	3	12	15 (3.5%)
11–15	5	14	19 (4.5%)
16–20	15	40	55 (13%)
21–25	12	26	38 (9%)
26–30	8	30	38 (9%)
31–35	22	58	80 (19%)
36–40	20	56	76 (18%)
41–45	13	33	46 (11%)
46–50	6	15	21 (5%)
51–55	3	9	12 (3%)
56–60	4	10	14 (3.5%)
› 60	2	4	6 (1.5%)
Total	113	307	420

From: EG Dowsett et al., *Postgraduate Medical Journal*, 1990, 66, p527.
Reproduced by kind permission of the Journal.

Sex

There is definitely a strong female bias in M.E. with a 3:1 ratio being reported by Drs Dowsett and Ramsay, and a 1.8:1 ratio in Dr Darrel Ho-Yen's more recent epidemiological survey amongst Scottish general practitioners (medical reference 50).

Outbreaks involving female nursing staff have frequently been reported over the years, though in other outbreaks the sex ratio was equal, and there have been a few instances where only men have been affected, for example in the Swiss army barracks. If women *are* predominantly affected, could there be any logical reasons for this?

First, mothers of young children are in constant contact with the very group that acts as a reservoir of enterovirus infection, passing it on in their faeces to susceptible individuals. Teachers and nurses, other groups commonly affected by M.E., are in a similar position.

Second, when women are ill and need to rest, their domestic and family commitments make it very difficult for them to do so. Unless their husbands can take time off work or extra help is drafted in to look after the family, they just cannot rest, no matter how ill they feel.

Third, women are more likely to know about M.E. and so get it diagnosed. Most of the recent publicity for the condition has been in women's magazines. No such information has been specifically aimed at men, so fewer of them have probably even heard of M.E.

Finally, there is the question of hormones. There is some experimental evidence to support the theory that female hormones can affect the body's immunity, and certainly many women sufferers notice a considerable alleviation of symptoms during pregnancy, when there are very significant shifts in the hormone pattern taking place.

In the laboratory, female mice may die young when introduced to a specific infection, but the males tend to survive. If, however, the sex hormones are removed from the males they will also succumb rapidly, and if the females are given the male sex hormone testosterone their resistance will significantly improve. In scientific experimentation one must be extremely careful about concluding that results from animals will also apply in the same way to human beings. However, these results do give some support to the theory that the sex hormones may be related to the risk of acquiring M.E. on meeting the 'right' virus at the wrong time in your life.

Physical and mental stress

One of the most significant co-factors in increasing susceptibility to developing M.E. appears to be undue physical or mental stress at the time of the original viral infection. Time and again I hear the same story of conscientious patients who struggle on in some stressful occupation or with family commitments, while feeling absolutely terrible, until they are finally forced to stop through sheer physical and mental exhaustion. Back at the Royal Free outbreak in 1955 it was the doctors and nurses, constantly on their feet, mentally and physically stressed, who were taken ill, while only twelve of the patients who were resting in their beds actually succumbed!

There is also some interesting experimental research to support the theory that exercise can be bad for one's health at the time of an infection. Athletes undergoing strenuous physical training programmes show decreased activity in various aspects of their normal immune response. Compared to a group of similar age, who are not undergoing such vigorous activity, the 'active' group is likely to develop more respiratory infections. There are also disturbing reports, from time to time, of sportsmen actually dying while carrying out vigorous exercise – particularly playing squash – at the time of an acute viral infection. The enterovirus Coxsackie can directly affect the heart muscle at the time of the acute illness, and may be the reason for some of these fatalities. In experiments in the laboratory, if the enterovirus Coxsackie B3 is given to two groups of mice, one exercising and the other living a sedentary existence, the exercising mice are more susceptible to the virus.

There are numerous reports of M.E. patients who, having started to make a degree of recovery, go and participate in some form of vigorous athletic activity. They join in a game of hockey or try a marathon run, only to find that this sudden burst of physical activity has left them completely poleaxed, and now their M.E. has relapsed again after a period of relative remission. This sort of activity is clearly *not* recommended for any M.E. patients – well or unwell – until they have remained in very good health for a considerable period of time, and even then only with great caution.

Of equal interest here is the similarity with polio infection: patients who were incubating this enterovirus and then went out and exercised were far more likely to succumb to its paralytic effects. Stress has also been shown to increase one's susceptibility to catching the common cold. In a recent trial reported in the *New England Journal of Medicine* (1991, 325, 606–612) nearly 400 healthy volunteers were given nasal drops containing common cold virus or a placebo. Individual stress levels were also assessed before receiving the virus, and it was found that those with the highest stress levels were far more likely to succumb to colds and chest infections following exposure.

It is not only physical stress that adversely affects the body's immunity. Mental stress and important 'life events' such as family crises, unemployment, bereavements and serious illness all seem capable of depressing the immune system, not only in the person affected, but also in those who are emotionally close. Any crisis could well help to tip the balance in the way someone copes with a viral infection in the first place, as well as influencing how they cope with the continuing illness.

Other forms of stress on the immune system including operations, pregnancy or even another type of infection, may also act as significant co-factors.

A western disease?

It has recently been suggested that in some cases of M.E., especially where there appears to be a gradual onset, the cause may not be a virus at all, but the result of an allergy, or possibly from chemicals and toxins in the environment. This is an attractive theory, and I have already discussed the possibility of organophosphorous pesticide chemicals being implicated.

Some scientists are now coming round to the idea that environmental pollution, along with the 'Western way of life', with its junk food, additives, cigarettes and excessive alcohol intake, may be steadily weakening the body's immune system over a long period of time. Then, when a particular infection comes along, the immune system has become so overloaded that it can no longer cope, and conditions like M.E. are triggered off.

There is not much evidence for M.E. occurring in non-

Westernised societies; maybe it is just not recognised in these parts of the world, but a more likely explanation is the fact that poor public health exposes children to far more enteroviruses, allowing a greater degree of immunity to develop before they reach the 'at-risk' age.

Allergic diseases, particularly hay fever and asthma, appear to increase in incidence when the Western way of life is introduced into primitive communities, so it may be that our environment does play some as yet undefined role in the disease process.

From the information so far gathered, it is still impossible to predict who might develop M.E., and how their particular disease is going to progress. However, the classic 'at risk' patient is female, in her mid-twenties to thirties, and coping with a fair amount of physical and mental stress. The majority of such individuals who contract the 'culprit' virus will *not* develop M.E. All we can say at present is that we have some of the explanations, but we still do not know them all.

Who can recover from M.E.?

'Will I ever get better?' is the first question the M.E. patient wants an answer to once the diagnosis has finally been established. Yes, you can recover from M.E.; it may take several years, but it is still possible after even quite long periods of time. Taking strict rest in the very early stages and readjusting lifestyle seem to have the most positive effect on outcome – which is why late diagnosis and inappropriate management can be so harmful. Until all doctors are able to recognise M.E. in its earliest stages, and to offer correct advice, many patients will not be taking the enforced rest they desperately require.

Any patient who makes steady progress during the first year or so of this illness can reasonably expect this to continue into the third and fourth years, although nothing is absolutely certain with M.E. Obviously the longer the condition remains chronic, without any significant progress, the less likely full recovery is.

M.E. is a very individual condition; some of the symptoms will come and go or vary in severity, whereas others will be there for most of the time. Patients will inevitably go through both good and bad periods during the course of this illness, so accurately assessing what will happen in the long term is very difficult.

Some patients want to know if having an acute or gradual onset to their illness affects chances of recovery. At present there are no accurate statistics available, but some doctors feel that those who develop M.E. in a more gradual fashion, with repeated infections producing a slow deterioration in health, may not do quite só well. One doctor researching M.E. wrote recently that most of his patients had improved over a year, and provided they can take adequate rest in the early stages of the disease, this will apply to many others. However, the attitude that the patient should be *better* by the end of a year is mistaken, though unfortunately still quite common among many doctors, who feel that when all you have had is a bit of post-viral debility you really cannot still be ill a whole year later.

The majority of M.E. patients tend to fall into four broad groups. Firstly there are the patients who, after months or years, make a full or significant degree of recovery, and so return to their normal pattern of life.

The second group of patients tends to follow a much more erratic course, with periods of remission and relapse. During periods of remission they may return to relative normality, even going back to work and starting to lead a normal social life once again. Then M.E. returns – it may be sudden and precipitated by another infection, or undue stress, or an excessive bout of physical activity. However, a few patients just seem to fall back into ill health for no apparent reason. For some, periods of remission can be shortlived, but I know of other M.E. patients who have enjoyed better health for years before succumbing to a relapse. For those whose remissions seem to be getting longer, and their relapses less severe, the eventual outlook is probably quite optimistic.

In the third group are those patients who have chronic unremitting M.E. Dr Melvin Ramsay has described this condition as 'a baffling syndrome with a tragic aftermath'. Follow-up studies of the outbreaks of M.E. described in this book have shown a significant number of patients who remain chronically disabled. Some of the nurses involved in the first recorded outbreak, in Los Angeles in 1934, were thoroughly reviewed nearly fifteen years later and found to be suffering the same muscle fatigue and brain malfunction. They had never managed to return to work. Similarly, over thirty years on from the famous outbreak at the Royal Free Hospital, many of those who were affected remain unwell today.

Sadly, a small but significant minority experience no significant periods of remission and may even start to deteriorate, although this latter course is fairly unusual. In Drs Dowsett and Ramsay's survey 31 per cent of patients reported steady improvement; 20 per cent fluctuating remissions and relapses; 25 per cent a steady level of disability, and 24 per cent had no remissions or experienced significant deterioration.

There is no doubt that some patients with M.E. will have to learn to live with a long-term illness that fluctuates in severity, and to cope with the same difficulties suffered by people with other chronic neurological disorders, like multiple sclerosis. Although some of their symptoms will undoubtedly come and go, and there will be good days to compensate for many of the bad ones, the cardinal features of muscular fatigue and brain malfunction will be present for most of the time. This group of patients will have to accept that life for the foreseeable future is going to be a plateau of ill health interrupted by recurrent exacerbations. The cold months of the year are often a particularly bad time.

Whichever group you seem to fit into, never give up hope. In the meantime accept your limitations, listen to what your body is telling you, and don't try to fight M.E. – it just won't work!

3. M.E. – The Cardinal Symptoms

The onset of M.E.

For the majority of M.E. patients, the illness tends to follow on in the wake of an acute infection. A previously fit individual contracts a mild and unremarkable flu-like illness – and from that point on never really feels well again. Sometimes the initial illness is specific, as in my own case, where M.E. was triggered by chicken-pox; occasionally it can be traced back to a gastric upset contracted while on holiday, possibly caused by bathing in infected water or eating contaminated seafood. But the initial symptoms of most patients follow a pattern we all recognise from bouts of ordinary flu.

There may be swollen and tender lymph glands in the neck and armpit, along with a slight rise in temperature and some general aches and pains. Some patients complain of an associated gastroenteritis ('gastric flu'), or respiratory symptoms such as a sore throat or cough. Marked dizziness and vomiting are an occasional prominent feature, which may lead the doctor to diagnose the illness as labyrinthitis – an infection in the inner ear. Occasionally severe chest pains are reported; patients are sometimes admitted to hospital with a suspected heart attack. The explanation may well be that the enterovirus is affecting either the lining of the heart, causing pericarditis; or the heart muscle itself, causing myocarditis; or that the muscles of the ribcage have become inflamed, which is known as Bornholm's disease. These presentations in M.E. are fairly uncommon but very important, and should not be missed by doctors, as it is now thought that enteroviruses may be one of the commonest causes of infective myocarditis.

As the initial flu-like symptoms start to subside there may

be a short period when the patient begins to feel a return to normal. However, most M.E. patients continue to feel unwell and tired. As they try to resume a normal life, the cardinal M.E. symptoms of exercise-induced muscular fatigue and brain malfunction become more and more apparent, and any undue stress from an early return to work quickly causes a marked exacerbation.

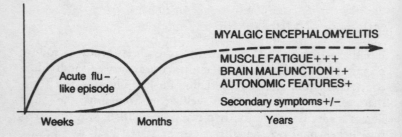

Although the majority of patients develop M.E. in this way, a few have an insidious or gradual onset of the disease, where there is no obvious triggering infection. The symptoms seem to develop over a longer period of time with recurrent mild infections, sore throats and swollen glands, resulting in a progressive deterioration in health. It may be that infection with the 'right virus' did initially take place, and that although it caused no obvious bout of illness at the time, it went on to persist in the body, eventually causing the characteristic features of M.E. to appear.

Muscle fatigue and pain

Exercise-induced muscular fatigue is the cardinal feature of M.E. – if this is not one of your symptoms then the diagnosis is *not* M.E. Rapid muscular fatigue, particularly in the arms and legs, will follow any physical exertion that the patient makes. The load-bearing muscles of the legs are always affected, and many patients notice that the effort of standing still for long periods may be more tiring than going for a walk. If the patient persists in physical activity after fatigue has set in, the result will be weakness and even total exhaustion. The activity involved may be very minimal, such as walking a few hundred yards or doing some light gardening, but for some severely affected M.E. patients even this is too much, and they can find themselves becoming almost housebound.

As M.E. is such an individual illness, different patients have widely varying capabilities as far as their exercise tolerance is concerned, but each soon learns to recognise his or her limitations and the dangers of exercising beyond such limits. Once the point of fatigue/weakness/exhaustion has been reached the M.E. patient will be forced to stop, rest and recover while energy levels return to normal, just like recharging a battery.

The arm muscles become fatigued and weak after lifting heavy objects or reaching up to put things on to a high shelf. Any repetitive activity using these muscles quickly produces weakness, and even a simple task like washing hair can leave some patients feeling thoroughly exhausted.

The highly characteristic recovery period in M.E., during which the energy starts to return to normal in the muscles, can take minutes, hours, even days – it all depends on the extent to which the patient has exceeded his or her capabilities. Exercising to the point of physical exhaustion can result in a very prolonged period of relapse.

Many M.E. patients describe how they have 'tired, aching muscles that wear out easily', and one lady recently described to me how she had spent a considerable part of her life literally crawling around on her hands and knees. A few patients notice that their muscle weakness seems to be worse on one side of the body, and this is often the side which they would regard as being their strongest. So, a right-handed person would find that the right side is predominantly affected. In general, though, muscular weakness will occur in any muscle that is being over-used. Even the very small muscles in the eye are affected, so that vision may become blurred after prolonged reading.

M.E. patients invariably find it extremely tiring trying to perform physical and mental activities simultaneously. This is partly why teachers, hairdressers and nurses with M.E. can find returning to work so difficult, and why pushing the supermarket trolley round to do the weekly shop can be such a debilitating experience. Equally, any sporting activity that requires concurrent physical and mental activity becomes an impossibility. Despite enforced inactivity, muscle wasting is unusual in M.E., and it should not occur unless the patient has been completely immobile for a considerable period of time.

There is no medical solution to muscular fatigue and weakness – the cardinal symptoms of M.E. Patients have to learn to perform within their individual limitations by balancing exercise with adequate periods of rest. My practical approach to exercise and rest is dealt with in further detail on pages 144–7.

Muscle pain and its management

Muscle pain (myalgia) affects up to 75 per cent of patients with M.E., and can become one of the most prominent and distressing symptoms in the whole illness. At first this myalgia is often confined to the shoulder, neck or chest muscles (especially following an attack of Bornholm's disease), but later on it may become much more generalised. It can also involve the tendons, which connect the muscles to the bones in the joints, especially the Achilles tendon in the ankle. Some patients only experience muscle aches and cramps which come on after physical activity. In a small but significant minority the pain takes on a severe and intractable burning quality resulting in loss of sleep and reactive depression, which obviously create further management problems.

Until we can understand much more about the mechanisms involved in pain production in M.E. within both the brain and muscle (perhaps due to a build-up of lactic acid or a disturbance in calcium metabolism), it seems unlikely that any really effective treatment will be made available. For the present, the current options to help with pain relief include:

Analgesics The response to mild pain killers bought over-the-counter in the pharmacy tends to be disappointing.

Aspirin remains an excellent anti-inflammatory drug provided you have no problems with side-effects – so do use it if it helps. Taking aspirin tablets after food helps to minimise stomach irritation, as do enteric-coated tablets. Do remember, though, that prolonged use of aspirin can lead to bleeding from the stomach lining, and that this drug should never be given to children under the age of twelve. There are also some preparations of aspirin which have a slow onset of action; these can sometimes be useful in providing relief from pain during the night.

Paracetamol is the main alternative to aspirin, but it has little in the way of anti-inflammatory action, making it less effective in the control of muscle and joint pains. The maximum safe dose of paracetamol for an adult is 8 × 500 mg tablets in 24 hours – never exceed this or take such quantities for a prolonged period of time, because it is now known that some people's livers are extremely sensitive to paracetamol, and fatal reactions have occurred at what were once thought to be fairly safe doses.

Codeine is another analgesic, sometimes combined with aspirin or paracetamol, which may be useful for mild to moderate pain relief. However, it is too constipating for long-term use, and may also cause dizziness, sedation and nausea. Caffeine is a weak stimulant that is sometimes added to analgesic tablets; it doesn't have pain-killing action and may aggravate any gastric discomfort. It is best avoided.

Stronger analgesics (e.g. Distalgesic, Fortral and DF118) are only available on a doctor's prescription and may only provide limited relief. The risk here is that you may become dependent, so most doctors are quite rightly reluctant to prescribe them without good reason.

An important point to remember with any of these analgesics is that when pain becomes severe and continuous, these drugs have to be taken *regularly* in order to build up and maintain an adequate level in the body. Taking them irregularly will not achieve a satisfactory effect, but do take care to keep well within the safe limits – if in doubt, ask your local pharmacist.

Anti-inflammatory drugs These new non-steroidal anti-inflammatory drugs (NSAIDs) are another type of mild analgesic which can help with muscle and joint pains, as well as headaches. Ibuprofen is sold over-the-counter as Brufen, or obtainable on a prescription. As with any analgesic the risk of side-effects also has to be taken into consideration, and these include stomach irritation and bleeding, rashes and blood problems. Unfortunately, some M.E. patients seem to be unduly sensitive to these particular drugs so they do need to be used with care. More worrying is the recent research which suggests that long-term use can result in thinning of the bones. NSAIDs are also available as ointments, which may be worth a try for localized pain. It should also be remembered that evening primrose oil is a very useful 'natural' drug for helping to alleviate joint pains (see pages 213–14).

Other drugs which are sometimes used in pain relief include anti-depressants and calcium blockers. A low dose of a tricyclic antidepressant, such as amitriptyline, has been found useful in a variety of painful musculoskeletal and neurological conditions, including fibromyalgia and post-shingles neuralgia (nerve pain). At night this can be combined with one of the mild analgesics or NSAIDs already mentioned. There are also reports of patients with severe exercise-induced muscle pain responding to drugs which interfere with calcium metabolism (see also page 149). These cases may be similar to the one described by the eminent neurologist, Sir John Walton, in *The Lancet* in 1981 (see medical reference 158). Drugs used in the treatment of muscle cramp are described on page 103.

Self-help measures which can be quite effective in pain relief include:

- The use of locally-applied heat in the form of a hot-water bottle, or by lying in a warm bath.
- Massage to the affected area using an embrocation from the pharmacy, such as Deep Heat; some patients even find horse linament warming and beneficial!
- Spray-on pain relief aerosols – these tend to provide only a very short period of pain relief.

Other approaches Alternative treatments such as acupuncture (see pages 184–5) or manipulation by an osteopath or chiropractor may be appropriate (see pages 218–20) for pain at specific sites. However, when pain becomes a continuous and disabling part of your illness, unrelieved by any of the above, it may be worth asking your GP to refer you to a pain clinic. Most of the large district hospitals now have such clinics, often run by anaesthetists, but with help from other specialists as well. Sometimes they offer alternative approaches like acupuncture, counselling and new ideas such as transcutaneous electrical nerve stimulation. This involves applying small electrodes onto the skin, directly over the site of chronic pain. A small current is then passed, which is thought to stimulate the production of endorphins – the body's own natural pain killers. Details of how to find a pain relief clinic are found on page 337. Lastly, there is the role of psychological treatments in the management of chronic pain. This is yet another rather controversial area in the management of M.E., because the treatment here may involve 'pushing on' despite increasing pain on the assumption that avoiding any activity which produces pain is counter-productive and only results in a further deterioration in pain tolerance.

Muscle twitchings (fasciculations)

The third quite common muscle feature is twitching of the muscles – referred to by doctors as fasciculation. This abnormality can occur in normal people who are run down, but its frequency in M.E. suggests that here it is probably related to the abnormal lack of co-ordination between the nerve messages and the muscle fibres. Fasciculations may just be noticed as ripples under the skin, or they can be quite coarse. They can appear almost anywhere in the body from large muscle groups in the arms and legs to the smaller muscles controlling the eyelids. Involuntary flickering of the eyelids is known as blepharospasm. This tends to vary in intensity from day to day and throughout the day, often being least severe in the morning, and less marked when the patient is concentrating. It also tends to be associated with sensitivity to bright light. Blepharospasm can occasionally become quite severe and even start to affect the vision. In such cases opthalmologists are now using injections which contain minute amounts of botulinum toxin which paralyses the tiny muscles around the eyelids. This particular treatment is very costly and has to be repeated every ten weeks or so. It is only available from specialist centres such as the Radcliffe Infirmary in Oxford.

Fortunately, fasciculations are usually only an intermittent problem, appearing at times of fatigue, or following undue muscular activity.

Muscle cell pathology in M.E. : a hypothesis

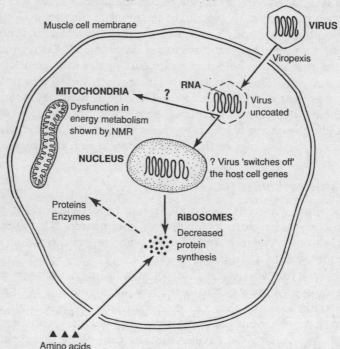

Research into muscle abnormalities in M.E. patients

One of the objects of research into M.E. has been to look for abnormalities in patients' muscles.

Muscle fatigue can have many different causes, depending on which part of the nervous system, or the muscle itself, is not functioning properly. Messages to move or contract a particular muscle group originate in the brain, from where they pass down the spinal cord to the peripheral nerves, which then control the individual muscles. Between the end of the nerve and the start of the muscle fibre is a very important gap, known as the neuro-muscular junction. The message to contract the muscle is conducted across the gap by chemicals known as neurotransmitters. When the message reaches its destination, the muscle fibre contracts and so the arm or leg moves. Muscle weakness can therefore originate anywhere along this pathway.

Patients with spinal cord injuries are obviously unable to pass on the messages below the site of the damage, and so may be unable to move both arms and legs. In conditions like multiple sclerosis the nervous system is also at fault, but in myasthenia gravis the weakness results from abnormalities in the chemical transmission of the messages across the junction. Diseases in which the weakness is purely due to a problem within the muscle are known as myopathies. In children these are usually due to inherited genetic defects (like muscular dystrophy) whereas in adults they can be caused by infections, hormone problems, alcoholism, steroid drugs and a variety of other ailments.

The big question as far as M.E. research is concerned is whether the muscle fatigue and pain are due to a problem in the actual muscle, the brain, or possibly a combination of both. On a very simple level it's rather like searching for a problem in a car that won't perform properly – does the reason lie in the engine (i.e. the muscle), or is it due to the fact that the driver issuing the instructions (i.e. the brain) is at fault?

Some doctors involved in the current M.E. debate, like Professor Richard Edwards from Liverpool, remain extremely sceptical about any evidence pointing to a primary muscle involvement. They argue that the microscopic changes described by Professor Behan are simply due to muscle disuse and inactivity. The real problem in M.E., they maintain, lies centrally in the brain, and involves the complex co-ordination of messages which pass to and from the muscle to maintain its power and activity. The fact that patients with M.E. invariably have normal muscle power when they are examined at rest is not in doubt – the muscle fatigue comes on as a result of exercise. Unfortunately, some of the critics have not always appreciated this fact, and they have also failed to distinguish between people who have chronic fatigue for a variety of reasons, and those who have a true post-viral condition (i.e. myalgic encephalomyelitis). I still believe that the various muscle abnormalities which are now described cannot simply be dismissed as being the result of inactivity.

As has already been discussed in the previous chapter, both Dr Len Archard and Professor Peter Behan have been able to demonstrate that enteroviral RNA persists in the muscle in a significant number of patients with M.E. (medical references 181 and 187). Using the polymerase chain reaction (PCR), the most sensitive molecular virology investigation currently available, Professor Behan and Dr Gow have found enterovirus particles in 53 per cent of muscle biopsies. The true percentage could well be much higher because it is a well-known fact that Coxsackie viruses tend to form patchy (focal) lesions in the muscle which could be easily missed by a needle when taking the biopsy. And, the PCR technique is still not capable of isolating extremely low levels of virus – in the case of M.E. it seems that this is somewhere in the ratio of one virus particle to about 2000 normal cells.

What effect this intracellular virus is having on actual muscle function has now become the subject of intense medical debate. The fact that it may be damaging the mitochondria and interfering with energy production is discussed later. Of equal importance is that Coxsackie viruses are known to multiply more readily in muscle which has been severely exercised (see medical reference 56); consequently, M.E. patients should always be advised to rest in the very early stages of their illness. There is also an important parallel here with polio – an enterovirus which had a predilection for attacking the nerves of recently active muscles, often leading to permanent paralysis. Lastly, there is the most recent finding from Professor Behan, suggesting that there may be abnormalities with calsequestrin – a vital protein that transports calcium around the cell.

To try and detect the ways in which these enteroviruses may be affecting the muscle in M.E., researchers have made use of three investigative techniques – single fibre electromyograms (SF–EMGs), muscle biopsies and nuclear magnetic resonance imaging.

Electromyograms (EMGs) These give the doctor a good idea of how a particular muscle group is responding to electrical stimuli which pass down from the brain and nerve fibres in the spinal cord instructing the muscle to contract. EMGs can show up abnormalities in the way the impulse crosses the gap between the nerve and muscle as well as within the actual muscle fibres.

Conventional EMGs are usually quite normal in patients with M.E. and have led most experts in this field to assume that there is nothing wrong within the muscle. Now, using a highly sophisticated technique known as single fibre electromyography (SF-EMG), Dr Goran Jamal, a neurophysiologist working with Professor Behan in Glasgow, has shown that about 75 per cent of M.E. patients have an abnormality known as 'prolonged jitter'. The unique feature about SF-EMG is that it enables researchers to study how an impulse is transmitted into two separate muscle fibres supplied by the same nerve. So, any abnormality in conduction can be picked up from the point at which the nerve divides, or across the neuromuscular junction, or in the muscle fibre itself. The lack of what is known as impulse blocking indicates that the problem does not lie in the neuromuscular junction (as in myasthenia gravis), and so the most likely site is, according to Dr Jamal, inside the muscle.

Increased jitter is not a specific finding in M.E. (it can also occur in various other nerve and muscle diseases), but in this case it does strongly suggest a definite conduction abnormality in the muscle fibres. It is also a finding that has been reported by Swedish researchers when they looked at the muscles of people during an acute viral infection. At the moment this technique has only been carried out on patients who are resting; but obviously as the muscle fatigue in M.E. comes on during exercise, it would be useful to know if the jitter is exacerbated by physical activity.

Single fibre electromyograms are still only available in a few specialist neurological centres, and they cannot be regarded as a test for M.E. More details of Dr Jamal's work can be found in medical references 102–104.

Muscle biopsies The second line of investigation into muscle involves taking a minute piece of tissue (this can be done almost painlessly using a local anaesthetic and a small needle) from the thigh and then examining it under a microscope.

Normal muscle is made up of two distinct types of fibre. Type I fibres are aerobic (oxygen requiring) and rich in mitochondria. This type of muscle is supposed to be fatigue-resistant, and thus able to withstand prolonged contraction, such as standing up for long periods of time. Type I fibres are also said to be more susceptible to the effects of muscle disuse than the type II variety.

Type II fibres are much more concerned with fine movements, such as performing delicate tasks with the fingers or moving the eyes.

Professor Behan's unit in Glasgow has now carried out muscle biopsies on several hundred M.E. patients. In their most recent series, 50 out of 60 biopsies showed a significant reduction in size (atrophy) of the type II fibres. Although this is not a specific finding in M.E., it cannot be simply explained away as being due to disuse because a leg which is immobilised in plaster does not show the same atrophic changes in the type II fibres.

Using high-powered electron microscopy, the Glasgow researchers have also been looking at individual structures within the muscle cell known as mitochondria. These are aptly named the 'power house of the cell' because it is here that glycogen is broken down to produce energy. Muscle cells are, of course, extremely rich in mitochondria, but these are also present in other tissues, and they have their own genetic codes in the form of DNA.

Under the electron microscope various changes have been noted which appear to be fairly specific to M.E. Firstly, the mitochondria were found to be abnormally situated in the cell clustering around its outer perimeter. Secondly, there appeared to be obvious damage to their internal structure. Instead of the normal convoluted pattern there was swelling, vacuole formation and the development of definite compartments. The significance of these changes has still to be evaluated, but it seems doubtful that such mitochondria can be performing their normal tasks in an effective manner. Once again, as with the SF-EMG findings, these are definite abnormalities which can be found during the acute stages of other viral infections. As mitochondria have their own genetic material

(DNA), it is possible that one effect of the persisting virus is to interfere and 'switch off' enzymes concerned with its normal energy-producing functions. These abnormalities could also fit in with the NMR findings which are described later.

A picture of one of these damaged mitochondria can be found in the *British Medical Bulletin*, October 1991, page 880. For further details of this work, please consult medical reference 100.

One additional test that can be carried out using muscle biopsy material is to stain it for the presence of enzymes which catalyse various functions inside the cell. Once again, several deficiencies have been observed in mitochondrial and cell respiration enzymes. Some of these changes are probably the consequence of relative inactivity in the muscle, whereas others (e.g. adenylate deaminase deficiency) do seem to be related to viral infections.

Professor Timothy Peters, from King's College Hospital in London, has been looking at yet another aspect of muscle cell function using biopsy material. He has been measuring the total content of genetic material (DNA and RNA) and protein in the patients' muscles. Professor Peters' results have shown a significant 17 per cent decrease in RNA, most of which is probably in the ribosomes – structures within the cell that actually manufacture proteins from dietary amino acids.

As a follow-up to this work, he has also been using a radioactively tagged amino acid (leucine C^{13}) to follow its uptake into protein manufacture within both the muscle and the whole body. The preliminary results, both showing decreased protein manufacture, suggest that there may also be a similar problem outside the muscle (see medical reference 108).

So, this is one further piece of evidence indicating that an intracellular virus may be 'switching off' selective aspects of the cell's normal housekeeping activities.

Nuclear magnetic resonance (NMR) This final piece of muscle research involved the co-operation of Professor George Radda and his team working at the John Radcliffe Hospital in Oxford. In the early 1980s they had started to use a new technique, NMR, which enabled them to measure energy production within the muscle by following various chemical changes which were taking place inside the cells. NMR is a painless non-invasive procedure in which the patient is placed inside a giant cylindrical magnet through which chemical changes and muscle acidity during exercise can be followed using a computer.

Dr Melvin Ramsay of the Royal Free asked if I could be the first M.E. patient to be investigated by this new technique, to see if there were any identifiable abnormalities in the way my muscles were producing their energy. I duly visited Oxford and the results confirmed that there was a unique biochemical defect in the way energy was being produced that was not observed in any of their healthy volunteers.

To understand the significance of this result, it is helpful to know how energy is produced inside the muscle. The initial source is provided by carbohydrates in food, which are first broken down by digestive processes, and then stored in the body as glycogen. This is the fuel which is burned up by exercise and, by a process known as glycolysis, converted into energy. For glycolysis to take place, two essential ingredients must be present.

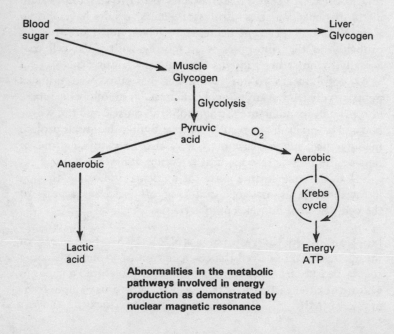

Abnormalities in the metabolic pathways involved in energy production as demonstrated by nuclear magnetic resonance

These are oxygen, brought to the muscles by the red blood cells, and enzymes, produced on site in the muscle cell, which act as catalysts in the burning process. When oxygen and enzymes are present in the right quantities, glycolysis takes place and energy is produced. This is known as aerobic metabolism. However, when oxygen is lacking, the result is anaerobic metabolism, in which excessive amounts of lactic acid are produced instead of energy.

All normal human beings produce lactic acid during exercise, but the results here showed a rapid and excessive acidity in the muscle, indicating a clear abnormality in the way the mitochondria were breaking down glycogen.

When these results were published in *The Lancet* in 1984 (see medical reference 98) it appeared that, at last, a primary defect in the muscle had been discovered. However, since then a further small group of classic M.E. patients has been referred to Oxford, but only about a quarter show this abnormality. At the moment it appears that these findings are probably only relevant to a small subgroup of patients with M.E. Once again this NMR abnormality cannot be regarded as a diagnostic test.

One other researcher who has been looking at the way the muscles perform during exercise is Dr David McCluskey from Belfast. Although he has not found any significant abnormality in lactic acid production, he did observe a reduction in the patients' oxygen requiring (aerobic) physical work capacity (see medical reference 138).

At present it remains uncertain which of these muscle abnormalities are really important in M.E. and how they might all fit together. My own feeling is that there is a muscular component which is not simply due to inactivity, although it is obviously not present in all cases to the same extent. At the same time there is no doubt that important mechanisms also exist in the brain for the production of fatigue. This is probably the explanation for the 'central' fatigue experienced by people with multiple sclerosis, and it may well be equally relevant in M.E. In the meantime the muscle research needs to be pursued as it may eventually isolate biochemical abnormalities which are amenable to treatment.

Further details on research into possible muscle abnormalities can be found in medical references 98 to 112.

How M.E. affects the brain

Brain fatigue and malfunction are invariably a major part of the illness, but just like muscle fatigue, they tend to fluctuate in severity according to exertion. For many patients the day their brains stopped functioning properly is the most distressing feature of M.E., and for those whose employment depends on mental abilities the results can be devastating.

Mental exertion from academic work, reading, attending meetings and any other kind of activity requiring a high degree of intellectual concentration soon causes a rapid deterioration in brain functioning, and patients describe how a cloud descends over the brain as their attention span rapidly shortens. Interestingly, excess physical activity will also cause intellectual fatigue, so at the end of say a walk or a spell in the garden it is not only the muscles that are not functioning – it is the brain as well.

The two commonest symptoms as brain function deteriorates are loss of concentration and loss of recent memory. Recent memory refers to any information that has entered the brain via ears or eyes within the past few minutes or hours. Longer-term memory loss for events in the past is not usually a problem, although a few sufferers do notice difficulties here. Inability to keep one's mind operating and correctly processing and storing incoming information makes mental activity possible for only short periods – few M.E. patients can carry on with a demanding mental task for more than half an hour; for most the period is much shorter. Even the plot of *Dallas* may become impossible to follow after the first thirty minutes! Once ability to concentrate has deteriorated patients (or their friends) may notice that they are using inappropriate or opposite words without realising it (e.g. saying 'hot' when they mean 'cold'), or are completely unable to remember a familiar word or name – what doctors call anomia.

The ability to perform previously learned and familiar procedures – even knotting a tie or doing up one's shoelaces – may become temporarily impossible during an episode of brain malfunction. Rest then restores the energy levels and relatively normal function returns. Clumsiness, especially when undertaking fine tasks like threading a needle, is very common, and many patients also experience difficulties in co-ordinating their legs on stairs, or coming off moving escalators – if they dare get on them in the first place! Handwriting often deteriorates in the course of writing a long letter – if the brain can supply the necessary information.

Whichever parts of the brain are involved in M.E., there certainly does not seem to be any dementing process, with a gradual progressive deterioration of mental abilities over the course of the illness. The features of intellectual malfunction characteristically tend to fluctuate in severity – the patient's mental functioning may be perfectly normal for a short period of time, and then deteriorate rapidly, usually after a burst of mental or physical activity.

What could be going wrong in the brain?

Brain symptoms in M.E. are often referred to as being the 'encephalitic' component of the illness, although there is no firm evidence that encephalitis (an inflammation of the brain tissues) is taking place. The explanation is actually far more complex, and involves the way in which brain cells function rather like a computer.

Although a number of explanations have been put forward as to the cause of this malfunction, my current view is that the primary disturbance involves a persisting virus. Other factors, such as increased lymphokine production and changes in blood flow or energy production, may also be playing a part, but they are probably of secondary importance.

As far as viruses are concerned, it is now well accepted that a number of common viruses, including measles, mumps, rubella, Epstein-Barr, chicken-pox and enteroviruses are all capable of entering, persisting and multiplying inside brain cells (medical reference 136). Areas of the brain that seem to be particularly affected include the hypothalamus (see later), the thalamus and the limbic system – the latter being a key area that co-ordinates hormonal and emotional responses to stressful signals. Once viruses have evaded the body's normal immune response and crossed what's known as the blood brain barrier, they have a remarkable ability to literally 'take over' almost every aspect of the cell's normal activities (see page 27), but particularly, the production of neurotransmitters – chemicals which transmit messages around the nervous system and so control mood, energy, sleep, well-being, etc. This is the reason why many researchers now believe that the main site for the production of fatigue in M.E. actually lies centrally in the brain, and not peripherally in the muscle. A similar situation probably occurs in multiple sclerosis where patients often have a lot of 'central' fatigue but quite normal muscles.

One neurotransmitter that is currently attracting a great deal of scientific attention is called serotonin (or 5HT/5 hydroxytryptamine). This is a chemical that is made in the nerve endings from tryptophan, an amino acid which forms part of our normal diet. As I describe later on page 170, there are now drugs available called reuptake inhibitors, which block the re-entry of 5HT back into the nerve endings and so enhance its activity in the brain. One part of the nervous system that is thought to be particularly rich in pathways controlled by this transmitter is the hypothalamus.

5HT is now known to have widespread effects in the body, not only on the nervous system, but also on the heart and digestive tract. In the brain it affects memory, temperature regulation, sleep, sexual behaviour and mood. It also appears that some types of depression may be caused by 5HT imbalance, and that it plays an important role in appetite control. 5HT activity is increased in anorexia and decreased in bulimia (binge eating), and so drugs which increase 5HT activity will reduce appetite and bring about weight loss. The fact that 5HT is made from tryptophan may also explain why some patients have cravings for carbohydrate foods which are rich in this amino acid.

Secondary explanations, that also need to be considered, include the possibility of persisting virus stimulating increased production of immune chemicals, such as interferon (see page 162), and disturbances in energy production due to mitochondrial dysfunction, as has already been shown to occur in muscle. It should be remembered that just as muscles run out of energy during activity, so does the brain. For the brain to function effectively, it requires large amounts of energy, just like the muscles.

Finally, there are the highly significant findings, from both the U.K. and America, of disturbances in the levels of various hormones controlled by the hypothalamus, some of which also have an important role in energy production.

Research into brain abnormalities

Because patients do not die from M.E., brain tissue seldom becomes available for examination under the microscope to help follow up these various theories as to what may be going wrong in the nervous system. However, in the past few years, some postmortem/autopsy material has been obtained from very sad instances where patients have committed suicide; there are now isolated (but unpublished) reports of enterovirus being found by the pathologists in these cases. For the moment, though, researchers have to largely rely on various investigative techniques and psychological testing to suggest where abnormalities in brain functioning might be occurring. These include:

EEG and BEAM scans The long-established method for looking at electrical activity in the brain is known as an electro-encephalogram (EEG). Here electrodes are placed on the scalp and changes in voltage are recorded which correspond to brain-wave activity. In the past, EEG measurements have only shown up occasional non-specific abnormalities in patients with M.E., with no evidence of active brain inflammation (encephalitis) despite the use of this term in the name. However, one group of neurologists are now re-evaluating the information obtained from EEGs to see if there could be specific diagnostic abnormalities present.

There are now some highly sophisticated forms of EEG equipment available from America which can extract more precise information. One such technique is know as a BEAM scan, but these are still few in number and only being used in specialist centres. One researcher, who has been making use of BEAM scans to map out the brain's activity, is Dr Marshall Handleman, a neurologist working at the University of Southern California Medical School. His results, presented to the 1990 Cambridge Symposium, suggest that there are abnormalities in parts of the brain known as the temporal lobes and hippocampus – the latter being an area that plays a key role in the formation of new memories.

Evoked Potentials Dr Leslie Findley and Dr Deepak Prasher at London's National Hospital for Nervous Diseases have been looking at what are called cortical evoked potentials – a way of measuring the way the brain reacts to and then processes all kinds of incoming information. Several different kinds of tests have been used, and those measuring auditory (hearing), visual and sensory evoked potentials were all found to be normal. (Incidentally, visual evoked potentials are often abnormal in multiple sclerosis, making this a useful test if there is doubt about the diagnosis). The important finding in the M.E. group of patients was an absence or delay in what is known as cognitive potential P3 – a finding which is probably consistent with the problems of concentration, memory and processing new information. Interestingly, this abnormality was not found in a group of depressed patients in whom concentration difficulties are also common and often quite severe. (See also medical reference 21).

MRI scans 'MRI' stands for Magnetic Resonance Imaging. Here, the part of the body being examined is placed in a high-powered magnetic field. A perfect picture of the anatomy can then be built up by measuring the amount of electromagnetic radiation being given off from the tissues. In the brain and nervous system this can give precise information about very small lesions which could never be obtained using conventional X-ray equipment.

American researchers, using an even more sensitive MRI scanner, have now detected small lesions in the white matter of the brain (medical reference 5). Dr Sandra Daugherty and colleagues from the University of Nevada School of Medicine have reported these findings in a group of fifteen patients with severe M.E./CFIDS, some of whom had also started to develop other neurological symptoms. Their scans revealed small but definite lesions in various parts of the brain which were not seen in 'control' patients or those with dementia or psychiatric disorders. Along with the abnormalities found on psychological testing, the team concluded that these MRI lesions could not be attributed to psychological factors and that they were, in fact, very similar to the disturbances seen in some adults with HIV infection affecting the brain.

The results of a much larger MRI study have now been reported in the *Annals of Internal Medicine* (medical reference 17). Here, Professor Tony Komaroff's team examined a group of patients who fell ill between 1984 and 1987 – many of whom were involved in the famous Lake Tahoe outbreak that I described in the first chapter.

These MRI scans revealed numerous pinpoint lesions in the white matter of the brain in 78 per cent of those examined. The authors concluded that the abnormalities were consistent with inflammation or demyelination (loss of the protective sheath that surrounds a nerve cell), and were very similar to findings sometimes observed in patients with multiple sclerosis or HIV infection involving the nervous system.

At the moment it is not yet possible to draw any firm conclusions from these MRI scans because similar findings occur in other neurological conditions, and occasionally in apparently healthy people. However, in view of the presence of larger and deeper lesions within the brain in this group, and the correlation of anatomical site to clinical symptoms, these do seem to be very important findings.

These type of MRI scans have not yet been done in the U.K., but this is obviously an important area of research that needs to be followed up and repeated to see if other researchers obtain similar results.

SPECT scans This acronym stands for Single Photon Emission Computerised Tomography. SPECT scans make use of the fact that specially labelled chemicals (radioactive isotopes) are taken by the patient. The radiation which is then emitted can be used to measure blood flow in various key parts of the brain. This technique has been used by Dr Ismael Mena, who is director of the nuclear medicine department at the Harbor–UCLA Medical Center in California. His results, again presented at the

Cambridge Symposium, suggest that about 70 per cent of the patients investigated had an abnormally low blood flow to one or both of the temporal lobes. Once again, this is not a specific diagnostic finding in M.E. – reduced blood flow can also occur in a variety of other neurological problems including migraine and strokes. However, these results certainly tie in with other neurological investigations looking at the temporal lobe area. It was also noted that, after being given drugs called calcium channel blockers (which help to dilate the blood vessels), there was an increase in temporal lobe blood flow.

The most recent results from Dr Mena's team (reported in *CFIDS Chronicle*, Fall 1991) involve a study to see if exercise makes any difference to brain blood flow because, as anyone with M.E. knows, physical activity can produce a rapid deterioration in mental functioning. In normal people, exercise increases blood flow to the brain, but in his group of patients there was a significant fall in supply to both the temporal and frontal lobes.

SPECT scans are an important new advance in the assessment of brain function rather than structure, and similar work is now under way at London's Middlesex Hospital and in Canada.

Psychological testing Clinical psychologists, by testing various mental skills, can to some extent show which specific parts of the brain are now working properly. Once again, most of this type of research is being carried out in America.

Dr Curt Sandman, a research psychologist at the University of California in Irvine, and Dr Sheila Bastien, a neurophysiologist from Berkeley, California, have both been studying how patients with M.E./CFIDS cope with mental performance tests.

Dr Sandman's results indicate that there are clear differences between M.E./CFIDS patients and people with a purely depressive illness. Firstly, most people, even those who are depressed, can improve their mental functioning with the aid of cues, but these seem to be of no value in M.E./CFIDS. This again suggests a specific problem with new memory formation. Secondly, he found that the ability of his patient group to learn new information was severely affected by any form of interruption – something which again is not a major problem in depression. Lastly, on specially devised mental ability tasks, the patients tended to overestimate their abilities, whereas those with depression tended to underestimate their abilities.

Dr Sheila Bastien has also been using a battery of complex psychological tests, and her results were presented to the Cambridge Symposium. She found that a patient group had a significantly reduced intellectual ability with particular problems in the areas of maintaining attention, concentration, problem solving and memories of recently spoken information. Again, her results pointed specifically towards temporal lobe dysfunction.

In the U.K. the principle research into this area of brain malfunction is being carried out by Dr Andrew Smith, who has been working with patients referred to Professor Behan's unit in Glasgow. Some of Dr Smith's preliminary results – which also confirm that patients with M.E. have problems with maintaining attention, retrieving stored information from the brain and carrying out logical reasoning – can be found in Dr Rachel Jenkins' book *Post-Viral Fatigue Syndrome* (see page 362). His results also appear to demonstrate clear differences between M.E. and depression. Dr Smith is now looking at similarities between the abnormalities seen in M.E. and those experienced by patients with HIV infection; these results are awaited with great interest.

A report giving detailed information on all the papers presented at the Cambridge International Symposium can be obtained from the M.E. Association (see Useful Addresses).

Further details of other papers which have been published on brain and nervous system disturbances can be found on page 347.

Hormone control and the hypothalamus

Probably the most important research findings to date concern the role of the hypothalamus, a tiny part of the brain which acts as the body's internal thermostat controlling appetite, sleep rhythm, temperature regulation and the autonomic nervous system – all of which may be affected in M.E. What is now becoming apparent is that there are clear abnormalities in these hypothalamic control mechanisms, as well as the way this gland provides a vital link between other parts of the brain and the various hormone-producing (endocrine) glands.

The way in which the hypothalamus finely tunes the blood levels of hormones like cortisol is best understood by following the diagram on page 69. Firstly, a number of factors such as sleep, exercise, emotions and levels of blood sugar all influence hypothalamic activity. As far as hormones are concerned, their blood levels are constantly monitored by receptors in the gland; should they rise or fall from normal the hypothalamus quickly responds by sending chemical messages to another hormone-producing gland, the pituitary or 'master gland', which is attached to the underside of the brain.

It is from here that hormone releasing factors are produced that stimulate glands such as the thyroid, adrenals and ovaries to start secreting their own individual hormones. These in turn enter the blood to carry out their various functions.

Researchers in both the U.K. and America have been looking at levels of three such hormones (ADH, prolactin and cortisol), all of which are controlled by the sophisticated feedback mechanisms of the hypothalamic-pituitary axis (HPA).

ADH (also known as the *antidiuretic hormone* or arginine vasopressin) is produced by the posterior part of the pituitary gland. Its function is to regulate the amount of water produced by the kidneys and excreted as urine. As I describe later (see page 94) many women with M.E. seem to have a problem with fluid retention, especially around the mid-point of the menstrual cycle when they may put on several pounds in weight. To study this further Professor Behan's team in Glasgow carried out various tests to see if there were any abnormalities in the hormonal control of water balance. One such test involved an overnight fast which was then followed by the intake of a large quantity of water. Normal people usually remove well over 80 per cent of such a load within four hours, but the M.E. group only managed about 60 per cent. They were also found to have an erratic release of ADH into the blood, and increased amounts of total body water when compared to a control group. The results indicate a definite abnormality in the way that water balance is being regulated by the hypothalamus and pituitary glands.

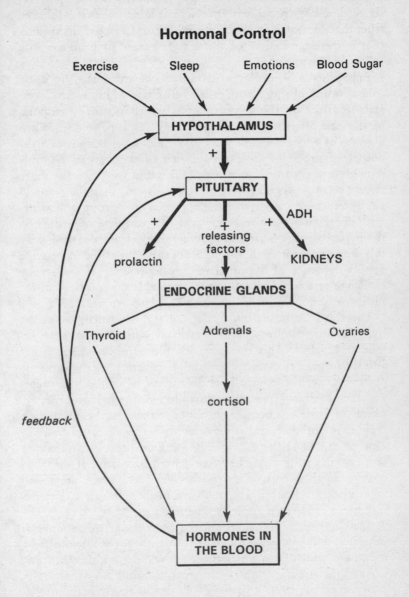

Hormonal Control

The second hypothalamic–pituitary abnormality being investigated in Glasgow concerns prolactin, a hormone that is released
from the anterior part of the pituitary gland, whose main function is the stimulation of the female breast to produce milk
following pregnancy.

Experimentally, prolactin release can be stimulated by using
a new tranquillising drug called buspirone. This locks on to
receptor sites on the hypothalamus which normally respond
to the neurotransmitter chemical $5HT_1$ (see page 62). When
a group of M.E. patients were given a dose of buspirone their
output of prolactin *far* exceeded that of the normal controls
strongly suggesting that their 5HT receptors were far more
sensitive (an 'upregulation' in medical jargon) than they should
be. Interestingly, when this test was used on a group of patients
with depression their response was the complete opposite. As
the hypothalamus is rich in nervous connections controlled by
this neurotransmitter chemical (5HT) these experiments provide
further evidence of hypothalamic dysfunction. The buspirone
challenge test could also become a valuable diagnostic tool for
distinguishing M.E. from depression. (Also see page 177.)

The third hormonal study looked for abnormalities in the
hypothalamic–pituitary–adrenal pathway which controls the release of cortisol. This hormone has powerful anti-allergy and
anti-inflammatory properties through its action on the immune
system, as well as controlling the way in which body proteins
and carbohydrates are broken down to produce heat and energy.
Levels of cortisol fluctuate throughout the day, being at their
highest in the early morning and lowest in the late evening.
One of the most important influences on cortisol production
is stress, and patients with severe depression often have marked
changes in their cortisol responses. Very low levels are found
in a condition known as Addison's disease, which is another
important cause of chronic fatigue (see page 119).

Cortisol production is stimulated from above by an anterior
pituitary hormone called ACTH (*a*dreno *c*ortico *s*timulating
*h*ormone) which in turn is influenced by feedback mechanisms,
particularly stress, acting on the hypothalamus.

In December 1991, a group of American researchers, including Drs Mark Demitrack and Stephen Straus from the National

Institute of Health, reported their findings on abnormalities in cortisol control in a group of 30 M.E./CFIDS patients.

This group had a *mild* decrease in blood cortisol levels which seemed to be present throughout the day. The results also indicated that the adrenal glands (which sit above the kidneys) had become oversensitive to a chronically low level of ACTH, and so the primary problem was at the level of the hypothalamus. Once again, as with the prolactin results, these are the complete opposite to what is found in depression.

It is also worth noting that a low level of cortisol could be altering immune function in such a way that it allows an exaggeration of allergic responses and the reactivation of dormant viral infections such as Epstein-Barr. This provides another possible reason for why some patients seem to show a rise in Epstein-Barr antibodies.

These three research projects should finally help to dispel any doubts about M.E. being a genuine organic illness, and the relevant medical references can be found under endocrinology research on page 349. Sadly, very few sceptical doctors will ever find the time to open their medical journals and study these results.

Management of brain malfunction

This second cardinal feature of the illness invariably becomes an extremely disabling and frustrating part of everyday life. However, on a more positive note, it's something that can definitely improve as time goes on, as I'm able to testify from personal experience. For some patients, though, their frequent and often severe episodes of mental incapacity bring sheer despair.

At present, there is no drug therapy that can be routinely recommended to help this particular aspect of the illness. Antidepressants may improve memory and concentration where there is co-existent depression, but I am not convinced of their value in its absence (see pages 167–9). The role of the new 5HT drugs mentioned earlier in this chapter looks more promising, but we must await the results of proper clinical trials before coming to any firm conclusions. In America some doctors are using drugs such as calcium blockers which may increase blood flow to the brain, but the claims are largely anecdotal. This type of approach does have theoretical advantages if the initial findings of the SPECT scans described earlier really do mean that there are significant reductions in blood flow and oxygenation to certain parts of the brain.

Self-help One of the biggest problems for anyone with M.E. is sustaining any form of intellectual activity. Here are a few practical suggestions which may help you to cope:

- Accept that mental activity is going to fluctuate widely from day to day, and even from hour to hour. Tasks which could be easily accomplished on one day may not be possible on the next.
- Totally abstaining from any kind of mental activity isn't a good idea even if your brain function may only feel like 20 per cent of normal. If you can't cope with a quality newspaper, then switch to a tabloid rather than reading nothing at all.
- Even when you are coping quite well with mental tasks, it's still a good idea to 'switch off', and relax completely for a few minutes each hour rather than pushing on to the point of mental exhaustion and confusion.
- Most people with M.E. tend to feel better at fairly predictable times during the day, so try to schedule activities which can be planned in advance to fit in with those times.
- As with physical activity, try to *gradually* increase the amount you decide to do on a 'day-to-day' basis, and accept that progress may be two steps forward followed by one step back.
- Make use of memory aids by keeping a pocket notebook to record a daily list of activities which need to be attended to, phone calls to be made, etc., etc., and then tick them off as they're completed. It's also a good idea to use a Filofax or keep a careful diary of forthcoming events, and write them all down before you forget.
- Mental confusion is always made considerably worse when there's too much activity going on around you. So, try to do the shopping at quieter times of the day and, if you do

have to concentrate on a mental task, then do it in a quiet environment.

● If you have to memorise some really important information, it can help by reading it out aloud. Seeing, hearing and reading something will reinforce your chances of retaining it.

● As far as leisure activities are concerned, if you can't concentrate on a favourite television programme at its scheduled time, consider hiring a video recorder rather than missing out on what may be one of your few sources of pleasure. Equally, active sports and hobbies which have been abandoned should ideally be replaced by something passive rather than doing nothing at all.

● If you're having severe difficulties with mental functioning, it may be worth asking to be referred to a clinical psychologist for an opinion and advice. These psychologists are often attached to neurological departments in hospitals or centres specialising in rehabilitation of stroke or head injury patients.

● Lastly, it's worth remembering that the brain needs feeding just like the rest of the body, so people with M.E. must take particular care to eat regular nutritious meals.

Headaches This symptom occurs in about 75 per cent of M.E. patients. My personal experience is of headaches which appear intermittently, but which are of sufficient severity to prevent any meaningful mental activity for a large part of the day.

If you have persisting or severe headaches it is always a good idea to check with your GP as they could be due to high blood pressure, a sinus problem, or something called temporal arteritis in the elderly age group. This latter condition is often accompanied by visual disturbances and quite severe muscle pain. It *must* be treated urgently with high doses of steroids to reduce the inflammation in the blood vessels.

As with muscular pain the response of headaches to simple over-the-counter painkillers is often far from satisfactory. I find that local heat (in the form of a warm facecloth or a hot water bottle) and some time resting in bed is the best solution. A warm bath can also be very relaxing if there is tension in the neck muscles. Stronger pain killers are best avoided unless really necessary. Some patients have reported relief by using evening primrose oil. For headaches that take on a migrainous character (i.e. one-sided, and associated with nausea and visual disturbances) there are specific and effective drugs available on prescription. One new one called Imigran (sumatriptan) affects blood flow in the brain by acting on the 5HT receptors that I have already referred to. In migraine it is also a good idea to try cutting out foods such as cheese and chocolate, as well as red wine and coffee for a while. The Migraine Trust (see Useful Addresses) are also very helpful.

How M.E. affects the nervous system

The human nervous system consists of millions of individual nerve cells, which store and pass on information and instructions rather like a computer. The various control centres for all this nervous activity are situated in different parts of the brain. From here the messages pass down the spinal cord and then out via the numerous tiny nerves to muscles, blood vessels and the body organs which are under nervous control. One particularly important part of the nervous system affected by M.E. are the autonomic nerves.

The autonomic nervous system

This consists of two complementary sets of nerves, known as the sympathetic and parasympathetic fibres, which both pass to the part of the body they are controlling, but have opposing functions. For example, the sympathetic nerves to the heart will speed up its rate, whereas the parasympathetic fibres will slow down the rate. These nerves are again controlled by 'higher centres' in the brain, particularly in the brain stem.

These nerves are called autonomic, because unlike the nerves which control muscle movements, we don't have much voluntary control over their actions. If we get very worried about something this will trigger activity in the sympathetic nerves and speed up the pulse rate quite automatically, but there's no way we can cancel out this automatic overactivity.

The autonomic nerves try to maintain a 'status quo' in the body, and exert control over a wide range of body functions. They pass to the heart, the intestines and the bladder where they control the emptying functions. They also have a very important role in body temperature control.

Temperature control and night sweats

One particularly important autonomic control centre in the brain is known as the hypothalamus, and it's from here that the body is programmed to maintain its constant internal temperature. It acts as an 'internal thermostat'.

M.E. patients invariably have various difficulties with their body temperature control, being abnormally sensitive to any extreme of temperature, be it a hot bath or climatic heat or cold. This is also quite a common finding in multiple sclerosis where marked fatigue follows a hot bath; some multiple sclerosis patients have reported significant benefits by using a special apparatus which helps to cool down the core temperature of the body.

Patients often feel cold and shivery, and may even want to wrap up when the external temperature is quite warm. It's not unusual to record body temperatures with a thermometer constantly a degree or so below normal. One strange aspect of this, which I personally experience, is that whenever I succumb to an infection I rarely have a raised temperature, but just feel cold and shivery, and so take to bed with a jersey and hot-water bottle.

One of the normal body mechanisms for losing heat is to sweat, and profuse night sweats (just like those some women experience during their menopause) are quite a common feature. Sweating may also be noticed by some patients when they try to 'push on' – mentally or physically – beyond their limitations.

Night sweats are also a prominent feature of a lymph node cancer known as Hodgkin's disease. Here the trigger factor is thought to be an increased production by the macrophages of one of the immune chemicals mentioned in the previous chapter (interleukin 1). Apparently, this can induce an abrupt increase in the manufacture of a substance called prostaglandin E2 within the hypothalamus, and this raises the body's thermostat. It is quite possible that similar mechanisms may be involved in M.E.

Unfortunately, there's no effective medical therapy for these problems with temperature regulation apart from avoiding, wherever possible, situations where they might occur. This is particularly appropriate if you go on holiday to hot climates and stay out too long in the sun, thinking it's bound to be beneficial.

The heart and blood vessels

M.E., through dysfunction of the nervous system, can also affect the heart and the small blood vessels. Overactivity in the sympathetic nervous system can cause a sudden increase in the pulse rate (a tachycardia) and this may be accompanied by the frightening sensation of actually feeling the heart beating inside the chest – palpitations. These palpitations will be exacerbated if the patient is also feeling anxious. If you experience either rapid pulse rates or palpitations, it's very important to avoid anything else which can overstimulate these nerves, including coffee, alcohol and even the contents of some cold cures and nasal sprays. If in doubt do ask your pharmacist.

There are drugs available, known as beta-blockers, which can dampen down this overactivity and help to control symptoms, and where palpitations are particularly bothersome such treatment may be worth trying. Before using these drugs your doctor may wish to check the heart rhythm using an electrocardiogram (ECG), just to make sure that there's no other problem with the heart itself. One of the disadvantages of using beta-blockers is that like all drugs they have side-effects, some of which can be similar to the symptoms already caused by M.E. It is also interesting to note that one of the findings in Professor Behan's placebo-controlled trial of high-dose evening primrose oil (see page 214) was a significant reduction in the incidence of palpitations and other heart rhythm disturbances. Similar benefits have also been described in animals with experimentally induced rhythm problems.

The sympathetic nerves also alter the size of the tiny blood vessels which supply blood to the hands and feet. The ghastly facial pallor which may be noticed before a patient feels grossly fatigued may be part of this malfunction, if blood supply to the skin is reduced. Cold hands and feet are a common accompaniment to M.E., and are often brought on by cold weather, when these tiny blood vessels seem to be unduly sensitive and clamp down. Inhalation of cigarette smoke can also worsen the problem. Beta-blockers can exacerbate these symptoms, as well as the feelings of fatigue. So, the exact drug needs to be chosen with care, and this usually means using one whose effects are primarily on the nerves to the heart (a cardioselective one), and at a low enough dose to be both effective, and hopefully free from side-effects.

The most effective way of dealing with the problems of cold hands and feet is by the following simple practical advice:

- In the house, try to make sure that at least one room is as draught free as possible; to save on heating bills in winter keep at least one area of the house constantly warm.
- At night have a warm drink before going to bed, and take a hot drink in a flask upstairs in case you feel cold in the night. A nightcap, bedsocks, gloves and pyjamas should all help to keep you warm, along with an electric blanket or covered hot water bottle if necessary.
- Lack of physical exercise isn't very good for the circulation, so do try to avoid sitting still for long periods of time. If you are going through a relapse and are very inactive it's still worth keeping up with some passive exercises in bed.
- Never warm up cold hands or feet by putting them straight on to a radiator or under hot running water – they *must* be warmed up gradually.
- It's vital to keep the trunk warm, this is best done by wearing several layers of thin clothing rather than one very thick layer. Air becomes trapped between the various layers and helps to insulate the body.
- Before going outside in winter always wear a hat (a considerable amount of heat is lost from the scalp and face), a scarf and thermal clothing if it's really cold.
- Hands and feet must always be adequately covered. Woollen tights, leg warmers and thick woollen socks are all ideal. Footwear can be insulated by lining it with aluminium foil or thermal 'space age' inner soles.

- Don't forget that the body needs plenty of warm 'fuel' on cold winter days. A bowl of hot porridge is an ideal way to start; then try to have regular small meals throughout the day to maintain energy levels.
- Avoid touching cold surfaces and objects, and don't go into the fridge or freezer without wearing insulated gloves.
- Don't smoke cigarettes (nicotine constricts the tiny blood vessels even further); avoid other people's smoke wherever possible.
- Try using a Mycoal Warm Pack which acts as a portable body warmer. These come as sachets, which when exposed to the air will generate heat from 50°–70°F. They can then be used to insulate gloves, shoes etc. Hand and Foot Warmers last up to six hours, Body Warmers up to twenty hours. If cold hands and feet are causing a lot of difficulties, especially outdoors in winter, it may be worth taking more radical measures, and purchasing some battery-heated shoes and gloves. The Raynaud's Association Trust (address on page 338) deals specifically with this condition, and can give further practical advice and details on how to obtain the Mycoal Warm Packs.

Although many patients experience palpitations and rapid pulse rates from time to time, this doesn't mean that the heart has become affected by the illness. The most likely reason is an overactivity of the sympathetic nerves which are telling it to start beating faster.

However, there are a few patients with M.E. who do have associated heart disease, because, as mentioned earlier, the enteroviruses can affect both the heart muscle (the myocardium = myocarditis) or the heart lining (the pericardium = pericarditis). In these cases the patient is often quite seriously ill at the beginning, due to the effects on the heart, and may have to be admitted to hospital. In many cases this heart involvement will completely settle down, but in a few these problems will continue. Previously doctors explained these patients' fatigue as being the result of poor output of blood from the damaged heart tissues. Although this is an important factor, it's now recognised that some of these 'heart patients' do have M.E. as well.

I must stress that this direct involvement of the heart is very unusual, but it can occur. If you are having persistent chest pains and palpitations your doctor will probably want to do some tests (e.g. an electrocardiogram to trace the heart rhythm), just to be sure there's nothing more serious going wrong. Medical references 52 to 60 refer to papers which specifically discuss the effects of enteroviral infection on the heart and its possible implications in M.E.

Feeling faint or fainting

One further important function of the autonomic nerves is that of controlling our blood pressure by their effect on the size of the larger blood vessels. If these vessels are too dilated, then the pressure in the system falls, not enough blood reaches the brain, and we either feel faint or actually faint. When we move from lying or sitting to a standing position these vessels should contract to keep blood flowing to the brain, but some M.E. patients find they feel faint on suddenly standing up, and this is what doctors call postural hypotension – a fall in blood pressure on standing.

Postural hypotension probably isn't the only reason why you may feel faint at times. In some of the earlier outbreaks of M.E., a few patients were found to have very low blood sugars (hypoglycaemia) and were even admitted to hospital unconscious because of this. Another factor may be related to any drugs being taken. Antidepressant drugs can lower blood pressure as a side-effect, as can alcohol and excessive heat. Lastly, there's a special type of fainting attack, known as micturition syncope, which tends to affect men when they have to get up in the middle of the night to pass urine. It seems that the combination of postural hypotension and the autonomic nerve activity involved in bladder emptying combine to cause a faint.

If feeling faint is a particular problem it's worth asking your doctor to check your blood pressure, to see if it does fall significantly when you change from lying to standing.

Whatever the cause, there are measures *you* can take:

- If postural hypotension is the problem, be very careful

about how you move from lying to standing. Learn to exercise your stomach muscles by pulling them in several times before changing position – this helps to raise the blood-pressure – and get up slowly.

- If you're getting hypoglycaemic take regular meals, and carry a supply of glucose tablets to take if necessary (see also page 148).

- With micturition syncope do make sure that you get out of bed very slowly at night, and always sit on the toilet when passing urine.

If feeling faint becomes very troublesome you should ask your doctor to check that there is nothing wrong with your blood cortisol level (see earlier in this chapter). There are also some drugs which can be prescribed, but they require very careful consideration, and are outside the scope of this book.

Problems with balance

The almost constant unsteadiness experienced by many patients is one further example of how M.E. can affect the way in which both the inner ear and parts of the central nervous system help to maintain our balance. This disturbance in equilibrium is often reported as being very similar to feeling 'drunk all the time' or even 'walking on rubber'. However, most patients don't experience the typical spinning sensation that doctors associate with the term vertigo.

For a significant minority, especially where the illness started with a viral labyrinthitis (an infection involving the inner ear), the problems with balance can become far more disabling. Tripping over in the dark is a common consequence, and the result can be a serious fall.

These problems with balance are often dismissed by doctors as being due to anxiety or hyperventilation (overbreathing), particularly when tests for balance have all turned out to be relatively normal. The doctor's examination is likely to include asking you to stand up with your eyes closed (the Romberg test), and you may well be referred to the ear, nose and throat clinic for more complicated hospital tests.

In my own case, it was only after being referred to the special balance unit at the National Hospital for Nervous Diseases in London that I was finally able to convince the doctors at the DSS that I did have a genuine problem with balance – this showed evidence of viral damage to a part of the brain, the cerebellum, which is involved in maintaining normal body equilibrium.

As far as management of unsteadiness is concerned, I have not found any of the prescription drugs used in the treatment of vertigo to be particularly beneficial. Drugs such as prochlorperazine (Stemetil) may be very helpful in an acute or severe attack, but they must *not* be used continually because they can cause additional neurological problems as a side-effect. A more recently used drug called cinnarizine (Stugeron) does appear to be very safe and can be purchased in the pharmacy without a prescription. Again, it's unlikely to help with persistent unsteadiness, but it can be useful for preventing motion sickness developing on car journeys or sea crossings.

Neurologists interested in the practical difficulties associated with vertigo have devised a series of exercises (Cooksey-Cawthorne); on a personal level I haven't found them to be helpful.

Bladder dysfunction

This can form an additional part to the other disturbances occurring in M.E. Some of the autonomic nerves help to contract the muscles of the bladder wall and cause emptying, whereas others help to keep the bladder exit sphincter closed till the body wishes to pass urine.

Symptoms such as frequently wanting to pass urine, getting up in the night to pass urine or the feeling of having an 'irritable bladder' seem fairly common in both men and women with M.E.

Poor muscle control may be the reason some men have a poor urinary stream and dribble at the end, but there is also a small group of men under the age of 40 who develop definite symptoms of prostate gland enlargement and inflammation (e.g. perineal pain and various difficulties in passing urine). This may well be due to the fact that enteroviral infection is persisting within the prostate gland tissues and causing chronic inflammation. This is an extremely difficult complication of M.E. when it comes to treatment. I now know of several men who have had prolonged courses of various antibiotics and prostate gland massage all to no avail. In the end the only solution has been to have a prostate operation, but again the results have often been far from satisfactory. Another problem with some men is fainting when passing urine in the middle of the night (micturition syncope) – this is covered on pages 79 and 80.

In women there may be weakness of the pelvic floor muscles and this may produce what's known as stress incontinence. Here sudden abdominal pressure from coughing, straining or exercise can suddenly produce an embarrassing leak of urine, as the pelvic muscles fail to contract properly around the urethra. If this is happening, a properly taught course of pelvic floor exercises will probably help. Also, a recently researched method is now being taught which involves the patient inserting cones of varying sizes into the vagina for short periods each day, and the effort of keeping the cones in place specifically strengthens the weak pelvic muscles.

If you do want to pass urine frequently, your doctor will probably want to exclude any infection by sending a specimen to the laboratory, but this would usually be recommended when some pain is present as well (dysuria). If no infection is present then the reason may well be to do with the nervous control of bladder function. The doctor may also decide to carry out a full investigation of the whole urinary tract from kidneys to bladder, by doing an IVP test (intravenous pyelogram), but with M.E. patients this is very unlikely to show up any abnormality.

More sophisticated techniques are now available in specialised urological units to accurately assess the nerve-muscle control of bladder function. It would be interesting to now examine some M.E. patients who have bladder problems using these techniques to try and get a better idea of what's going wrong in this aspect of M.E.

If bladder symptoms such as frequency are becoming very incapacitating there are some drugs which may be of help, but again would only be prescribed after careful consideration.

Disturbances involving sensory nerves

One last part of the nervous system which seems to be affected in some patients are the sensory nerves, which carry information on sensation, pain, pressure and temperature change back to the brain. If there are problems here, such symptoms as numbness (hypoaesthesiae), 'pins and needles' (paraesthesiae) or sometimes an increased awareness of sensation (hyperaesthesiae) can occur.

I'd had M.E. for about five years before ever experiencing any of these changes. Then one very cold November day I'd been out walking my dog, and on returning home I noticed that my right foot had started to feel cold and numb. Over the following few days I also started to develop pins and needles in my fingers. These symptoms continued intermittently all through the winter till spring arrived, and now they return each year, in varying degrees of severity according to how cold the weather is.

Many other M.E. patients also notice that these sensory changes tend to come and go, and particularly affect the hands and feet, but are not necessarily related to the cold. A few patients also notice altered sensations on their tongues and inside their mouths.

There are no obvious medical solutions to these abnormal sensations. They can have many other different causes, some of them treatable, and it's important, that if such symptoms come on after M.E. has been present for some time, the doctor carries out some investigations to exclude all other possibilities. Those which should always be considered include:

- Diabetes (increased thirst, weight loss, calf pains and skin infections).
- Pernicious anaemia (sore tongue, anaemic symptoms, previous stomach surgery).
- Multiple sclerosis (balance and speech problems, eye pain and visual disturbances).
- Porphyria (stomach pains and mental disturbances).

Various vitamin B supplements and injections are often prescribed by doctors for these sensory symptoms, but their value in M.E. is very doubtful because no specific deficiencies or problems with absorption have, as yet, been demonstrated. See also vitamins in the chapter on Alternative Approaches.

Appendix: Symptoms and signs in 420 patients with ME

Commonly found (> 50%)	No.	%
Muscle fatigue	420	100
Emotional lability†	411	98
Myalgia††	336	80
Cognitive disturbance†††	323	77
Headache	310	74
Giddiness, disequilibrium	302	72
Autonomic dysfunction††††	289	69
Auditory disturbances*	289	69
Reversal of sleep rhythm	268	64
Visual disturbances**	260	62
Paraesthesia, hypo & hyperaesthesia	256	61
Intercostal myalgia/weakness	247	59
Fasciculation, spasm, myoclonus	239	57
Clumsiness***	235	56

† Includes frustration, elation, depression; †† characteristically affects limbs, shoulder girdle, spinal muscles; ††† memory, concentration, anomia, dyslexia; †††† especially circulation and thermoregulation; * hyperacusis, deafness, tinnitus; ** mainly loss of accommodation, photophobia, nystagmus; *** usually due to impaired spatial discrimination.

Less commonly found (> 50%)	No.	%
Gastrointestinal symptoms ****	205	49
Disturbance of micturition§	160	38
Recurrent lymphadenopathy§§	152	36
Arthralgia	118	28
Orthostatic tachycardia	88	21
Recurrent abacterial conjunctivitis	68	16
Orchitis/prostatism in young males	15/113	13
Seronegative polyarthritis	42	10
Vasculitic skin lesions	42	10
Myo/pericarditis	34	8
Positive Romberg sign	25	6
Thyroiditis in female patients	15/307	5
Mesenteric adenitis§§§	5	1
Paresis and muscle wasting	3	1

**** nausea/disturbance of intestinal motility; § frequency incontinence, retention; §§ enlargement, recurrent after prodrome; §§§ surgical intervention for abdominal pain.

From: E G Dowsett et al. Myalgic Encephalomyelitis – a persistent enteroviral infection. *Postgraduate Medical Journal*, 1990, 66, 526–30.
Reproduced by kind permission of the Journal.

4. Secondary Problems

The cardinal symptoms of M.E., discussed in the previous chapter, are joined in some patients as the disease progresses by secondary symptoms affecting other parts of the body.

Although you may have cleared the first hurdle and got your doctor to accept that M.E. really does exist – causing muscle fatigue and brain malfunction – you may once again be facing an uphill struggle persuading him or her that these seemingly unrelated problems are also part of the disease process, and aren't due to the fact that you've now become depressed because you've got M.E. Many members of the medical profession have forgotten most of what they learnt about viruses back at medical school, and just aren't aware of the diverse range of body tissues that they can affect. However, both doctors and patients should remember that it is unwise simply to blame the development of any new symptom on M.E. – there may be a completely unrelated problem which requires investigation and specific treatment.

The ears and hearing problems

M.E. patients quite frequently remark on three particular problems connected with hearing:

- The presence of abnormal noises in the ear – tinnitus. These sounds can be high-pitched whistling or hissing, and particularly occur at times of stress or undue fatigue.
- Being unable to cope with constant chatter in a room full of people, or a lot of loud noise (hyperacusis). Hyperacusis may alternate with periods of deafness or normal hearing.
- Pain in or around the ear.

Sound is normally transmitted in waves through the various components of the outer and middle ear to a structure called the cochlea. This is a fluid-filled chamber with thousands of tiny hair cells lining its walls. Sound vibrations pass through it moving the tiny hairs, and thus the message is transformed into a nerve impulse, which passes along the auditory nerve (or nerve of hearing) to the brain, where it is decoded. It seems that in M.E. patients the ability of the auditory nerve to conduct sound waves suffers from interference – rather like a faulty telephone wire.

Tinnitus is an extremely distressing accompaniment to M.E. – especially if present for much of the time, which makes any form of concentration even more difficult. There is no effective drug treatment for tinnitus, although some doctors will prescribe tranquillisers where stress is a factor, but these drugs are not a long-term solution. Fortunately, in many cases, the symptom is intermittent, and in my personal experience it can disappear altogether for quite long periods of time.

If tinnitus is persistent and troublesome then an ENT (ear, nose and throat) surgeon may recommend trying what is known as a 'masking device'. This acts rather like a hearing aid, and masks the unpleasant noise with a pleasant background sound. An alternative do-it-yourself method for masking tinnitus is using a personal stereo to play soothing music. The Tinnitus Association (see page 341) can provide further information and practical advice if necessary.

Eyes and visual disturbances

M.E. is capable of causing several visual disturbances:

- **Blurring of vision (defective accommodation)** This is very common, especially after prolonged periods of watching television, reading print in a newspaper or book, or when having to switch from near to far vision. The printed words become increasingly difficult to focus on and may start to appear double (double vision = diplopia). The cause is probably related to the fact that correct focusing of the eye is controlled by tiny muscles – ciliary muscles – and just like other muscles in M.E. they are prone to fatigue after prolonged use.

Some patients make repeated visits to the optician to try and get the problem sorted out. The optician, not surprisingly, finds nothing wrong. So, for M.E. patients, it is important not to visit your optician on an 'off day', feeling exhausted, with your vision worse than usual.

- **Photophobia** – dislike of bright lights – is also quite common, and this may stem from increased sensitivity to light in the brain. If patients cannot avoid shops, working areas, etc., where there are very bright lights, they should try wearing dark glasses when necessary.

- **Pain** in and around the eyes can be quite severe, and become localised behind one eye (retro-orbital pain). The doctor may query a diagnosis of migraine, but the pain is not usually associated with the sickness or visual disturbances seen in migraine. This type of eye pain does not tend to respond well to analgesics, and often all you can do is rest quietly until it goes away.

- **Nystagmus**, an involuntary rolling movement of the eyeball, is an occasional complication that is picked up during a neurological examination. There is no specific treatment. (See also page 336).

- The problems of **blepharospasm** (involuntary spasm and flickering of the eyelids) is discussed on page 51, and **dry eyes** on page 47.

Irritable bowel symptomatology

M.E. patients seem to have a lot of problems with their digestion and bowels, and some people can get unduly worried about such symptoms, which is only likely to make them worse. So, if you have gastric problems, do discuss them with your doctor, and get any tests done that seem appropriate to rule out other causes such as coeliac disease and Giardia (see also page 120).

In a few patients food sensitivity or allergy may be a problem, but please do not embark on any drastic dietary alterations without expert supervision (see pages 147–9).

M.E. seems capable of causing a wide variety of digestive problems, with a large number of patients having persisting or fluctuating symptoms, including nausea, vague colicky stomach pains, bloating or feeling abnormally full after a meal, and alterations in bowel habit, which can veer towards diarrhoea or constipation. Vomiting, progressive weight loss or blood in the motions should *not* be ascribed to M.E., and a search *must* be made for an alternative explanation.

Trying to establish the reason for these symptoms so that a treatment can be devised is not easy, but a number of explanations have been put forward. The whole gastrointestinal tract consists of a long hosepipe-like tube which starts at the oesophagus. From here, food enters the stomach where digestion takes place, then it continues its journey through many feet of intestines where nutrients are absorbed and waste products excreted. The lining of the intestine is made up of cells which form a membrane called the mucosa. Surrounding the mucosa are layers of muscle fibres, whose function is to rhythmically contract in a wave-like manner to propel the food and waste products along. Like any other muscle this is under nervous control, and may therefore be affected by M.E.

Where there is a combination of colicky stomach pain, bloating or wind, and alteration in normal bowel habit, the explanation may be what doctors term the 'irritable bowel syndrome'. This seems to be a common problem not only in M.E.; it has been estimated that about 15 per cent of all adults suffer from irritable bowel. Even when this syndrome is not seen in patients with M.E. it is commonly associated with headaches, joint pains and fatigue.

One suggested cause for irritable bowel is an overactivity of the nerves controlling the propulsive movements of the muscle in the bowel wall, and as these movements become uncoordinated muscle spasm and pain result. It has been shown in experiments that if a balloon is introduced into the intestine, and the pressure inside it is increased, the characteristic colicky pain can be reproduced. As a result of this abnormal or increased propulsion of bowel contents there may also be diarrhoea. It has been suggested that gastric infections may initiate the development of irritable bowel, and it is not unknown for this condition to develop after a nasty stomach upset caught abroad on holiday.

Abnormal nerve-muscle control of the bowel wall may be only part of the explanation for the diverse range of gastric upsets seen in M.E. patients. We now know from the research work at St Mary's Hospital, London, that many M.E. patients have a persisting enteroviral infection in the gut, and this reservoir of infection may be inflaming the lining mucosa to produce food sensitivities, intolerance or allergy.

Treatment of irritable bowel symptoms

Whatever causes irritable bowel in the first place the symptoms will inevitably be exacerbated by any associated anxiety about the condition, so it is worth emphasising that it has no serious consequences, cannot lead to cancer, and frequently resolves or improves in the course of time. The way the medical profession treats irritable bowel is by trying to alleviate the individual symptoms. The colicky pain may be helped by drugs that have a direct relaxing effect on the muscle. Colofac, taken twenty minutes before meals, is one such drug, but it requires a prescription from your doctor. A course of capsules containing peppermint oil (Colpermin, available over the counter with one or two capsules being taken half an hour before meals) is an alternative that may be worth trying. This also relaxes the intestinal muscles to help with colic and bloating, though some patients find it causes side-effects including gastric irritation and heartburn.

The most popular method of managing irritable bowel symptoms is an increase in dietary fibre. This means ensuring that the diet is rich in fruit, vegetables and wholemeal bread, or even adding bran directly on to food, such as the morning breakfast cereal. This sort of dietary change has to be introduced *gradually* (especially if you are going to try added bran), as a drastic change in diet may exacerbate symptoms, and increased fibre does not suit all patients. In a few patients, where nerve-muscle control seems to be at fault, increasing fibre can lead to more pain and bloating. In this case one of the now unfashionable stimulant laxatives (e.g. Senna) may be helpful.

However, many doctors are now seriously questioning whether a high fibre diet really is the best way to manage the symptoms of irritable bowel syndrome. There is growing evidence that food intolerance may be a significant factor in up to half of all cases. The main provocative foods appear to be dairy produce (particularly milk in people with a defect in an enzyme called lactase which helps to break up milk and aid its absorption), corn, wheat (unfortunately, the main constituent of a high fibre diet), fried foods, chocolate, caffeine (which acts as a laxative) and citrus fruits. So, it may well be worth experimenting with an exclusion diet, and completely cutting out *all* these foods for a period of two to three weeks to see if any improvement occurs. Then, groups of foods can be reintroduced one by one to see if any obvious reaction occurs. If it does the 'culprit' food(s) should be totally excluded from the diet. This sort of dietary manipulation should only be carried out with careful thought and with the help of an interested doctor or dietician – after all, people with M.E. have quite enough restrictions imposed on their lives without having to cut out all their favourite foods as well.

Wind and bloating or flatulence can often be helped by a preparation containing dimethicone, which helps to make the wind bubbles in the stomach coalesce. Alternatively, it may be worth trying one of the preparations containing charcoal.

When constipation is the predominant symptom, it may help to use a laxative that increases the bulk contents of the stools, such as Fybogel or Isogel. These drugs help the stool to retain water, so expanding the size, and thus increasing the motility.

If diarrhoea accompanies the pain, then management is rather different. The diarrhoea of irritable bowel is not usually like that of true infective diarrhoea – it has the consistency of toothpaste, and may alternate with normal stools, or constipated pellet-like motions. In a phase of diarrhoea, a prescribed anti-diarrhoeal drug such as codeine phosphate or loperamide (Imodium) may be useful. If you have persisting watery diarrhoea a stool sample should be sent to the local laboratory to check for Giardia although enteroviral infection cannot be detected by standard techniques. Your doctor may also wish to arrange further hospital investigations including a sigmoidoscopy (a look inside the lower bowel using a long flexible tube) or barium examination, just to make sure there is nothing more serious going on.

Blood in the motions is *not* part of irritable bowel (or M.E.); if this occurs you *must* go to your doctor – it may simply be piles, but it could indicate something more significant.

A couple of new approaches to the management of irritable bowel include hypnotherapy and the use of anti-allergy drugs. Self-hypnosis centres on the idea that the spasm inside the intestines can be overcome by producing a mental picture of 'knotted muscles' in the gut. Then, with hands on the stomach, soothing massage movements and concentration is used to reduce the knot.

Researchers from Italy have also reported some success in severe cases of food intolerance by using a drug called sodium cromoglycate which seems to help make the gut lining less sensitive to various foods.

If you are having problems with any of these irritable bowel symptoms, and your own general practitioner is finding it difficult to know what to do next, you could always ask to be referred to a gastroenterology specialist who is interested in this topic.

Weight changes in M.E.

Some patients, especially children, lose a significant amount of weight in the very early stages of the illness, and then experience considerable difficulty in putting it back on again no matter how hard they try. Unfortunately, a few of them also go on to develop a true anorexic state which is very worrying. It should be noted that significant or progressive weight loss is not a normal feature of M.E., and when it occurs alternative explanations (e.g. an overactive thyroid gland) should always be excluded.

Other patients experience quite the opposite problem and find that their weight is gradually increasing. The relatively inactive lifestyle imposed by the illness obviously decreases energy requirements quite substantially, so some patients may find that they have to cut down their calories accordingly. This should be done by reducing the sugar and fat content in the normal diet, not by any dramatic starvation-type diets involving a very low calorie intake.

Weight gain can occasionally be associated with a hormonal problem, and if underactivity of the thyroid gland is suspected your doctor will want to take some blood tests to check the thyroid function. It can also be a fairly common side-effect associated with the use of tricyclic antidepressant drugs.

Some women find that they have a marked cyclical weight gain, around the mid point of the menstrual cycle. This is known as cyclical ideopathic oedema, and several patients studied in Professor Behan's unit in Glasgow have been found to put on an extra 10–12 lbs over this period. This type of menstrual weight gain may be related to a disturbance in the hormonal control of fluid retention.

Nausea

Some patients experience intermittent feelings of nausea (sickness), though this is not usually associated with vomiting. Why this should be is not certain – there is an area in the brain, which if disturbed, can cause a feeling of sickness; nausea can also be associated with anxiety. If necessary there is a variety of drugs that can help, including metoclopramide (Maxalon) and a phenothiazine like Stemetil, which is probably more helpful in acute attacks. This latter drug should not be used continuously over long periods of time because of its side-effects on the nervous system. There are also some new anti-sickness drugs being developed which are proving to be particularly useful in cases associated with cancer treatment where nausea can be severe and continuous. These drugs act on chemical transmitters in the brain (5HT/5 hydroxytryptamine), and may also turn out to be useful in other illnesses associated with nausea. They are, however, very expensive. Two natural solutions reported as being effective are root ginger and acupressure. Acupressure is similar to acupuncture but involves pressure to a precise point on the wrist (the Neiguan point). This is achieved by an elasticated wrist band and a stud which presses on this acupressure site, about three fingers above the first wrist crease.

Oesophageal spasm

Spasms in the oesophagus (throat) tend to come and go and may cause difficulty with swallowing. Such spasms may be related to those elsewhere in the gut which cause irritable bowel. Any continual difficulty with swallowing is a symptom you must see the doctor about, as it will require further investigation. If oesophageal spasm is the difficulty then there are drugs that can help, but you must take the advice of an experienced gastroenterologist.

Proctalgia fugax

This is the name given to a severe cramp-like pain in the anus. It often comes on suddenly, but may then last for up to half an hour or so before gradually starting to subside. Some relief may be obtained by going to the toilet, or having a warm bath, otherwise there is no effective treatment. Tranquillisers should be avoided if possible. The connection with M.E., as with oesophageal spasm, is muscular and nervous disturbance.

Hypoglycaemia

It is widely assumed that episodes of hypoglycaemia (abnormally low blood sugar) can be a problem in M.E. However, apart from one or two isolated reports, there is very little good objective evidence to back up these claims. In fact, when Dr David McCluskey and his colleagues in Belfast actually measured blood sugar levels in a group of M.E. patients during exercise, the results turned out to be no different to the control group or people with a pure irritable bowel syndrome (medical reference 138). What I suspect may be happening is that people with M.E., just like many women with premenstrual syndrome, become *more sensitive* to lower levels of blood sugar, and this is why they develop hypoglycaemic symptoms (e.g. sweating, light headedness, headaches and tremor). Once again, if this particular problem becomes severe it is worth being referred to a diabetic specialist who can rule out any other possible causes of low blood sugar if such a finding can be clearly demonstrated on blood tests. Advice on how to prevent these types of hypoglycaemic symptoms occurring is contained in the chapter including nutritional advice – see pages 147–9.

Pre-menstrual tension (PMT)

If you're unlucky enough to have both M.E. and the symptoms of pre-menstrual tension, the two conditions are going to interact and make each other seem worse. PMT symptoms characteristically start towards the latter part of the cycle from the time of ovulation, and then rapidly improve within a day or so of starting the period. There is a long list of symptoms, both mental and physical, associated with PMT, but among the commonest are irritability, depression, stomach bloating, breast enlargement or pain (mastalgia) and fluid retention. Although there are now a large number of treatments being advocated for PMT, very few of them have been scientifically proven to be of value. The most popular ones include:

- Vitamin B6 (pyridoxine) which can be taken at a dose of 50–100 mg daily. Do not exceed 150 mg per day as this vitamin can damage the sensory nerves (see medical references 163 and 168).

- Vitamin E and magnesium supplements are widely promoted by health magazines but are of doubtful value.

- Efamol (evening primrose oil) can be taken at a dose of eight × 500 mg capsules per day from day 15 till the onset of menstruation. Unfortunately, this can become very costly as this supplement is not yet available on the NHS. It can, however, be prescribed as Efamast for cyclical breast pain (mastalgia).

- Diuretics (water losing tablets) in small doses may help when bloating or fluid retention is a particular problem.

- Relaxation techniques can also be extremely useful – see Relaxation for Living in Useful Addresses.

- Dietary changes advocated include the reduction of refined sugars, salt and fat. It may also be beneficial to cut out coffee, cola drinks and chocolate. Taking a regular snack of a complex carbohydrate (even just a Ryvita biscuit) sometimes seems to help prevent the rapid swings in blood sugar and resulting hypoglycaemic type symptoms.

- Hormonal treatments are sometimes necessary when symptoms become more severe. These include the use of oestrogen skin patches and implants which prevent ovulation – apparently now regarded by some gynaecologists as the most effective way of dealing with PMT. It also seems that the contraceptive pill is not all that effective in alleviating this condition. More potent types of hormonal drugs such as Danol are also effective, but they are invariably accompanied by unpleasant side-effects (e.g. sickness, dizziness, more fluid retention and headaches) making them not very suitable for someone with M.E. Some gynaecologists recommend the use of natural progesterone hormones which are given by vaginal or rectal suppository, but there is no universal agreement on this particular approach.

There is no simple solution to PMT; what suits one woman may not help another, so trying several different treatments may be necessary before relief is obtained. Further help and advice is available from the Premenstrual Society (see Useful Addresses).

The menopause and osteoporosis

The menopause is the time of life when the ovaries start to decrease their production of the hormone oestrogen. The first sign may be an increasing irregularity in the pattern and blood loss of periods – though this should not automatically be ascribed to the menopause. Some women start to experience menopausal symptoms as early as forty, whereas others may be over fifty before anything changes. Many women go through the menopause with no problems at all, but in some the falling levels of oestrogen produce definite symptoms such as hot flushes, sweats and aching joints. Vague emotional symptoms may also occur, including irritability and depression – just as with PMT.

The problem for any woman with M.E. who is approaching the menopause is that many of the symptoms overlap, particularly vasomotor instability (hot flushes, night sweats, palpitations), which is probably due to the autonomic nerve malfunction described on pages 74–5. Consequently the two conditions will interact to exacerbate one another.

If there is any doubt as to whether the vasomotor symptoms are due to M.E. or to the menopause, the latter is the likely cause if there are associated changes in period pattern, with vaginal dryness and a rise in the hormone FSH, which can be measured by your doctor. Vaginal dryness may cause pain during sexual intercourse and this can be helped by increasing the lubrication with KY Jelly (from the pharmacy) or a locally applied oestrogen cream available on prescription.

Another problem related to the menopause is osteoporosis – loss of calcium and consequent thinning of bones – a natural ageing process, but one that accelerates in women going through the menopause because of the dramatic fall of oestrogen levels. Osteoporotic bones, especially in the wrist and hip, become fragile and susceptible to fracture.

Female M.E. patients of any age who are already thin and inactive (which also increases calcium loss), and who do not get outside in the sunlight to absorb vitamin D, are increasing their chances of developing osteoporosis, especially if they are also on a diet excluding milk and other dairy products – foods rich in calcium. Cigarette smoking is another contributory factor.

To try and minimise the risk of developing osteoporosis, any M.E. patient who is not taking adequate calcium in her diet should be taking some form of calcium supplement (e.g. Sandocal tablets, which can be made into a fizzy drink, or ordinary calcium tablets from the pharmacy), but *do not exceed* the recommended doses, as excess calcium can be harmful.

Hormone Replacement Therapy (HRT) involves using a

low dose of oestrogen which is available in pill form, skin patches, or implants which are inserted surgically (a very minor operation) under the skin. This is something to be seriously considered by any M.E. patient entering the menopause, as it not only helps the vasomotor symptoms, but slows down the calcium loss caused by the falling oestrogen levels. In addition, it is believed to give increased protection against heart disease. HRT should be discussed with your doctor, and may be a viable option provided there are no medical contra-indications – e.g. heart disease, previous cancer of the breast or uterus.

If you require further information about the symptoms of the menopause and the various treatments available contact the Amarant Trust (see Useful Addresses). The Osteoporosis Society (Useful Addresses) provides further information on this particular menopausal complication.

Thrush

Candida albicans, or thrush, is probably the commonest cause of vaginal discharge in women. For some, though, it is not just an occasional 'one-off' problem, but a recurring nuisance which never seems to go away.

The yeast candida often lives quite happily in our bodies without causing any problems. Then, from time to time, it gets out of control and multiplies to start causing definite symptoms. In the vagina this is a creamy discharge along with external soreness and irritation, but other parts of the body, particularly the skin and nails, can also be affected.

A variety of explanations have been put forward as to what 'tips the balance', and allows the yeast to start multiplying. These include courses of antibiotics, diabetes and immune-deficiency. Many gynaecologists now doubt that there is any link between thrush and taking the oral contraceptive pill. The fact that it is a latent organism prone to periodic reactivation has caused some doctors to link it with M.E., but in my personal view the incidence of thrush is not much higher among M.E. patients than elsewhere in the population. I am dealing with it here for the benefit of those patients who do believe there is a link.

Treatment of an acute episode of thrush is usually very

effective; it is preventing recurrence that causes the problem. Pessaries are the commonest prescribed treatment – these used to have to be inserted for a week or more, but now there are new types of pessary which are equally effective in a few days, or can even be taken in one 'megadose'. Some women prefer the anti-fungal creams, which can be prescribed along with an applicator, and are also very effective. Your male partner may also have the infection on his penis, and without any symptoms, so it is usually a good idea to get him to use some cream twice daily also.

Self-help measures can significantly reduce the chances of a recurrence:

- Avoid tight-fitting jeans, nylon pants and tights – in fact any clothing that helps to create a warm, moist environment in which the yeast thrives.
- Wipe your bottom away from your vagina as reinfection can come from the bowels.
- Do not 'traumatise' the vagina by using chemicals like bubble baths in the bath or vaginal douches; if you are dry during intercourse use some KY Jelly.

Some patients find the use of natural yogurt prepared with Lactobacillus helpful, although recent research from Sweden has questioned its value.

If you do keep getting recurrences of thrush your doctor may be willing to give you a further supply of medication, or a prescription, so you can start treatment yourself as soon as any symptoms recur.

If none of this seems to help then a prolonged course of anti-fungal treatment may be necessary.

Pain in the joints

In addition to the muscle pain (myalgia) which may accompany the fatigue in M.E., some patients also experience a variety of joint and bone pains. This kind of pain – arthralgia – is not usually as severe as the muscle pain, and is not associated with any permanent disruption to the joint, which can occur in purely rheumatic diseases.

If the joints are carefully examined by the doctor it is unusual to find any restriction in their range of movements and there are no changes seen with X-rays. For these reasons the cause may well be due to involvement of the supporting structures – muscles and tendons – which surround the joint. However, it is also recognised that a variety of viral infections can cause a temporary arthritis, with rubella being particularly common. And it has been suggested that viruses may persist inside cells known as chondrocytes, which produce the joint cartilage.

If you are experiencing joint pains, particularly if there is any associated swelling, a search should be made by your doctor to exclude one of the rheumatic diseases before ascribing this symptom to M.E. Conditions such as Sjøgren's syndrome and systemic lupus erythematosus (SLE) which are occasionally confused with M.E. are described in more detail on page 120.

Treatment of arthralgia is normally with one of the anti-inflammatory drugs, whichever seems to suit the individual patient best. Aspirin, taken four to six hourly, is still a very effective drug if it does not upset the stomach. If this is unsuitable one of the new anti-inflammatory drugs (NSAIDs) can be purchased (e.g. Brufen) or prescribed, but they do not suit all M.E. patients. Paracetamol is not a very effective drug for arthritic pain, and steroids should *definitely* be avoided.

One useful alternative approach is Evening Primrose Oil (Efamol), which has been shown in scientifically controlled trials to be as effective as conventional drugs in some patients. It is free from any side-effects (see also page 213–14).

Another 'natural' product which has been shown to have similar anti-inflammatory effects to evening primrose oil is a daily dose of olive oil (*British Journal of Rheumatology*, October 1991).

Sore throats and enlarged glands

These two symptoms form a common initial presentation of the illness, and in some patients go on to become a persistent and recurring problem, possibly due to reactivation of the virus or an oversensitivity of the immune system to any 'new' infection in the throat.

Throat swabs taken by a doctor seldom reveal any organisms which are sensitive to antibiotics. These drugs are best avoided in M.E., and should only be used where a specific bacteria has been grown by the pathology laboratory, or where there is a marked general illness with fever and noticeably enlarged glands in the neck.

Antiseptic mouth washes, gargles and throat pastilles are probably a waste of money in this situation. A soothing warm drink made from glycerine, honey and lemon, or sucking a boiled sweet is a much cheaper alternative, and probably more soothing. Recurrent sore throats are not an indication to have your tonsils removed, although this will be considered if there are several attacks of genuine tonsillitis throughout the year.

Disordered sleep

Normal adults vary widely in their nightly sleep requirements. Some people, like Mrs Thatcher, are bright and alert after only five or six hours, whereas others must have their statutory eight hours or more of good solid sleep.

A common occurrence in all M.E. patients is their greatly increased sleep requirements (hypersomnia). This is especially so in the very early stages of the illness, when sleeping for 14 or 16 hours a day is not unusual. Those who are recovering seldom seem able to cope with being up and about for a full twelve-hour day without some form of rest period, unless they're going through an extremely good patch. Even after a full night's sleep, someone with M.E. will still wake up feeling unrefreshed.

It's important to remember that the commonest sleep problem in M.E. – that of requiring too much sleep – isn't something to fight against. This is your body's way of instructing you to rest and slow down, and it's also a very important healing mechanism, which allows the body to repair its damaged tissues and aid recovery. So don't feel guilty about having a short sleep in the afternoon, or going to bed early if you feel the need to. If your body says 'sleep' then this is what you really must do.

Normal human sleep is divided into two quite distinct components, each occurring in alternate periods throughout the night.

Dream sleep occupies about a quarter of the total time asleep, coming on in bouts of gradually increasing length. This type of sleep is technically known as rapid eye movement (REM) sleep.

The other type of sleep – orthodox or non-REM sleep – occurs in rather longer periods between each block of dream sleep. During these periods you gradually pass from light sleep into deep sleep and then re-enter a period of dream sleep.

As far as the benefits of sleep are concerned it's the first four or five hours of deep sleep that are really important. Any interruption in these first few vital hours has now been shown to significantly affect mental functioning and the ability to learn new tasks the following day. The final few hours of sleep are far less important.

Control of sleep is thought to centre in parts of the brain known as the brain stem and hypothalamus. As I've already mentioned, the latter may turn out to be a key part of the brain that is affected by M.E. Whether people with M.E. have significant changes in the ratio of dream sleep to non-dream sleep is an area that warrants further research in sleep laboratories.

Another possible explanation for these sleep disturbances has been put forward by one of the world's leading authorities on sleep, Professor Harvey Moldofsky. He has suggested that some of the immune system abnormalities (e.g. increased production of cytokines such as muramyl peptides), which are triggered by viral infections, may be affecting sleep control centres in the brain. In fact, some of the patients he has looked at have increased amounts of non-REM sleep (medical reference 39).

Besides the generally increased requirement for sleep there are several other disturbances in sleep pattern which commonly occur. Some people with M.E. find themselves falling asleep at inappropriate times of the day, and in children it is not unusual to find a complete reversal of the normal pattern with sleeping during the day and being awake at night. However, the three commonest types of disturbed sleep are:

(1) Difficulty getting off to sleep This often coincides with a rise in mental activity after retiring to bed. Thoughts of unachieved plans for that day, coming events, or a range of unsolvable anxieties may all start to surface and prevent the initiation of sleep.

(2) Waking up once asleep Here the cause can often be associated with distressing physical symptoms which disturb normal sleep, e.g. sweating, muscle aches and cramps, needing to pass urine, restless legs or jerking movements. These sort of physical ailments may continually interrupt sleep throughout the night, and breaking this vicious circle can be extremely difficult.

Night cramps in the calf muscles can affect anyone, and if massage or local heat won't provide relief a simple stretching exercise can often be very effective in relieving the pain.

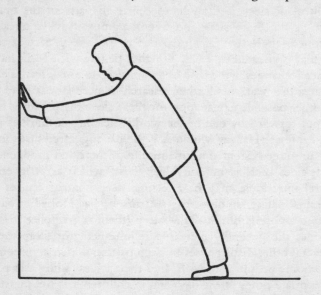

Stand and face the bedroom wall, with feet about three feet away from the skirting board. Then lean forward using hands and arms to act as support against the wall, making sure that the heels don't move off the ground. This will stretch the calf muscles: keep them stretched for about ten seconds, then relax for a while and repeat the exercise.

If cramp is occurring regularly try repeating these exercises three times a day as well.

A wide range of drugs have also been tried for treating night cramps (Quinine sulphate is frequently prescribed), but there's no general agreement as to their value.

Restless legs are another cause of restless nights, whereby patients complain of a variety of strange sensations, which seem to be more in the muscle than in the skin. (Doctors sometimes refer to this condition as Ekbom's Syndrome.) Tickling, pricking, burning or crawling feelings are frequently mentioned, and some patients also experience jerking movements in the legs. This strange activity is usually confined to the lower parts of the leg; the thigh and ankle areas are not usually affected.

The symptoms seem to gradually increase in intensity, till the only way of obtaining relief is to get out of bed and walk around the room. Unfortunately, this may have to be repeated several times in one night.

Doctors don't know what causes 'restless legs'; it's certainly not confined to M.E. patients, and has also been linked with rheumatoid arthritis, iron deficiency anaemia and an excessive intake of caffeine – so perhaps it's worth trying decaffeinated coffee. Sometimes warming (or cooling) the affected leg may help; other sufferers try exercises before going to sleep, but there doesn't seem to be any effective treatment which suits everyone.

As with night cramps, a variety of drugs have been tried, but the results are not impressive. Fortunately, for many people awoken by this strange phenomenon it's a transient problem which seems to come and go.

Vivid dreams, or even nightmares are also reported by some M.E. patients. These dreams are often described as being in vivid colours and involving various 'pressures' which seem to be worrying the patient, e.g. getting back to work again, or the frustrations of trying to achieve some other impossible task.

(3) Early morning wakening This is when you wake up at, say, 4 or 5 a.m., and then have great difficulty in getting back to sleep again. This type of sleep disturbance is very characteristic of clinical depression, which would obviously require expert medical advice.

Helping yourself to a better night's sleep

Here are some useful tips which may help in promoting a better night's sleep, without having to resort to sleeping tablets.

- Try not to involve yourself in stimulating mental activity or watching exciting television programmes in the hour or so before you normally retire to bed. Reading a small amount from a good book is a much better way of 'switching off'.
- If you don't feel relaxed last thing at night try the relaxation techniques I describe on pages 177–8, especially if you have any painful 'trouble spots'. An audio cassette programme (e.g. *Sleep Well!*, from Lifeskills – see address section) can also be very helpful. You could also try creative visualisation techniques to quieten the mind.
- Don't embark on heavy meals, alcohol or caffeine-containing drinks late in the evening. A glass of warm milk or a herbal tea such as camomile or lime blossom is a much better alternative.
- Inhaling an aromatic oil, such as ylang-ylang or orange blossom added to a warm bath are both soothing and relaxing – see also aromatherapy in the chapter on Alternative Approaches.
- If pain is waking you up in the night or preventing you from getting off to sleep, try taking a mild pain killer before retiring.
- If you're not feeling too tired, sex is a very good way of sending people off to sleep!
- Homeopaths often recommend arnica for those who feel over-tired and restless, or Coffea if you're dwelling on the following day's problems.
- Finally, don't forget the importance of sleeping in a room with some fresh air coming in and a warm comfortable bed. A good firm mattress could be a very sound investment!

How can the doctor help?

Unfortunately, all too often this leads to a prescription for 'sleeping pills'. These may well help to break a vicious circle but are not a long-term solution. If used, this type of medication should only be taken for a very short period (preferably not longer than a week) or intermittently – say every third day over a slightly longer period.

Sleeping tablets The most commonly prescribed drugs are called benzodiazepines which are chemically very similar to tranquillisers like Valium. They all carry the same serious risks of dependence and side-effects which include headaches, drowsiness, light-headedness, confusion and dizziness the following day. So, they should *only* be used when a sleep problem becomes severe and disabling. Benzodiazepines are divided into three main groups. Short-acting drugs last for less than six hours. However, after prolonged use, they can start to produce disturbing anxiety symptoms the following day. They are best used when there is difficulty in getting off to sleep. One commonly-prescribed drug in this group called Halcion (triazolam) has now been banned in the U.K. and Holland.

Intermediate-lasting benzodiazepines last for about 6–10 hours and may cause mild residual effects the next day. Examples include Loprazolam, Lormetazepam, Normison, Rohypnol and Temazepam.

The long-acting drugs all produce sedating effects which persist well into the following day. After repeated use they also accumulate in the body, especially in the elderly where they may lead to confusion. I would *not* recommend their use in M.E. Examples include Dalmane, Mogadon and Nitrazepam.

Other drugs which are occasionally used include antihistamines, which are relatively safe and a better choice for children. Heminevrin is claimed to be useful in the elderly as it has less of a 'hangover' effect the following day, although it can cause nasal irritation and congestion. Barbiturates should no longer be prescribed for insomnia.

One new drug called Zimovane is said to produce a better quality of sleep than the benzodiazepines, and it may also have much less in the way of side-effects – apart from producing a metallic taste in the mouth. Whether it is a more appropriate choice in M.E. remains to be seen.

One final alternative is to use one of the sedating tricyclic antidepressant drugs, and I know of several patients who have found this approach helpful.

When researchers finally unravel the workings of the biological clock that regulates normal sleep, it seems highly likely that safe and more effective drugs will become available. Dr William Dement, director of the world's first sleep disorders clinic at Stanford University, California, predicts that such products will become available within the next ten years. If they do so, we may well be able to help patients whose sleep disturbance is a major obstacle on the road to recovery.

Lastly, I'd like to briefly consider two important sleep disturbances – sleep apnoea syndrome and narcolepsy – which are both associated with severe daytime fatigue, and are occasionally misdiagnosed as M.E.

Sleep apnoea

Although not strictly related to M.E. this problem is worth including here because it is yet another cause of chronic fatigue that is often overlooked. I know of several patients with suspected M.E. in whom this turned out to be the main reason for their ill-health.

Sleep apnoea is a condition of disordered breathing which occurs during the night. The result is a very low level of oxygen reaching the brain. Common causes include obesity (a collar size of more than 17½" is said to be an important clue!) and large tonsils or adenoids. These obstructions to the airway in the throat cause it to collapse during the night, and sleep is constantly disturbed by a series of 'attacks' where abortive breaths are followed by loud snorts and near-wakening. In the morning the bed looks like a battlefield, and the constant lack of satisfactory sleep produces severe daytime drowsiness.

Serious sleep disorders like this are best diagnosed in hospitals that have established sleep laboratories. Well-known ones include the City Hospital in Edinburgh, the John Radcliffe Hospital in Oxford, Leicester Infirmary, and one at the department of psychiatry, St George's Hospital, London.

Narcolepsy

This is a rare sleep disorder which is inherited, and almost always starts before the age of 30. Disturbances in sleep control mechanisms within the brain result in periodic and embarrassing attacks of suddenly going off to sleep during the day, each one lasting for about fifteen minutes. These attacks commonly occur after meals, while travelling, or at times of boredom. Some people with narcolepsy have up to 20 such attacks during the course of a single day. Narcolepsy is sometimes associated with terrifying hallucinations and sleep paralysis.

Periods of excessive sleep can also occur in another rare condition known as the Kleine Levin Syndrome which predominantly affects young men. These may last for days or even weeks, and on recovery there is a phase of abnormal eating.

Part 2

PRACTICAL STEPS TOWARDS
COPING WITH M.E.

1. M.E. And Your Doctor

My personal experiences over the past few years, both as a doctor and as an M.E. patient, have made me appreciate the fact that in many chronic diseases doctors only play a relatively small role in any recovery process. What is far more important in conditions like M.E. is how patients learn to help themselves, and the actions which other individuals and agencies can carry out, both to help and hinder recovery. When doctors discuss the management of such conditions they tend to concentrate on the medical side of the treatment, often failing to take into account the humanising factors which are so important when trying to cope with something like M.E. So, unless the patient, the illness, the family and the environment are all taken into consideration progress won't be made. Fortunately, many doctors are now becoming increasingly convinced that this holistic approach to illness, where the humanising aspects are regarded as being equally important as the purely medical treatment, is a far better way of managing patients with conditions like M.E.

The current trend towards high-tech medicine has also falsely raised the expectations of many patients, as to what doctors can actually do in 'curing' disease. The attitude the patient takes towards his or her illness is going to be far more important. A positive approach to recovery, making appropriate changes in lifestyle, sympathetic support from doctors, family and friends are all essential components.

Equally, external factors will all have an important role to play in the recovery process, and if M.E. patients are battling to obtain social service benefits, or having to give up their jobs

because they can no longer cope, this will obviously have a very
adverse effect on the outcome.

In any disease where doctors and orthodox medicine are
at present so limited in the help they can offer, it's hardly
surprising that many patients are keen to try one of the numerous
alternative approaches, and these are dealt with in detail on pages
182–225.

Getting M.E. diagnosed by your doctor

Why do some doctors find it so difficult to cope with their M.E.
patients, their diagnosis and management? It's very instructive
to place yourself in their position. In order to understand how
your doctor sees you – the patient with M.E. – it's necessary
to go right back to the onset of your M.E.

Your first consultation was probably along the lines: 'I had
this dose of flu a few weeks ago, but I'm definitely *not* getting
over it. I'm tired all the time, and I've got tired, aching muscles
which soon get weak after exercise, and then my brain won't
work either.'

At this point the GP's role is essentially trying to work
out some sort of 'label' for your condition. If he can do that,
he can then suggest some form of management, which may be
via the prescription pad. Your doctor would very much like to
'cure' the condition which has just been diagnosed, but if that's
not possible at least try to alleviate some of the symptoms. If
he can't decide what's wrong, and you don't seem to have any
complaints which suggest something seriously wrong, he may
well conclude it's a 'self-limiting condition', i.e. it will go away
in its own time. And, like so many patients he sees – where it's
not possible to make a firm diagnosis – he'll be hoping that both
you and your strange symptoms will now go away without any
further investigations or treatment!

Now, if doctors can't actually recognise a particular pattern
of symptoms and associate them with a specific disease, they're
not going to diagnose that condition, and that's why so many
patients come unstuck at the first hurdle – getting a diagnosis.
Patients who present with characteristic M.E. symptoms will
find that their GP is all too familiar with them as individual

symptoms, but put them all together and he's probably quite baffled, unless he's already become aware of M.E.

At this point the patient is often informed that 'You've got a bit of "post-viral debility", or "post-flu flop"; take it easy for a while and you'll soon feel better.' In fact, if you have got M.E., it's really crucial in this very early stage that you should now be resting, for it seems that this may well have a very positive effect on your chances of recovery. Far too many M.E. patients return to work or household and family duties, struggle on, and make their condition gradually worse until they can't cope any longer.

On the second or third visits you're 'still not well', can't cope with your normal daily routine or work, sleeping whenever you can, and you've got the characteristic overwhelming muscle fatigue and brain malfunction.

With all these persisting symptoms how does the doctor go about trying to make a diagnosis? They have to rely on key pieces of information – medical clues.

The first key piece of information comes from what you tell the doctor – what's known as your clinical history – and in general practice this is where the most important clues come from. If the diagnosis of M.E. isn't fairly obvious to the doctor after a patient has given a good description of M.E., then information from the rest of the consultation isn't likely to provide the answer.

The second part of the assessment, the physical examination, may well reinforce the doctor's belief that you're not physically unwell, because he or she may find the patient's muscle power relatively normal. Only the astute physician who goes to the bother of exercising an M.E. patient to the point of fatigue will find that muscle weakness does indeed occur.

Doctors who are prepared to thoroughly examine their patients, may well find, as Dr Melvin Ramsay has repeatedly observed, that very careful fingertip palpation of particular muscles (especially the trapezius in the neck and the gastrocnemius in the leg) can demonstrate tiny foci of exquisite tenderness. Unfortunately, this art of clinical examination is all too often being replaced by spending time looking at bits of paper from the laboratory.

M.E. patients also complain of unsteadiness. Doctors use a test to assess this symptom (Romberg's test), where they ask you to try and stand still with the eyes closed. The results of this may be quite normal. Unsteadiness is a very common symptom which GPs deal with frequently, but if they can't find an obvious cause they may think anxiety, only, is the cause.

If you are having difficulty in persuading a GP or specialist that M.E. is a real disease then ask the M.E. Association to send the doctor a copy of Professor Peter Behan's booklet on diagnostic and clinical guidelines. You could also suggest that they look at some of the more important medical papers which have been published in the journals (see medical reference section on pages 345–61).

Blood tests
Your doctor may next decide to see if any abnormalities show up in blood tests. With M.E. patients these routine blood tests often come back from the lab relatively normal, so their value is partly in excluding other possible causes for the symptoms.

Typical blood tests which your GP may carry out include:

The ESR (erythrocyte sedimentation rate) Healthy individuals have red blood cells which do not tend to stick together. However, in a wide range of illnesses – particularly infections and inflammatory conditions – this stickiness increases so that the cells clump together (agglutinate) and hence sediment more easily.

The ESR test measures the speed at which such sedimentation occurs, and if raised indicates that 'something is wrong somewhere'. In M.E. the ESR is almost always within the normal range and this may suggest to the doctor that the patient has no serious health problem.

Haemoglobin (Hb) contains the iron in the blood, and if decreased, shows if any anaemia is present. M.E. patients shouldn't be anaemic – if you are there must be some other cause apart from M.E., and this requires further investigation by your doctor.

White Blood Count (WBC) measures the number of cells in the blood which are primarily produced to fight infections. There are several different types including neutrophils, lymphocytes and eosinophils. In the early stage of an infection the lymphocytes are often raised in number – a lymphocytosis. As the condition becomes chronic there may be no significant abnormalities, even though the virus is persisting, although a few patients do then seem to show a decrease in their white cell counts. Sometimes M.E. patients have a few abnormally shaped lymphocytes under the microscope, suggesting the presence of persisting infection. T lymphocytes can't be seen on this sort of routine blood examination requested by a GP. They need to be examined at specialist centres.

Immunoglobulins are the antibodies in the blood, and minor abnormalities are quite often found. These are described in more detail in the section dealing with immune system disturbances on page 126.

Enzymes are proteins which are released from inside a cell when inflammation or damage occurs. The different body tissues all produce their own characteristic enzymes which can easily be measured once they spill into the blood, so that actual site(s) of damage can often be identified. Coxsackie infections can sometimes inflame the liver (hepatitis) during the early stages of M.E., so raised levels of specific liver enzymes might be found using such a blood test.

Muscle enzymes are also released into the blood in a variety of muscle diseases. Creatine kinase is the one most frequently measured, but only about 5 per cent of M.E. patients have raised levels, usually early on in the illness. Unfortunately, having a normal muscle enzyme profile may yet again lead the doctor to the assumption that there is nothing wrong in the muscle.

Liver function tests measure the amounts of specific liver enzymes and chemicals in the blood such as bilirubin – the pigment that turns the skin yellow during an attack of jaundice. Raised levels of these enzymes indicate that some form of inflammation or malfunction is taking place inside the liver. The most common causes for this are infections, drugs such as antidepressants and too much alcohol. In some M.E. patients these changes in liver enzymes are very similar to those seen in Gilbert's syndrome, an inherited form of mild liver dysfunction. If your liver function tests remain permanently and significantly abnormal it is probably a good idea to ask to be referred to a specialist who can decide if further hospital investigations are necessary. This might involve taking a small liver sample (a biopsy) for microscopic examination, and an ultrasound scan to see if there is any form of obstruction taking place.

Thyroid function tests Some doctors will also want to check the function of the thyroid gland. There are two reasons for this.

Firstly, in an older patient, partial failure of the gland may already be occurring and this can produce a range of symptoms which have many similarities to those of M.E., e.g. fatigue, muscle aches, poor brain function, etc. (If there is any co-existent thyroid malfunction it is likely to make any M.E. symptoms worse.) Secondly, although rare, the Coxsackie viruses are capable of causing a painful inflammation of the thyroid gland which in the early stages causes overactivity (hyperthyroidism) and then may be followed by underactivity (hypothyroidism or myxoedema) – although the latter usually resolves in time. This condition is known as de Quervain's thyroiditis.

Cortisol A severe deficiency of this stress hormone occurs in a condition known as Addison's disease; researchers in America have also shown that some patients with M.E. have reductions in their blood cortisol levels (see pages 156–7).

Calcium Although not strictly relevant to M.E. this is still worth checking if there is any doubt about the diagnosis because a raised blood calcium is a rare but well recognised cause of fatigue.

Urea and electrolytes The amount of urea in the blood gives a rough and ready guide as to how well the kidneys are functioning. Levels of electrolytes (body salts) such as potassium and sodium are also measured at the same time. Both of these tests should be normal in M.E. A raised level of potassium in the blood suggests the possibility of Addison's disease.

Although I'm not in favour of over-investigating patients who have a clear cut history of M.E., the tests I've listed so far are all worth checking, especially if there is any doubt about the diagnosis. However, the chances are that the results will all come back completely normal, and so the doctor who doesn't believe in M.E. is then left with a diagnostic problem: a patient with symptoms that he or she doesn't recognise; nothing wrong on physical examination, and a whole range of normal laboratory results.

Testing for the presence of persisting viral infection

There is still no definitive test for M.E. – what we do have are further blood tests which either show the presence of antibodies to enteroviruses such as Coxsackie B, or the 'VP1 test', which if positive, demonstrates the presence of a persisting enteroviral protein.

The antibody tests merely state that the body has reacted in the past (neutralising antibodies) or is probably still reacting (IgM antibodies) to the Coxsackie virus. Although providing useful information, these tests are of limited value, and even when positive don't 'prove' someone has M.E., and at the same time if negative won't disprove the diagnosis. The problems associated with these antibody tests and the value of new diagnostic procedures such as the polymerase chain reaction are discussed in more detail on pages 24–5.

The VP1 Test VP1 stands for Viral Protein One. It is one of four different proteins which form the outer capsule of any enterovirus. One specific portion of VP1 is present in *all* of the seventy-two different enteroviruses.

The researchers at St Mary's Hospital, London, have developed an antibody which can identify this common portion of VP1 and have used it to develop this blood test. A positive test indicates the presence of enterovirus in the blood, but not which one. It is *not* a 'test for M.E.' or an indicator of disease activity. It can also be positive in someone who has picked up an enteroviral infection and just has a cold, so it has to be interpreted with caution. As far as M.E. is concerned a positive test will support the diagnosis, and in patients tested so far, about 55 per cent are positive. A negative result does not exclude the diagnosis of M.E., but means another type of virus (possibly Epstein-Barr) may be responsible. Further details about this test are contained in medical reference 194.

Epstein-Barr virus tests These are much more difficult to interpret because 90 per cent of all adults will have already developed antibodies to this virus by the age of 30 from previous contact with the infection. Any such rise in antibody levels may therefore be simply due to a reactivation of a latent virus. However, several studies have shown that about 20 per cent of patients with M.E. do have raised levels of an antibody known as anti EA (EA = early antigen), and this suggests an increased production of Epstein-Barr virus. Further information on these type of antibody tests is contained in the medical references on pages 345–61.

Other investigations used in M.E.

X-rays of the chest and joints are usually perfectly normal. A trace of the heart rhythm (an electrocardiogram) sometimes reveals abnormalities in patients who start off their illness with an infection involving the heart muscle (a myocarditis). The results of a lumbar puncture – which drains off some of the fluid surrounding the spinal cord – are usually quite normal. Electroencephalograms (EEGs), which monitor electrical activity in the brain, may reveal minor non-specific abnormalities, the significance of which remains uncertain.

As has been described in earlier chapters, there are now a wide range of high-technology investigations which can identify viruses (e.g. polymerase chain reaction) and pick up subtle abnormalities in muscle (e.g. single fibre EMGs), brain tissue (e.g. MRI scans) and the immune system (e.g. T lymphocyte analysis). Unfortunately, the results are not always very consistent, and their significance in M.E. has yet to be fully assessed. None can be regarded as being diagnostic and they are seldom available outside the specialist teaching hospitals. You are unlikely to be referred for any of these investigations unless you are seeing a consultant who is involved in a particular research project.

So, at present, there is no reliable objective way of confirming that someone has M.E. – it is still down to the doctor's basic clinical skills and intuition. This can result in a very long wait before the diagnosis is finally made.

Other causes of chronic fatigue

It's also important to remember that M.E. is not the only cause of chronic fatigue. Other possible explanations, which may even be successfully treated, must not be overlooked, especially when the illness does not follow a clear-cut viral infection.

Obviously, it's not always necessary for a doctor to exclude every single one of these possibilities, but when a particular symptom – say, joint pains – predominates then the rheumatic disorders I describe later really ought to be excluded. Equally, for anyone living in the countryside, 'rural infections' need thinking about; and in the case of more elderly patients, disorders such as hypothyroidism and Parkinson's disease must be seriously considered.

I'd now like to look at a number of conditions, all of which have been initially misdiagnosed as being M.E.

Neurological disease The most common cause of confusion here lies with the illness multiple sclerosis (M.S.) which can be difficult to diagnose in the very early stages. People with M.S. commonly have fatigue (especially after exertion and temperature extremes), tingling/numbness in the skin, and problems with balance. They can also experience similar episodes of depression and mood change. However, optic neuritis – a rapid onset of painful blurred vision in one eye – does not occur in M.E. If there is any confusion between the two conditions, there are three neurological tests which often reveal abnormalities in cases of M.S. which are not seen in M.E. These include delays in visually evoked potentials (see page 86); abnormal proteins in the spinal fluid; and characteristic lesions in the brain shown by magnetic resonance imaging (MRI).

There are also several rare disorders of muscle which can produce pain and weakness. These should certainly be considered if the history is not typical of M.E. or when there is actual *wasting* of the muscle – something not usually seen unless an M.E. patient has become very inactive. Myasthenia gravis is one specific muscle disease that occasionally causes confusion. Here the weakness is *painless* and almost always starts with the face, causing eyelid weakness, double vision, and difficulties with speech and swallowing. The arms and legs tend to become involved at a later stage. Once again, there are special diagnostic tests available.

Early Parkinson's disease should always be considered in anyone over the age of 50, especially when the deterioration in health comes on gradually. In this disorder there is a progressive slowing down in all body movements followed by muscle rigidity and tremor. Once all the classic symptoms are present the diagnosis is unlikely to be missed, but in the very early stages it is often overlooked. Researchers now think that viral infections may also play a part in the development of Parkinson's disease.

Infections Apart from the viruses already discussed, there are several other important non-viral infections which may need excluding. TB is once again on the increase, especially within ethnic communities, and must be considered if there is persisting fever or weight loss.

For anyone in regular contact with farm animals (or has been consuming unpasteurised milk or cheese), brucellosis and leptospirosis hardjo (caught from cattle urine) can both cause a flu-like illness followed by persisting malaise. Toxoplasmosis can be acquired via cats, or by eating undercooked meats from infected animals. It produces an illness very similar to glandular fever with enlarged glands, fever and muscle weakness. There are specific blood tests for all these infections. The possibility that agricultural pesticides, particularly those used in sheep dips, may produce an M.E.-like illness is also considered on page 29.

If your M.E. started off with a gastroenteritis which does not seem to have ever cleared up (especially if it followed a foreign holiday), you may have picked up an infection called Giardia lamblia. This causes continuing diarrhoea, weight loss, stomach pains and wind. In addition there may be headaches, skin rashes, arthritis and muscle pains. Once diagnosed (from a series of stool specimens), Giardia can be successfully treated with a course of antibiotics.

Lyme disease is a relatively new infection which is transmitted by tick bites. The ticks live on sheep and deer; this infection is becoming increasingly common in parts of Southern England – particularly the New Forest area. Symptoms include a character- istic circular rash, arthritis, muscle pains, neurological problems (paralysis of the facial nerve) and fatigue. Once diagnosed (by a blood test), Lyme disease can be treated with antibiotics.

Lastly, it's important to remember that HIV infection (the AIDS virus) can produce fatigue, concentration problems and enlarged glands well before more serious consequences occur. If you feel that you may have put yourself at risk of catching HIV, you ought to discuss this with your GP. Alternatively, you can visit one of the NHS sexual disease clinics for a confidential test.

All the infections I've described are fairly uncommon, but if you genuinely have a persistent raised temperature (keep a proper diary of this to show your doctor), these are infections which do need excluding.

Hormonal There are two important hormonal disturbances which should never be missed. Thyroid gland failure (myx- oedema) usually occurs in later life and produces a variety of symptoms including puffy dry skin, loss of hair and eyebrows, hoarse voice, weight gain, cold intolerance and fatigue. Myx- oedema is easily diagnosed by the blood tests described earlier in the chapter, and is treated with replacement tablets. Overactivity of the thyroid gland (thyrotoxicosis) can cause muscle weakness, along with anxiety and weight loss. The muscle weakness here can be very similar to that seen in myasthenia gravis. Addison's disease is a much rarer hormone deficiency which occurs when the adrenal glands stop producing the stress hormone cortisol. This causes increased skin pigmentation in the mouth and hand creases, lowered blood pressure, stomach pains, diarrhoea and hair loss. Again, it is easy to diagnose with blood tests and can be treated with cortisone replacement.

Gastrointestinal Besides the problems of Giardia there are several other gut conditions which also produce significant fatigue. They should always be considered when stomach pain and changes in bowel habit are the prominent features. Food allergy, irritable bowel syndrome and coeliac disease are all covered elsewhere in the book.

Rheumatic disorders Although rheumatic pain may be a feature of M.E., there are no obvious abnormalities in the joints themselves. However, when arthritic symptoms become marked, it is always worth considering the possibility of a co-existent rheumatic disorder; or an infection such as Lyme disease where, at a later stage, there are migratory joint pains, often in the larger joints such as the knees.

Fatigue can be a prominent feature in rheumatoid arthritis (diagnosed by blood tests and X-rays) along with two more unusual conditions known as Sjøgren's syndrome and systemic lupus erythematosus (SLE).

Sjøgren's syndrome should always be suspected when there are accompanying problems with a dry mouth or eyes. SLE produces a very diverse range of symptoms, many of which overlap with M.E. These include muscle pains, arthritis (small joints), Raynaud's phenomenon (cold hands and feet) and neurological problems. In addition, patients with SLE usually have a characteristic red 'butterfly' rash on their cheeks along with patchy hair loss. There shouldn't be any confusion with M.E. because there are now some very specific blood tests used in the diagnosis of SLE. The most valuable is to look for antibodies to double stranded DNA (ds DNA).

Fibromyalgia is a newly recognised rheumatic disorder with several features that again seem to overlap with M.E. The syndrome consists of widespread aching and stiffness which is accompanied by chronic fatigue and sleep disturbances. Other common symptoms include headaches, irritable bowel disturbances, feelings of swelling around the joints, tingling in the skin and anxiety. One important diagnostic feature is the presence of numerous well-defined tender spots in the tissues. The cause of fibromyalgia remains uncertain, but it has been suggested that the basic problem lies in a disturbance of normal sleep pattern – possibly due to decreased levels of a brain chemical called serotonin that helps to control both pain and normal sleep. Although there is no really effective treatment for fibromyalgia, many patients seem to benefit from a combination of gradually increasing physical activity, small doses of antidepressant drugs, and occasional injections of steroids into the most tender spots. For more information follow up medical references 41 and 44.

Other conditions A complete list of all the remaining medical disorders producing fatigue would be endless; however, there are a few which continue to cause confusion with M.E.

Alcohol abuse is obviously something that few patients would ever admit to. This toxic substance not only damages the liver – over a long period of time it can also affect the brain and heart and produce chronic ill health. If you have raised levels of the liver enzymes described earlier then your doctor may well query if this is the reason. *Anaemia* should be easily picked up on routine blood testing, but I'm always particularly careful to check for pernicious anaemia – which damages the nerves in the spinal cord producing pins and needles (paraesthesiae). If this particular symptom is present, you should ask your doctor to check and make sure there are no signs of Vitamin B12 deficiency in the blood. *Hodgkin's disease* is a form of lymph node cancer which normally affects young adults in the M.E. age group. Symptoms include enlarged glands in the neck and groin, night sweats, fever and weight loss. It's essential that Hodgkin's disease is recognised as early as possible because modern treatment is remarkably successful. *A raised blood calcium* produces gradual loss of appetite, sickness, constipation, excessive thirst, muscle weakness and depression. The symptoms tend to come on insidiously, and so a blood calcium check should be mandatory whenever the diagnosis is in doubt. *Sarcoidosis* can present acutely with fever, arthritis, a disc-shaped rash on the legs and fatigue. Later on there are chronic chest problems when the disease spreads to the lungs. This is something that should be considered (along with TB) if you have persisting chest problems. Up until recently, doctors in the U.K. have always refused to accept that *low blood pressure* (hypotension) could be a cause of ill health. However, a recent large scale survey published in the *British Medical Journal* (medical reference 42) suggests that it may well be a significant factor in causing fatigue and a variety of problems with mental functioning. Anyone who has fatigue which dramatically improves at the weekends may be suffering from a newly recognised occupational disorder known as *sick building syndrome*. This is thought to be related to faulty air conditioning systems in new office buildings. The syndrome consists of headaches, lethargy, dry skin, chest tightness, a runny nose and watering eyes. Two sleep disturbances, namely *sleep apnoea syndrome* and *narcolepsy* are covered on pages 106–7. Lastly, there are several important *psychiatric disorders* (anxiety, hyperventilation, depression and somatisation) in which fatigue forms a major component. These are all dealt with in detail in the chapter on Mind and Body.

How to deal with your doctor once M.E. is diagnosed

People with M.E. don't make easy patients – you've got what is probably a long-term illness that can't be 'cured'; you have a wide variety of symptoms which modern medicine is very limited in its ability to help, and you may also have a whole range of social, emotional and employment problems which require help. So, from your GP's point of view M.E. patients are not the easiest of people to manage successfully.

Despite all these hurdles, an increasing number of doctors are becoming interested in M.E. and consequently diagnosing the illness correctly in the vital early stages. This is borne out by a survey conducted by Dr Darrel Ho-Yen, a consultant interested in M.E., who recently sought the opinions of nearly 200 general practitioners (see medical reference 50). Overall, 71 per cent accepted the diagnosis; 22 per cent remained undecided, but only 7 per cent did not. This survey also suggested an incidence of M.E. of 1.3 cases per 1000 patients with women

Conditions which can be mistaken for M.E.

Neuromuscular Disease	Multiple Sclerosis Myasthenia Gravis Parkinson's Disease Rare muscle disorders
Chronic Infections	Brucellosis Giardia Hepatitis B HIV+ Leptospirosis hardjo Lyme Disease Toxoplasmosis
Gastric Disorders	Coeliac Disease Crohn's Disease Food Allergy Irritable Bowel Syndrome
Hormonal Imbalance	Addison's Disease Hypothyroidism (Myxoedema) Thyrotoxicosis Pituitary Tumour
Psychiatric Disorders	Anxiety +/− hyperventilation Depression Somatisation
Rheumatic Disorders	Fibromyalgia Lyme Disease Sjøgren's Syndrome Systemic Lupus Erythematosus
Miscellaneous	Alcohol abuse Anaemia Hodgkin's Disease Hypercalcaemia Organophosphate pesticides Sarcoidosis Sick Building Syndrome Sleep Apnoea and Narcolepsy TB

outnumbering men by about 2:1.

Unfortunately, some doctors still remain ignorant of the recent research advances. So, if you are convinced that M.E.

is the cause of your symptoms don't be fobbed off with explanations that 'the disease does not exist', and try to obtain an
opinion from a doctor who is aware of the condition.

Some physicians are becoming increasingly aware and involved in what is termed the holistic approach to medicine
and patient care. This means they take into account not only
your physical illness, but also your attitude to it, the interaction
between you and your family and any environmental factors
which may be having an effect.

It's this sort of approach, where everything is considered,
and the patient's family fully involved, that is particularly
appropriate to conditions like M.E.

What can the doctor prescribe?

Although there are a growing number of specific treatments
under investigation, the results are far from conclusive. Any
sort of 'cure' for M.E. still seems a long way off. To date the
only drugs, which have been subjected to properly controlled
clinical trials, are magnesium, evening primrose oil (both of
which are covered in the chapter on Alternative Approaches),
and injections of immunoglobulin. Drugs which may provide
symptomatic relief are discussed under the relevant symptom
in the preceding chapters.

Antidepressants These drugs may well be of considerable
benefit where there is associated depression; lower doses of
which have been used for treating sleep disturbances and pain
– sometimes quite successfully. Otherwise, their use in M.E. is
very debatable, and many patients seem particularly susceptible
to their side-effects. The detailed use of antidepressants is covered in the chapter on Mind and Body.

Antiviral drugs The problems associated with the development
of new drugs which can act against specific viruses have already
been discussed on pages 28–29, and to date there do not appear
to be any effective products in the case of M.E.

Acyclovir, which is effective against some *active* herpes virus
infections, has been tried in America without any success (see

medical reference 157) where it was thought that Epstein–Barr virus (one of the herpes group) may be a causative organism.

Although there has been some experimental research into the development of specific drugs against enteroviruses (see medical reference 134) none are available for human use; the major pharmaceutical companies are unlikely to plough resources into research in this area unless they are fully convinced about the enterovirus link to M.E.

Amantadine (Symmetrel) is a drug which was originally developed for treating Parkinson's disease. Then it was discovered that it also had some weak antiviral properties as well, particularly against influenza viruses and herpes zoster. Amantadine is now being used by some doctors to treat M.E., but there have been no clinical trials to properly assess these anecdotal claims. Also, there is no evidence that it has any significant effect on enteroviral infection. Although this drug is generally well tolerated, it can cause fluid retention, skin rashes along with adverse effects on the nervous system which include sleep disturbances, dizziness, convulsions and severe psychiatric reactions. It should not be given to anyone who has had convulsions, gastric ulcers or kidney disease. At the moment there is not enough evidence to recommend the use of amantadine in M.E., especially in view of its potential side-effects. However, one small trial has looked at the possible role of using amantadine in relieving the fatigue which is commonly associated with multiple sclerosis (see medical reference 154).

Immunotherapy A wide variety of treatments directed at correcting disturbances in the immune system have been tried in America, Australia and the U.K., many of which are extremely costly and not without unpleasant side-effects. At the moment I would not recommend this particular approach until the researchers have some more reliable information as to their benefits.

Treatments which have been tried and failed include plasma exchange (removes immune complexes from the blood); thymic hormone (supposed to boost T cell production); Imunovir (a drug with weak antiviral properties as well); and high doses of steroids (which should *not* be prescribed in M.E.). Neverthe-less, in view of the abnormalities now described in hormone production (see pages 119–20) the role of drugs which influence cortisol levels needs to be assessed.

One particular form of immunotherapy, which is claimed to work, involves injections of immunoglobulin. It is possible that this drug neutralises persisting viruses or corrects a defect in the immune system. In the U.K. immunoglobulin is usually given in fairly small doses into the muscle. Some patients do seem to improve but may well relapse when it is stopped. Others gain no benefit and may even feel worse.

In November 1990 the *American Journal of Medicine* pub-lished the results of two separate trials which both used much higher doses of immunoglobulin G given directly into the vein. Unfortunately, the results were conflicting. Dr Andrew Lloyd's Australian trial involved 49 patients who were given three monthly injections (dose 2g/kg) or a placebo. Improvement in physical, psychological and immune status occurred in 10 out of 23 being treated compared to only 3 out of 26 in the placebo group. Dr Dan Peterson's American trial involved 30 adults who were given six injections monthly (dose 1g/kg) of immunoglobulin or a placebo. About 25 per cent in each group reported some improvement. For further details see medical references 145, 151 and 153.

Clearly, further trials need to be carried out to see if there really is a distinct sub-group of patients with specific immune abnormalities who benefit from this approach. The problem with high doses of immunoglobulin is that it is extremely costly and not without side-effects. These include headaches, inflammation of the vein (phlebitis), and the possibility of transmitting hepatitis C virus.

In America and Australia various experimental forms of immunotherapy are also being assessed including Ampligen and transfer factor. Ampligen is claimed to be capable of either 'up regulating or down regulating the immune system': There have been some initial reports of success in a small number of patients, but once again it is very costly and unlikely to be used in the U.K. unless properly controlled trials confirm its potential. A recent report in the *Journal of the American Medical Association* (medical reference 146) reported initial data from a double-blind, placebo-controlled, multi-centre, 24-week trial of ampligen in 92 severely ill patients who all met the U.S. definition of M.E. The treated group showed significant improvements in both physical and mental functioning; the ones most likely to respond were those with abnormalities on MRI brain scans and markedly raised levels of interleukin 1. Apart from minor skin rashes and fever most patients completed this trial without serious adverse effects, but there have been concerns expressed about the drug causing liver damage. At the moment the American Food and Drug Administration have placed Ampligen on 'clinical hold' until more data on its side-effects becomes available. Further information on Ampligen can be obtained from H.E.M. Research, 1 Penn Center, Suite 660, 1617 JFK Boulevard, Philadelphia 19103, USA. Tel. 0101-215-9880080.

Another drug currently being used in America is called Kutapressin, and this is described in further detail on page 217.

Transfer factor is another type of immune chemical which is present in white blood cells. It can be extracted from the white cells of a close relative and then transferred to the patient. In theory this should then transfer some degree of natural immunity from one person to another – hence the name. So far the only properly controlled trial of transfer factor has been carried out by Dr Andrew Lloyd's team in Australia which involved 90 patients taking either active treatment or a placebo drug. After a follow-up period of three months there was no difference between the two groups. It would not appear that this particular form of immune therapy is going to be of value in treating M.E.

5HT drugs are a brand new group of pharmaceutical compounds which are arousing tremendous interest, and may well turn out to have an important role in the management of M.E. There is also accumulating evidence that they are useful in a whole range of conditions as varied as severe nausea, anxiety, depression (see page 170), migraine-type headaches, schizophrenia, and coronary heart disease.

5HT is medical shorthand for a vital brain transmitter

chemical known as 5 hydroxytryptamine or serotonin. Both animal and human experiments indicate that serotonin is involved in a whole range of body functions including sleep, appetite, sexual desire, mood control, as well as the way the brain regulates various hormonal responses.

It is also becoming apparent that there are several highly selective receptor sites in the brain which respond to different types of 5HT drugs – so far designated as $5HT_{1-3}$. For example, $5HT_1$ sites are being linked to migraine; $5HT_2$ to depression and schizophrenia; and $5HT_3$ to a nausea and vomiting control centre in the brain.

As more information accumulates on the role of this important neurotransmitter, and the way it interacts with other brain chemicals, hormones and the immune system, the result could well be one of the most important pharmaceutical breakthroughs this century. As far as M.E. is concerned trials with 5HT drugs are now under way, and the results are awaited with interest.

Vitamin and mineral supplements Apart from magnesium sulphate injections there is no published evidence to suggest that supplementation with these products is of any value. The pros and cons of such therapy is considered in greater detail on pages 201–11. It should also be noted that the NHS regards many of the commercial supplements as 'borderline substances' meaning that they should not be given out on prescription unless there is a very good reason for doing so.

As you can see it's not easy for doctors when patients with M.E. demand that 'something must be done' in the form of specific drug treatment. There are undoubtedly a few drugs which do now seem to help some groups of patients, whereas others will just experience their side-effects. The only way forward in this area is for properly controlled clinical trials to take place involving more than one group of patients (multi-centre trials) who have well defined M.E. As the various pieces of the M.E. jigsaw all fit into place I have no doubt that effective treatments will eventually materialise.

A full list of medical references describing the various treatments that have been tried in M.E. – both orthodox and alternative – can be found on pages 346–61.

Referral to consultants

Is there any need for you to be referred to a consultant? Obviously, yes, if your general practitioner has any doubt about the diagnosis. But as many patients know from bitter experience, this can still be counter productive, and even harmful if you then end up seeing a specialist who isn't familiar with M.E. The diagnosis is missed and thoughts of a 'psychiatric problem' then become foremost in the GP's mind. Having had one specialist opinion who 'can't find anything wrong' your GP may then feel very reluctant to send you to other specialists for further second opinions, and so the psychiatrist becomes the only option. And so the merry-go-round of general physician–neurologist–psychiatrist goes on until someone finally makes the correct diagnosis.

As M.E. symptoms cross a whole range of medical boundaries (virology, infectious diseases, neurology, gut problems, immunology, etc.) specialists in a wide range of subjects have become involved. It should now be possible, in most parts of the country, to find a specialist interested in M.E., although this may mean travelling to the local teaching hospital.

Your own GP may know of a local specialist interested in M.E., but if he doesn't there'll be an element of pot luck involved, if you're just referred to a local general physician. One useful source of information in these circumstances are members of the local M.E. group, who are often very well informed about who's worth going to see – and not worth going to see.

NHS consultants don't generally like seeing patients privately unless they're first referred by their GP, so it's always best to ask your family doctor to write a referral note. Some GPs actually get very upset when their patients go off to see private consultants without their knowledge or 'permission' – and they do have a valid point. Even if a consultant is prepared to see you without a referral letter, it's still regarded as being unethical if they don't then keep your GP fully informed about their diagnostic opinion or treatment.

If you're really not happy about the way your GP is managing your illness, do think very carefully about going off for other opinions without discussing it, as it's quite likely to put an additional strain on your relationship.

In Britain, there's nothing to prevent your GP referring you on to an NHS specialist outside your usual health district, although many hospitals actively discourage such referrals. The other problem in doing so is that those specialists who are interested in M.E., particularly in London, have at times become so overwhelmed by such requests, that they've become practically unable to cope with any further outside requests.

M.E. really is a condition which is ideally managed by good and interested general practitioners – provided you can find one!

The private medical sector

There are now a growing number of private medical practitioners and clinics who claim to specialise in the treatment of M.E. Some are willing to accept referrals without the knowledge of your own GP, but this is neither ethical nor wise. Although their approaches vary considerably, a great deal of emphasis tends to be placed on identifying and treating allergies (using the sort of techniques described in the chapter on Alternative Approaches), anti-candida regimes and dietary modification. One or two are much more orientated towards the current psychiatric view of M.E. and concentrate on behaviour modification techniques and psychological therapies. Some of these approaches have come in for considerable criticism and few have been subjected to good clinical trials to assess their value. Equally, there are no tests available in the private sector that can diagnose M.E. If you do decide to obtain private treatment, please take advice from your own GP first, and try to find out how much the consultations and treatments will cost before making a firm commitment. Unfortunately, there is no doubt that anyone with the time and money will eventually find a doctor in the private sector who will give them a diagnosis of M.E. provided they search hard enough!

Uninterested doctors

What can you do if your general practitioner just isn't interested or sympathetic towards M.E., and can't accept that you really do feel as ghastly as you claim?

Your doctor may well be one of those who is just not interested in chronic illnesses, where there's very little he can do to alleviate the symptoms or change the course of the disease by writing out something on the prescription pad. He may be one of those doctors who doesn't really like talking to his patients for more than ten minutes, and feels that emotional problems aren't his concern – whereas for the patient they're an extremely important part of the illness.

If you have got a doctor in this category, and his attitude doesn't seem to change, even after you've gone to the bother of getting him all the latest medical references on the subject, there's probably no other option but to try and find someone else. If you belong to a group practice it should be quite easy to see another partner, and you may not have to actually change on to their individual list. Any good practice should have a flexible policy for patients who find they don't have any rapport with their doctor and want to see another member of the team.

Alternatively, you might try the practice 'trainee' if they have one – a good sign that the practice has come up to standard when it was selected for such a purpose. Trainee general practitioners are often bright young doctors, fresh from doing three or four years in hospital medicine, but are now intending to enter general practice. They work for an introductory year under the supervision of one of the senior partners in the practice. Trainees often have more time to devote to their individual patients, and are often encouraged to take on unusual or 'difficult' conditions – even writing them up as part of their examination – so if you find a trainee taking considerable time and interest in your case, stick with him or her. Unfortunately, they're only with the practice for one year, and only rarely progress on to a job in the same practice, so this isn't a long-term solution.

As a last resort you may have to consider finding another GP altogether. Try and find out from friends and neighbours (or other M.E. patients) about the local doctors, and possibly go round and ask if the one you choose is prepared to take you on to the list. Some doctors are even quite happy for prospective patients to come to the surgery for a quick chat before joining the practice.

In Britain, however, it's worth remembering that the GP is paid on a capitation fee system – about £15 every year for each patient on the list, no matter how many times he sees or visits you – so there's no great incentive to encourage people with chronic illnesses to join the list!

As many M.E. patients are already too well aware, some doctors tend to be very wary of patients who 'swap' doctors in the same area, and may view you as a potential problem. Also, practices have fairly well-defined geographical limits on who they're prepared to take on, so outside large towns such action may be practically very difficult or even impossible.

If you do decide to change doctor try not to leave it to your Family Health Service Authority (FHSA) to allocate you a new practice. This really is the last resort, and a very bad start to any new doctor–patient relationship. No doctor likes having patients allocated to them by an anonymous administrator, whether they like it or not. Your local Community Health Council or FHSA can help you further with the technical details of how to change.

The final option is to opt out of the NHS altogether and go privately, but do take advice and think very carefully about who you go and see, or you could end up spending a lot of money on unnecessary drugs and investigations and just getting the wrong advice. In many large towns there are now a few purely private general practitioners, but you're not supposed to remain on an NHS practitioner's list at the same time. A private GP, although he may obviously be able to spend more time with you, may not know any more about M.E. than your NHS one.

There aren't any easy answers about how to establish a good doctor–patient relationship; a lot depends on pure luck and where you happen to live. At the end of the day it's like any relationship – some doctors just don't hit it off with some of their patients and vice versa. You've really got to treat it like a marriage – if both partners don't contribute it won't work.

Some of your 'rights' from the NHS

Patients don't have many rights when it comes to the NHS – just reasonable requests. This is a summary of the most important ones which relate to M.E.

General practitioners Everyone is entitled to join a GP's practice. You can choose from any local NHS general practitioner, provided he or she is willing to accept you. Some GPs even allow prospective patients to come and have a chat before joining their list to see if both parties are going to be suited! Lists of all the local GPs can be found in main post offices, libraries, the local family health service authority (FHSA) or at a citizens advice bureau. All GPs should now be producing a leaflet giving details of their staff, hours of clinics and other services which are provided.

During normal working hours you have a 'right' to be seen by a GP in the practice, but not necessarily your own. If the practice runs an appointment system you should be given a space as soon as possible, provided the delay isn't harmful.

Patients do not have a 'right' to demand a visit at home from a G.P. This all depends on the doctor's individual judgement as to whether it is necessary. Doctors are becoming increasingly reluctant to do home visiting for the chronic sick, and prefer their patients to visit the surgery whenever possible. However, your GP is obliged, under the NHS contract, to come out and visit in any true emergency. Anyone aged 75 or over is entitled to one home visit each year.

If you're temporarily away from home on holiday, you can visit one of the local GPs and be seen as a temporary resident. This shouldn't cause any problems as it attracts an extra fee!

When you move to another area (or if you become unhappy with your present GP) it should be quite easy to change to another doctor or practice, and you don't have to give any reason for doing so. Ask the new GP if you can be accepted on to their list and then send your medical card to the FHSA. Equally, it's also possible for GPs to remove patients from their list without giving any reason; although few doctors would do this just because of a chronic illness. The usual reason is a breakdown due to a clash of personalities, or disagreements over treatment. In this case the FHSA must find you another doctor.

Drugs As far as drugs are concerned, you can't demand to have a new treatment which you may have heard about, but which your GP isn't yet aware of. Doctors are quite rightly reluctant to start prescribing new drugs until their benefits have been proved and long-term side-effects fully established. If your GP is unfamiliar with the use of a drug in M.E. such as the gammaglobulin injections or magnesium, he or she will probably want to discuss this with a specialist before giving it. It seems that long legal actions against doctors, for side-effects from drugs they've prescribed, are going to be increasingly common, so such caution will very likely increase.

Hospital treatment Once again, you don't have any 'right' to a second opinion from a specialist, but it would be unreasonable if a GP refused such a request when there were doubts about either the diagnosis, or how the illness should be managed. Under the NHS you can't choose which specialist you want to be referred to, but there's nothing to stop you suggesting a particular name if you're heard that this consultant is sympathetic to or interested in M.E.

If you are admitted to hospital you can discharge yourself at any time if you are unhappy with either the treatment or the investigations being carried out. Obviously, this will cause a great deal of upset, and won't make you very popular with either the hospital or your GP. The ward staff will almost certainly make you sign a form to say that you left hospital against medical advice. However, this does not necessarily relieve them of legal liability if anything goes wrong following such treatment.

You can only be detained in hospital against your will if the doctors decide to use their powers granted under the 1983 Mental Health Act. This is really only relevant to severe psychiatric illness and does contain an appeal procedure. The best organisation to provide further help in this area is MIND (see page 335).

Consenting to treatment and investigations All patients should fully understand what their treatment and tests entail before they commence. If you end up being treated or examined without such consent it could, in legal terms, be regarded as assault. This is particularly important where doctors are using treatment regimes which are unproven or as part of clinical trials for new drugs.

In theory you are free to decide whether or not to accept any particular treatment option, but as we all know different specialists take opposing views as to which is the best way to manage patients with M.E. I have no doubt that some patients are being pressurised into following advice which they are not happy about and may well be doing them harm.

It's essential that when a specialist wants to involve you in any unusual or risky new treatment/investigation that all the possible hazards are fully explained first. Otherwise the doctors could be laying themselves open to legal action if something goes wrong. Most hospitals now have ethical committees which are supposed to vet any clinical trials, and it's worth asking whether this has happened if you are at all concerned.

In the large teaching hospitals it's also quite likely that you'll be examined by medical students. Most patients are only too happy to co-operate in this learning process, but if you'd rather not then do tell the consultant.

Access to medical records From November 1991 all patients were given the right to inspect their medical records under the 1990 Health Records Act. You also have a previous right under the 1984 Data Protection Act to inspect any health records which are held on computer.

Although far from perfect, this new legislation does give patients the opportunity to check what has been written about them by GPs and specialists. In theory it also provides a means of correcting any inaccuracies. Unfortunately, one of the loopholes in the Act is that the holder of the records does not have to clearly state that part of the information has been withheld, so you may never even know what's been left out!

The Act covers information held by both the NHS and private sectors, except for Northern Ireland which is covered by a separate law. So, in theory, you can inspect anything that has been written about you by a doctor, dentist, optician or clinical psychologist. Unfortunately, you only have legal access to information recorded after 1 November 1991; before that you will have to rely on the doctor's willingness to comply.

If you wish to make use of the Act you should apply in writing to your GP, or to the local health authority (health board in Scotland) in the case of NHS hospitals. With 'trust' and private hospitals you should apply directly.

After this you should be given access to your medical records within 40 days. It is also permissible to ask someone else to look at your notes or for you to take photocopies. If you notice any mistakes, you can ask for them to be corrected. If the holder (doctor or hospital) disagrees with this request, a note of your views should still be recorded.

Access can only be refused on three grounds: where it will cause *serious harm* to your mental or physical health; where it comprises a third party, such as a relative; and where the information was recorded before 1 November 1991.

If you have difficulties in persuading your doctor or hospital to comply, do contact your local Community Health Council. There is also a right of appeal to the courts if access is refused; but it may also be possible to pursue such a dispute by using the established hospital complaints procedures.

If your GP writes a medical report to your employer or an insurance company, you also have a right to see this before it is passed on – unless the doctor decides the information could be harmful. If necessary, you can refuse to let your employer or insurer see this report, and may even add your own comments.

Medical confidentiality Doctors should never pass on medical information without your permission. The only exceptions are to other health professionals involved in your treatment, and in certain circumstances your close relatives. If you don't want a doctor to discuss your condition with a spouse or partner, do make sure that this fact is clearly written down in your medical notes.

Complaints about doctors

If you want to make a complaint about your GP this has to be done in writing within 13 weeks of whatever incident prompted the complaint. You should write to the family health service authority (FHSA), but remember they only deal with formal complaints about GPs who do not comply with their NHS contract. If you need any help about how to complain or to write such a letter, contact your local Community Health Council.

Most NHS hospitals now have a senior member of staff who looks into complaints that cannot be resolved after direct contact with the specialist concerned. If this process proves to be unsatisfactory you can then ask for the matter to be investigated by a regional medical officer (or medical officer for complaints in Wales).

Doctors who behave unethically or unprofessionally can be reported to the General Medical Council in London (see page 331). They deal with complaints about neglectful care, or where a doctor appears to be incapable of providing satisfactory care. They will also look into treatments which are obviously fraudulent or harmful.

If you're still not satisfied about the way a complaint has been handled, you can take your case to the Health Service Commissioner (see pages 331–2). This should be done within a year of you realising that you have something to complain about.

As a last resort you can go to court, but you must have a strong case and be able to prove that negligence occurred. This will obviously involve taking expert legal advice from a solicitor who is experienced in this aspect of the law. You could also ask an organisation called Action for Victims of Medical Accidents for advice (see page 323).

The Patients Association (see page 337) are also very helpful when it comes to advice and information on complaints or queries about your 'rights' as a consumer in the National Health Service.

Insurance problems

With an increasing number of claims now being submitted, M.E. is starting to cause concern amongst the insurance companies. There are five types of policy in which problems may arise.

Motor vehicle insurance Most policies now ask very careful questions about any illness or disability which could impair one's ability to drive. Obviously, the fact that you have M.E. cannot be ignored when filling in such a form, and failure to disclose this information could result in problems if an accident occurs – even if it is not your fault. The fact that you have M.E. may result in the insurer requesting a medical opinion from your GP on your fitness to drive, or asking you to report your circumstances to the medical department at the DVLC in Swansea.

Life insurance This is one piece of important financial planning that should not cause any great difficulty. I am not aware that any of the reputable major insurance companies are refusing life cover on the grounds of M.E.; although the cost of the policy might be slightly loaded and a medical examination requested if the cover is high. M.E. is not a life-threatening condition, although for the small minority who have persisting heart problems following an initial myocarditis the insurers are likely to be far more cautious.

Permanent health insurance (PHI) This type of policy pays out a regular monthly income as long as the policyholder is unfit for work. Because of the high cost of premiums, most PHI policies tend to come into operation after several months of ill health, often when sick pay from an employer has been terminated or reduced.

As long as your GP is willing to issue DSS sick notes confirming that you are 'unfit for work', there shouldn't be any difficulties. However, problems will arise if the DSS stops sickness benefit or recommends that you are now fit to resume 'suitable alternative work'. In the latter case the policy may be such that it will 'top up' any loss of earnings as a result of switching to lower paid employment or part-time work. When a PHI claim continues for a prolonged period of time the insurer may well ask for an independent medical examination.

Permanent disablement insurance This type of policy pays out a lump sum 'or a regular monthly income when the company is fully satisfied that the claimant is fully and permanently disabled. In the case of M.E., permanent disablement is not always easy to define especially in the early stages of the illness when outcome is very unpredictable. And, it is not unknown for some degree of recovery to occur even after a prolonged period of ill health. So, in view of the large sums of money often involved, the insurers are unlikely to settle unless they are fully satisfied that there is no real chance of recovery taking place. In practice this almost certainly means that several years of ill health will have to occur before a settlement is reached. It is also quite likely that the insurer will require a specialist medical examination, and this may not always be carried out by a doctor who views the condition favourably.

Private medical insurance Once again, some of the insurers specialising in this type of cover are becoming concerned about the very high cost of investigations and speculative treatments being advocated by private doctors and clinics who claim to treat M.E. I know of one private hospital where bills running into several thousand pounds are not unknown. Some of these insurers are already making it clear that they will no longer reimburse high charges for an ongoing illness like M.E. over an indefinite period. So, if you are embarking on expensive private care using insurance cover it may be wise to check with the company before doing so. It is also possible to purchase private health insurance which covers several types of alternative therapies.

Travel insurance Policies which provide medical cover for travel abroad shouldn't cause any problems providing you are not travelling against medical advice. However, it's always a good idea to check the small print on any package holiday cover well before departure.

When problems with insurance companies arise with a claim relating to M.E., do make sure that you keep carbon copies of all correspondence with the official involved. If you're not making satisfactory progress, then write to either the Chief General Manager or the Chief Medical Officer and send your letter by recorded delivery. As a last resort you can ask the Insurance Ombudsman (see page 333) to intervene and arbitrate.

Miscellaneous problems

Jury service could involve a very unpredictable amount of time in court, and would obviously require periods of sustained concentration making it a most unsuitable task for anyone with M.E. If you are still unwell and receive such a request to report for jury service you should write to the court and state that you have M.E. You should also explain that this causes severe problems with any kind of intense or prolonged concentration as well as short-term memory loss. It's highly likely that the court will accept this explanation and not pursue the request. In the unlikely event of the court not accepting your word it will then be necessary to ask your GP to write out a certificate stating that you are not fit for jury service. This may involve payment of a small fee.

2. Self-Help

So long as conventional medicine seems to be of relatively little help in altering the natural course of recovery in M.E., the onus lies on patients themselves to try and create the optimum conditions for progress to take place. A period of slow, steady convalescence is essential – something which has gone out of fashion in modern medicine.

Coming to terms with the many restrictions imposed by this illness; remaining positive about the chances of recovery; and adopting sensible changes in lifestyle are the three most important areas of self-help that require careful consideration. Inevitably, this will mean 'redefining your boundaries' in all aspects of everyday life, and not pushing yourself to the point of physical or mental exhaustion. For many previously fit young adults these are changes which can be very difficult to accept and put into practice – as I know all too well from my own personal experiences of the illness over the past twelve years.

Rest and relaxation

Rest is definitely the most important factor in promoting recovery from M.E. Without rest, recovery will *not* occur, and those patients who continually struggle on, either at home or at work, to the point of regularly reaching mental or physical fatigue stand very little chance of making any form of positive progress.

Rest means not only relaxing physically, but mentally as well. Every single day needs to be carefully planned ahead to make sure that activities are spaced to allow a period of rest in between. Ideally, rest periods should be taken in quiet surroundings where there is freedom from interruption. Take the phone off the hook; let friends and neighbours know that you don't want to be disturbed, and probably won't answer the doorbell.

Nobody with M.E. should feel guilty about taking a period of bed rest in the afternoon. For many patients it's the only way they can manage to complete the day. You don't have to go to bed, just have a quiet lie down for an hour or so, and listen to the radio or tape if you don't feel sleepy. Alternatively, make it the time of day you carry out the relaxation techniques described on pages 177–8.

In the very early stages of M.E. (i.e straight after the initial viral infection) I have no hesitation in recommending a period of *total bed rest* before a very gradual return to normal activities. This may mean two or three weeks in bed and several months getting back to normal: by doing so you will, hopefully, avoid the progression of M.E. into a chronic condition lasting for years.

However, prolonged bed rest can also damage your health, and once the disease has become established, it requires careful thought. (In my own case a period of three weeks' bed rest, two years after the original illness when the diagnosis was first made failed to produce any benefits.) Besides the obvious problems of constipation, prolonged immobility from bed rest can produce rather more serious consequences. Doctors now refer to an 'immobility syndrome' which can occur after such extended periods of rest, with decreased oxygen intake to the lungs, risks of venous thrombosis in the legs (another good reason for taking some form of passive exercise) and loss of calcium, increasing the risk of osteoporosis later. If you put a perfectly healthy person to bed for a couple of weeks, he or she will feel very weak when trying to get up and about again. It's hardly surprising that people with M.E. experience much greater difficulties when trying to return to relative normality.

Complete bed rest is only to be recommended at the time of a relapse (e.g. with another unrelated infection) or if you seem to be on a downhill patch, possibly from trying to do too much physically or mentally. At the time of relapse I immediately go to bed, and try to rest as much as possible, for say forty-eight hours, or a little longer. After that I try to start a gradual recovery process – even if it only means getting out of bed to sit in my chair for half an hour. I know it's not always possible, but the longer you do stay on bed rest during a relapse, the harder it's going to be to 'get going again'.

Some M.E. patients may find themselves confined to bed for quite long periods. If this is so, do try and make sure that either you or your family help with some passive exercises with your arms and legs whilst in bed. This involves carrying out the normal movements you'd make when up and about. Some people find it quite comforting to do these sort of exercises while in a warm bath. If you're not sure about what you could be doing, a physiotherapist might be willing to come in and help.

There will be times when long periods are spent confined to the bedroom – especially during a relapse. It may be worth making some significant alterations to the bedroom's layout to make it into an all-purpose room, in which you can eat, work, see visitors, as well as relax and sleep. During a period of relapse, a trip up and down the stairs can be quite shattering, so make the bedroom as comfortable as possible, with the phone by the bed. Have some shelves close by to keep books and other essential items on. Try also to transfer a few kitchen essentials, so that you don't go downstairs continually to the kitchen to get a drink or prepare a snack. It may all seem very strange to friends, relatives and visitors, but it is a very practical solution to trying to make sure you get rest when necessary.

It's a good idea, if you can afford it, to invest in a comfortable firm mattress and good pillows for the bed – after all, you're probably spending more of your life there than anywhere else. It's also quite helpful to have a comfortable armchair in the bedroom, so you can get up and sit for a while, if you don't want to venture downstairs.

Try not to get bothered about seeing your visitors in the bedroom. If the room is large enough, have a couple of fold-up chairs for visitors to use. Socialising with friends and relatives can be a tiring experience when you're not well, and this works as a compromise to not seeing people at all.

Make sure you have a good bedside light. If you like watching television consider buying a portable set for the bedroom, but try not to let it become your main interest!

During more stable periods you may still need extensive rest. If you get up in the morning and feel awful, knowing that body and mind aren't going to function effectively, do try resting or even going back to bed for a bit, and possibly start again after lunch. Don't struggle on with what you intended to do – you'll only end up making mistakes, and making yourself feel worse in the process. On the other hand, if you do start the day off well, and accomplish all that you planned to do, follow this by considering very carefully how much extra you can now do. It's far better to build up your activities gradually during a good spell, than overdo it on the first few days, and end up feeling bloody awful because you tried to do too much.

No two days are going to be the same with M.E., and predicting how one is going to feel tomorrow or the following week is quite impossible. This is why forward planning of any sort of activity becomes so difficult, and arrangements frequently have to be cancelled at the last minute.

It can be very helpful to make a written list of all planned activities for the coming week – nothing too ambitious – and then tick them off as you go along. It does help self-esteem to actually plan to do something and then carry it out, and keep some record of what you've actually done, even though it may be a shadow of your previous performance.

Exercise

One of the most difficult aspects of coming to terms with a new lifestyle is striking the right balance between taking an adequate amount of rest on one hand, and what might be described as 'beneficial exercise' on the other. All too often, one hears about M.E. patients – and here I include myself – who, in the earliest stages of the illness, before any diagnosis has been made, have tried to get better by overdoing exercise and not taking sufficient rest.

First, how much exercise should you be taking and in what form? Like everything else, exercise tolerance in M.E. varies considerably from patient to patient, but each individual soon learns to recognise his or her own limitations – be it walking, gardening or any other physical activity. The cardinal rule when

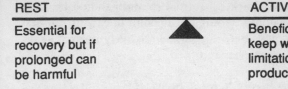

REST		ACTIVITY
Essential for recovery but if prolonged can be harmful		Beneficial, provided you keep within your own limitations - excess will produce a relapse

taking part in any sort of activity is to avoid pushing yourself to the point of fatigue, and *never* to the point of exhaustion. In practice this is probably best explained by using a diagram:

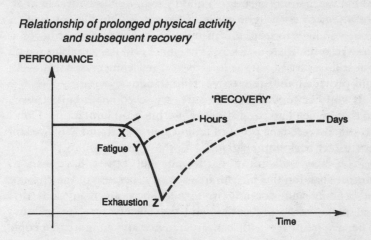

Relationship of prolonged physical activity and subsequent recovery

You know already from your own experiences that after starting to go for a walk you can carry on at a fairly steady pace till you reach **X** – when the muscles start to tire. For some people this may only be 100 yards, but for others it may be half a mile or so. If you then decide to push on beyond point **X** the fatigue becomes steadily worse, till you reach a point **Y**, where it's becoming very difficult to go much further. If you still decide to carry on beyond **Y** there is a rapid deterioration, and you're very quickly exhausted and weak at the knees, forcing complete cessation of activity – **Z**.

The aim in all physical activity must therefore be to learn how much you can usefully achieve before reaching the points of fatigue and exhaustion, and keep within those limits at all times. If you stop your physical activity at or before the point of fatigue your recovery period back to normal strength should be fairly short – minutes or hours. Going to the point of exhaustion may mean that it takes days before you feel relatively normal again, and the muscle strength has returned.

What sort of exercise is helpful in M.E.?

Few M.E. patients find that they can participate in any form of active sport, and certainly in nothing which involves both physical ability and rapid mental functioning. The great danger is that when going through a good patch, you may decide to go for a jog, or try a light game of tennis. Within a quarter of an hour you have to stop, exhausted, and you may now be heading for a relapse. There are, however, some physical activities which can still be carried out, as long as you're feeling reasonably well, and provided you stick to your limitations.

If you like to walk for pleasure, try to go on 'circular tours', so that you end up back at home, within your limitations. Don't set off and reach the point of fatigue half way round. You've still got to get back home again!

You may still enjoy gardening, but others have had to almost abandon this pleasurable activity, because of the amount of bending and stooping involved. There are many aids that can make gardening easier, and the Society for Horticultural Therapy (see page 340) can give advice and support to people with disabilities, who find gardening very therapeutic.

Another enjoyable form of exercise is a short period of swimming in a *warm* pool. You may find that your local authority pool has a special weekly session when the water is heated up a little extra. The Association of Swimming Therapy promotes and teaches the art of swimming to people with disabilities using a special technique called the Halliwick Method (see page 341). The buoyancy of the water in a swimming pool makes it an ideal medium in which to exercise weakened muscles in a gentle fashion, and also to mobilise any painful joints. Your local hospital may also have a hydrotherapy pool, and a physiotherapist may be able to arrange a regular session on the NHS.

Some patients also find yoga beneficial, but do take guidance from an experienced teacher, and stick to positions which are not too fatiguing.

In the end it all comes down to listening to what your body is telling you. If you're going through a good patch don't overdo it, but gradually try to increase your activities on a day-by-day basis. Don't push on at a faster pace than you can adequately cope with, or you'll just end up relapsing again.

Nutrition

It goes without saying that all aspects of healthy eating should be encouraged, taking into account any personal allergies or sensitivities to foods.

A wide variety of digestive problems can become a part of this illness, but the cause remains uncertain. One factor could be the presence of a persisting enteroviral infection in the bowel wall which, in turn, interferes with enzymes that aid the digestion of food. Certainly, one well-recognised after-effect of a gastrointestinal infection is the development of milk intolerance. This is because the infection reduces the jejunal mucosa's ability to produce an enzyme called lactase which helps to break down milk and aid its absorption. Common symptoms include pain, wind and diarrhoea. The diagnosis of lactase deficiency can be confirmed by finding what are known as reducing sugars in the motions. There should then be a dramatic improvement in symptoms so long as milk and all milk products are removed from the diet.

It has also been suggested that bowel problems such as bloating, pain and diarrhoea may be connected with a chronic candida infection, but the evidence here is not at all convincing (see pages 193–9). Another explanation, put forward in *The Lancet* (medical reference 172) by Dr John Hunter from Addenbrooke's Hospital in Cambridge, is that food residues are broken down by organisms in the gut to produce chemicals which, in susceptible people, are not properly dealt with by the liver enzymes, and so pass into the general circulation to produce symptoms – a so-called enterometabolic disorder.

Problems with the absorption of vitamins, amino acids and trace elements, such as magnesium and zinc, are often quoted, but there is still no reliable published evidence to back up such claims. Vitamin and mineral supplements won't do any harm provided they are from a reputable manufacturer and not taken in excess (see pages 200–201).

A well-balanced diet should be low in sugar and fat as well as containing plenty of fish, fruit and vegetables. Try to take regular meals of energy-rich foods which contain good quality proteins, fibre, vitamins and minerals. Good examples include wholemeal bread, pasta, brown rice, peas, beans, lentils, nuts and dried fruit. Foods which contain complex carbohydrates are digested slowly and so release a constant supply of energy into the blood which minimises the risk of hypoglycaemia. Again, hypoglycaemia is frequently quoted as an important feature of M.E., but the evidence to support this is very flimsy (see page 93).

Green vegetables, citrus fruits, tomatoes, potatoes and dried apricots all provide essential vitamins, minerals and fibre. Much of the goodness lies in the skin, but I'd recommend that fresh fruits are always peeled. Citrus fruits and fruit juices are excellent sources of Vitamin C. Bananas are very useful as a between-meal snack, and are often used by cyclists because they allow a slow release of fructose into the body. They're also a good source of fibre and contain an essential amino acid called tryptophan, which has a calming effect on the brain.

Some alternative therapists now advocate a much more radical change in diet, but this is not without its dangers and should only be carried out under strict supervision. I have now seen several patients who have made themselves very ill on such a regime. My own feeling is that people with M.E. have quite enough restrictions placed on their lives without adding a vast range of foods to that list. Equally, I would never recommend fasting as a treatment for M.E.

The relationship between food allergy and M.E. remains a very controversial topic and most doctors feel that it is all too often being diagnosed by tests which are not reliable (see pages 186–90). Even so, many people with M.E. believe that they have multiple food allergies and cut out dairy produce and wheat in particular. As far as wheat is concerned, I do know of a few patients who seem to have benefited quite considerably, and I wonder if they may have some form of mild adult coeliac disease. If you go on to remove all dairy produce from the diet, there is inevitably going to be a severe lack of calcium. This, along with physical inactivity, is an important risk factor in the development of osteoporosis (thinning of the bones) in later life. So, it's essential for anyone under the age of forty, especially if you're female, to make sure that there is an adequate intake of calcium in the diet. Calcium supplementation may well be advisable here, usually with tablets, although milk, sardines and shellfish are excellent sources of natural calcium. If you do take calcium tablets, *never* exceed the recommended dose as too much can be just as dangerous as too little.

Lastly, as I've already pointed out in the previous chapter, anyone with a large number of gastric symptoms may need investigations to rule out the possibility of coeliac disease or Giardia infection. The specific management of irritable bowel symptomatology is dealt with on pages 89–91.

Hobbies

Family and friends may wonder how M.E. patients keep themselves occupied throughout their long days stuck at home. A non-energetic hobby can be both entertaining and rewarding.

Before I got M.E. many of my interests had started to gather dust, but the stamp collection has been sorted out, and I've become interested in photography once again. Writing isn't the sort of thing that everyone can do easily, but I now know several friends with M.E. who have taken this up – it's the sort of activity you can do without much physical effort. Some people have invested in a word processor, which is also great fun, and very helpful when you can easily correct all the mistakes!

Starting a new academic course from home might be something to think about. Open University courses can be taken over a period of several years, and the organisers are keen to help people with disabilities wherever possible (see page 336).

Pets are a very good source of companionship. They don't chatter away all day, but can be there as a friend. Remember, a dog will need exercising. A cat (Siamese are great friends), a budgie or even a guinea pig would do just as well.

Avoiding a relapse

Whatever the current state of your illness, be it static, recovering, or even now in remission, there's always the possibility that a relapse may occur. Most M.E. patients quickly learn to recognise the things which seem almost guaranteed to worsen M.E., but avoiding them isn't always easy. Undue physical and mental stress are probably the commonest causes of relapse, and these factors, along with the adverse effects of temperature extremes have already been covered. However, there are other important factors which all patients need to take care with.

Alcohol

Alcohol intolerance is extremely common in M.E.; I rarely see a patient who doesn't volunteer this fact, and if you're not affected by large amounts of alcohol M.E. seems an unlikely diagnosis.

Some patients who previously enjoyed and tolerated regular consumption of alcohol, without any adverse effects, now find that even small amounts make them feel extremely unwell. This isn't an allergy but a hypersensitivity to the effects of alcohol, possibly related to two important facts.

First, the soporific effects of alcohol are partly explained by the fact that it increases the effects of one of the brain's chemicals (neurotransmitters) – gamma amino butyric acid (GABA). This in turn reduces the availability of calcium, which is responsible for triggering nerve cell activity, and so brain function is depressed.

Second, alcohol can also dilate the small blood vessels in the skin, so it helps to divert blood flow away from the brain and other vital organs. So, anyone who is particularly susceptible to the autonomic/vasomotor effects of M.E. (feeling faint or dizzy on standing up) will probably find this made worse after alcohol.

It's difficult to say whether alcohol consumption, even in moderation, causes any harm in M.E. If there's any evidence of inflammation in the liver it should be avoided altogether.

However, most patients find that they no longer want any alcohol, so the problem doesn't arise.

I have come across the occasional patient who has used alcohol to try and 'blot out' their symptoms of M.E.; but this is alcohol abuse. It's a very dangerous path to start on; you only end up feeling ten times worse the next morning, and run a serious risk of becoming an alcoholic.

One final reason for avoiding alcohol is the fact that it can damage muscle, but this is usually only associated with heavy drinking.

Cigarettes and environmental pollution

Any form of environmental pollution, and that means both active smoking and inhaling other people's smoke (passive smoking) is best avoided if at all possible. Do explain to your friends and relatives that *their* smoking might be damaging *your* health, and try to make your house or office a no-smoking zone.

Smoking cigarettes decreases the capability of the red blood cells to carry vital oxygen around the body in an efficient manner. M.E. research has already suggested that there may be problems with the red cells themselves, as well as lack of oxygen to vital muscle and nerve cells. It doesn't seem sensible to go and exacerbate this problem further.

Many M.E. patients undoubtedly feel a lot better in a non-polluted atmosphere, and it's also wise to clean up the environment at home by banning (like Prince Charles) the use of aerosols and spray-on chemicals.

Drugs

All medication, both prescribed by your doctor, or purchased over the counter (and this includes vitamins, minerals and herbal preparations) should be taken with caution, and only with good reason. M.E. patients seem to experience increased sensitivity to many drugs. These don't seem to be true allergic reactions and may well be due to problems with the way that drugs are broken down in the body.

Antibiotic sensitivity may be a problem in some patients, but if you succumb to a serious infection which requires treatment with a specific antibiotic, then do take it – unless, of course,

Drugs and M.E.:

1 *Drugs which may exacerbate pre-existing M.E. symptoms:*
   Antidepressants   – worsen autonomic/vasomotor
                              symptoms, and can cause further sedation.
   Tranquillisers   – increased sedating effect.
   Beta-blockers   – fatigue in higher doses.
   Some asthma drugs   – worsen autonomic symptoms.
2 *Drugs to which patients seem more sensitive:*
   Antibiotics
   Some analgesics and NSAIDs
3. *Drugs which are best avoided*
   Steroids   – depress the immune system.

you have a true allergy to something like penicillin.

Infections

Picking up any new infection will almost certainly cause a relapse. Patients who are in regular contact with small children may find it difficult to avoid such infections. It's obviously sensible to try and avoid close contact with any friend or relative who has an infection, particularly anyone who is coughing or spluttering, even though this may seem anti-social.

Good dental care with regular check-ups is also very important, as a nasty grumbling tooth or gum infection can make you very debilitated.

If you do get any sort of infection and start to feel off-colour, rest immediately and perhaps go back to bed for forty-eight hours. It depends on how severe the infection is. Rest as necessary, and then start a recovery plan.

If you have an infection and temperature and are not sure why, it's wise to consult your general practitioner after about forty-eight hours. It may be a urinary infection or chest infection, which is producing little in the way of obvious symptoms, but may need antibiotic treatment.

A severe infection is likely to leave anyone with M.E. feeling extra-debilitated for many weeks, so be patient while gradually returning to your usual state of health.

Surgical operations and general anaesthetics

For an M.E. patient, having an operation will be a major event, so try to do everything possible to minimise the upheaval. To start, to be in the best physical state possible, try to get a period of forty-eight hours' solid rest before the day of admission.

Let both your consultant and anaesthetist know in advance that you have M.E. and the effect that it has on you. Surgeons and anaesthetists probably may not know very much about M.E., so you may have to explain that it is a genuine medical problem which can be exacerbated by surgery and anaesthetics. Often, when a patient is admitted to hospital with a co-existing medical problem, and the surgical team don't know much about it, they'll ask one of their physician colleagues to come and look you over as well.

The actual surgery is probably inevitable, but there is a trend towards using less drastic methods wherever possible. Kidney stones, for example, can now be dissolved, which doesn't involve any surgery on the kidney at all, and some gall stones can be dissolved by new drugs. Such alternatives aren't available for everything, but ask your surgeon if the operation is really necessary, and whether there are any alternative approaches available.

Local anaesthesia is also being used increasingly for a whole range of operations (some of them quite major), and again this is a possibility which you can discuss with the anaesthetist.

Explain to the sister on the surgical ward that you have M.E. and what you can and can't do for yourself. It's quite likely that they haven't nursed a patient with M.E., and like the surgeons they work with, know little about the illness. It might be worth taking in a medical article on M.E. for them to read, but the response may be very varied!

Your recovery post-operation is likely to be slower than usual. Everyone feels weak and tired after an operation, but the M.E. patient will probably experience increased fatigue for a much longer period. Hopefully the ward will be sympathetic, and will not try to get you going at too fast a pace. If you're not happy about things, do speak to the sister or one of the surgical doctors.

You may require a considerable degree of help when you return home, from both the family, and possibly the community nursing services. Try and make sure this sort of help is organised before you go into hospital, so that everything runs smoothly on your return home.

Vaccinations

Some M.E. patients experience a quite severe reaction or relapse in symptoms following vaccinations. So, it's always a good idea to arrange with your GP for a vaccine to be given at a time when you're feeling reasonably well or can take things easy for the next few days. In the case of schoolchildren this may mean postponing a non-essential booster to a time during the holiday period. Obviously, any such risk will always have to be carefully weighed up against the chances of contracting whatever disease you are being protected against. For example, maintaining up-to-date tetanus protection would be vital for anyone working on a farm. And, for anyone whose job places them at risk from catching hepatitis B (e.g. theatre nurses), vaccination against this serious liver infection must be considered. On the other hand, flu vaccinations may be better avoided, unless there is a good medical reason for having one. It's certainly important to avoid crowded public places when there is a flu epidemic in progress. The value of high doses of Vitamin C in preventing or curing colds and flu remains unproven.

Foreign travel occasionally involves compulsory vaccination, as well as those which are just recommended. Always try to plan a course of holiday vaccinations well in advance, and do make sure that you are not having any final boosters the day before you actually set off! Polio is still a common disease in underdeveloped countries and it would be very unwise to go there without full protection. Hepatitis A vaccination doesn't usually produce any serious adverse effects, and gives very good short-term protection for anyone planning to travel in an area where sanitation is likely to be unsatisfactory. Typhoid and cholera vaccines offer less protection and can cause bad reactions in quite healthy people. Taking sensible precautions with food, drinking water and where you bathe is probably just as important as the vaccination. Reactions here can be reduced by having the injection just into the skin (intradermally).

Antimalarial tablets *must* be taken if advised.

For a small fee MASTA (Medical Advisory Services for

Travel Abroad, Tel 071-631 4408) operates an individual advice scheme on the prevention of illness abroad.

Dr Richard Dawood has written an excellent book called *Traveller's Health* (Oxford University Press) which covers all aspects of health care in detail for anyone planning to travel abroad.

Summary of how to cope with a relapse of M.E.

- Try to avoid any of the factors which are known to worsen M.E.
- At the first sign of a relapse in your state of health, start to increase your ratio of rest to activity. If you've got an infection and temperature go to bed. Aspirin is still a very good drug to use, provided you can tolerate it.
- If you have a serious infection let your general practitioner know, and take any antibiotics prescribed.
- Organise your bedroom into a living area, so you're not struggling up and down the stairs all day.
- Try not to prolong the strict bed rest for more than a few days, and don't be afraid to commence a gradual rehabilitation programme, keeping within your limitations.
- Try to do some muscle exercises during bed rest, either by yourself or with help from family or a physiotherapist.
  Don't repeat any exercise to the point of fatigue.
  Don't exercise painful muscles and joints – let them settle down first.
- Don't neglect your diet – if you can't face solid food try to take some liquid nourishment (e.g. Complan), and don't let your fluid intake fall.
- Organise the family, friends, neighbours into helping out as much as possible.

Your body can recover from a relapse of M.E.; but you've got to give it the best possible circumstances in which to do so. And remember, it's far better to regard these relapses as setbacks on your road to recovery, rather than a 'step down the ladder'.

3. Mind And Body

'If you don't think that you're ever going to get better, then you probably never will.'

Taken literally, such a dramatic statement is not entirely applicable to something like M.E., but there's no doubt that there's more than a grain of truth in it. Attitude of mind – both positive and negative – is going to have a very significant effect on many aspects of M.E., as it can with other similar conditions.

The primary effect may simply be on your 'coping mechanisms' – i.e. how you're able to deal with all the frustrations, anxieties and problems associated with M.E. It also seems quite likely that some of the physical symptoms associated with the illness can be equally affected by your mental attitude to them, and there's accumulating evidence that the body's immune system can be either improved or weakened by the effects of 'the psyche'. This is not to say that M.E. is a purely psychosomatic disease, one where the physical symptoms are *largely* under the control of the mind. But there is, for some people, a psychosomatic element to their M.E., just as in other physical illnesses like asthma, where both physical factors (infections and allergies) can combine with emotional ones to exacerbate or cause relapse.

The relationship between the brain and the immune system is highly complex, and only just beginning to be understood by scientists interested in the subject – the study of what's referred to as psychoneuroimmunology. Several studies have now shown that T lymphocytes are often reduced in number in patients with severe depression; and that Natural Killer cell activity is altered by stressful life events. Equally, the amount of the stress hormone cortisol, regulated by the hypothalamus (see pages 67–71), has an important role in the regulation of T lymphocytes. It's not only the mind that can have an effect on body matter. The reverse process can also occur – what's known as somatopsychic illness, where the physical symptoms start to affect the emotional state, causing anxiety and depression as additional problems. These inter-relationships between mind and body are highly complicated, but in illnesses like M.E. they both probably occur in varying degrees of severity.

How can this knowledge be usefully applied to helping someone who's actually ill with M.E.? The obvious first step must be to try and take a 'positive approach'. I know it's not easy being optimistic when everything seems to be going wrong, but it's essential not to let your mind slip into the 'I'm never going to get better' approach, even when things are at their lowest ebb. Patients with HIV infection (AIDS) are now being taught to 'think positive' ('body positive'), even to the extent of imagining that the cells of their immune systems are actually being released 'into battle' against the persisting HIV infection, and killing off the virus (a technique called 'imaging'). There's no scientific proof that this approach actually reverses any of the immunedeficiency changes seen in AIDS, but it does stimulate a very positive approach of mind. I'm not suggesting that everyone with M.E. should sit down and meditate about their immune system killing off their persisting viral infection, but I am advocating that *all* M.E. patients take a very positive approach to getting better. You *can* and *will* get better from M.E., even if it takes a long time.

M.E. is a very individual illness, in its presentation, symptoms, the secondary problems it causes, and the way it progresses. If you sit down with a group of people with M.E. each one will probably have a symptom or a problem that no one else has. This is why it's essential to take an individual approach to the management in each case.

In the early stages (and in the case of M.E. this means anything up to the first two years or so after the illness started) when M.E. may not have even been diagnosed by the doctor, it's possible to remain optimistic, hoping that the mysterious symptoms can and will go away by themselves, given time. However, if time goes on and the symptoms don't improve, anxieties will naturally increase, especially if doctors are still searching for a diagnosis. Then, the day finally arrives when the patient gets a positive diagnosis of M.E. and this often creates a sense of tremendous relief.

At last, someone has produced an explanation for all these bizarre symptoms, and you have a 'genuine illness': something to be believed by your general practitioner (hopefully), your family and your friends. You've now got some idea of what's going wrong with your body, why you feel so ill all the time, and the sort of actions you should be taking to try and recover. Most importantly, you're no longer quite so alone. There are an awful lot of others who are suffering in a similar manner, who also find a trip to the supermarket a major effort, and have equal difficulties with friends and family when they're 'non-visibly' disabled.

However, this feeling of relief may only be temporary. After the diagnosis has been made, and the resulting consequences have started to sink in, a further change in attitude may then start to occur. Unfortunately, at this point, it's quite easy to become depressed and pessimistic about what may lie ahead. You start to realise that you're going to have to come to terms with the possibility of M.E. being a chronic illness, with the eventual outcome unpredictable, even to those who are looking after you. Both you and your family are now going to have to consider making very significant changes in lifestyle.

All kinds of questions will now arise: what to do about work, whether to put off starting or adding to the family, whether or not to move home. Making the correct decisions isn't going to be easy. At this point it's often quite helpful to arrange to spend some time talking on a one-to-one basis with another M.E. patient, who can give sensible practical advice about 'living with M.E.', which your doctor can't do. Then, hopefully, you can keep in touch, even if it's only by phone or letter – with someone who really understands how you feel, and can offer sound advice when nobody else seems to know what to do.

If you're in an occupation such as teaching or nursing, talking to someone in the same job about how to cope with difficulties at work or with sick leave, can also be very helpful, just as mothers with young children can pick up equally useful advice from others in the same position. If you're having difficulty finding someone in the same occupation the M.E. Association may be able to help (see pages 317–19).

If you're having trouble with social security benefits, then talking to someone else who's experienced the same difficulties and won in the end can be very supporting. Try not to get fed up and give up. It doesn't help you, and it won't help other M.E. patients in the same situation in the future.

You may also be wondering about whether to start or extend a family. M.E. comes along at an age when this sort of decision is often about to be made. If a woman has M.E., this can be a very difficult decision to make – just how long should one keep putting off getting pregnant, whilst hoping that significant recovery is going to occur? Once again, talking things through with someone else who's got M.E. and become pregnant is the most useful advice that can be offered. (Pregnancy and M.E. is also covered on pages 239–45).

At times when things aren't going too well, or you're going through a relapse or exacerbation of symptoms, try to think of this as being a set-back on the road to recovery – something that's only going to be temporary, which you *will* get over, and not an irreversible change for the worse.

Stress, anxiety and depression

There's no doubt that although M.E. is capable of producing a wide range of psychiatric and emotional problems, the illness itself is definitely *not* a psychiatric disorder. For a few patients, psychiatric and emotional problems can become an increasingly distressing part of their illness, and when the doctors and specialists have missed the diagnosis of M.E. these aspects may even start to dominate their lives.

Some patients, with classic M.E. symptoms, are still being referred in desperation to psychiatrists by their general practitioners who feel there can be no other explanation. Fortunately, many of these patients do return from the visit with a clean bill of mental health, along with the comment that 'X isn't psychiatrically ill. There's something going wrong, but I don't know what it is.'

Understandably, depression is quite common in M.E. patients. Non-sufferers who are depressed are very commonly 'tired' as well, but this isn't the type of overwhelming exercise-related muscular fatigue and weakness experienced in M.E. The brain malfunction problems of M.E., such as loss of concentration and short-term memory, can also form part of depression, but mixing up words, carrying out inappropriate actions, lack of co-ordination and clumsiness related to physical or mental exertion are not characteristic of a depressive illness.

The final part of the M.E. symptom triad – the problems with autonomic nerve malfunction – are, as described earlier, thought to be due to overactivity of the sympathetic nerves. Unfortunately, these are also the nerves that can overact as part of acute anxiety, so some of the symptoms can be very similar in both conditions. Complaints such as palpitations, sweating, feeling tense or faint are common to both, and if prominent in M.E., the diagnosis of pure anxiety may be made. Again, there shouldn't be any confusion when the classic symptoms of muscle fatigue are added in, and the unusual problems of temperature control experienced in M.E. are not seen with anxiety.

One particular feature which does seem to be a true part of the M.E. disease process is what doctors refer to as emotional lability. Here, the patient's emotional state and mood may fluctuate widely, often for no apparent reason, but sometimes related to the frustrations imposed by the condition. Patients may suddenly burst into tears, feel extremely low and depressed or become uncharacteristically irritable with their family and friends. Not all M.E. patients experience these sorts of mood swing, but they can even occur in patients who would have regarded themselves as being very stable individuals, not subject to showing emotions, before the onset of their M.E.

It's important to remember that it's a perfectly normal human reaction to periodically feel very fed up with M.E., especially when you seem to be going through a bad patch, either due to the symptoms or associated problems at work or with your family. Who wouldn't, with such a frustrating condition which was imposing so many restrictions on your life? The important thing is to be able to differentiate being fed up from being truly depressed, and not letting all your feelings of inner anger radiate out and make everyone around you feel fed up as well.

Why do some M.E. patients go on to develop significant emotional and psychiatric problems, whereas others don't? The most important underlying reason is probably connected with previous personality, before M.E. ever arrived. By this we mean to what extent you used to be a 'coper' – how you used to react to life's major upsets and crises. Those who were used to 'sailing through' before, not letting things get them down too much, and having a generally optimistic view of life and the future are probably going to fare much better from the emotional point of view than the opposite type of personality. For people who do not cope as well, the problems associated with having M.E. may well tip the balance and trigger any underlying susceptibility to developing anxiety or a depressive illness – especially if this has already occurred in the past.

There is some evidence that women patients are more likely to succumb to these aspects of M.E., especially when they're part of a conventional family grouping. They may be quite unable to take time off to rest when they are still trying to cope with bringing up the children, doing the housework and providing meals at the end of the day. Such women just don't get any chance to start the recovery process.

In contrast, the conventional husband who develops M.E. is still likely to be at work, and if he then goes on sick leave problems with the children and the home can be delegated while he initiates the major changes in lifestyle so necessary for recovery.

So, the M.E. patient's underlying personality may be the central factor in deciding how he or she manages to cope with this illness. Unfortunately, many other aspects of the condition may then start to interact and form a vicious circle which exacerbates the basic emotional problems.

Initiating this circle of events is the fact that the actual disease process in M.E. – the persisting viral infection – may be having a direct effect on parts of the brain which control emotion and mood, particularly the frontal lobes. It's already well known that an important cause of a true depressive illness is the aftermath of a viral infection. One possible explanation is that levels of neurotransmitters in key areas of the brain may be

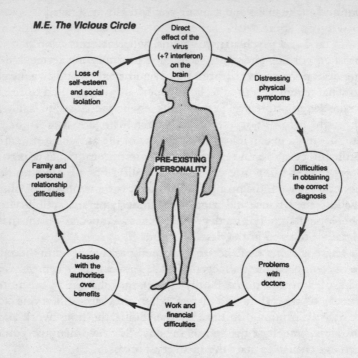

M.E. The Vicious Circle

at fault, and secondly, the persisting virus may be causing the continued production of excess interferon, a substance which seems capable of having direct effects on various aspects of mental functioning.

Proceeding round the circle, the frustrating and disabling physical symptoms, and the constant feeling of being unwell are depressing in themselves. This can only then be increased in those who are still trying to get a diagnosis. The circle is completed, as time goes on, by the social, family and financial problems which so commonly become part of M.E., and these in turn aren't helped by battles with the authorities to obtain various sickness and disability benefits. All these social factors interact and may place a great strain, not only on the patient, but also his or her family. A resultant loss of self-esteem, even feelings of worthlessness, when all aspects of one's life seem to be falling apart, can place a tremendous pressure on the most stoic of individuals, and they may eventually find they just can't cope any longer.

So, it's not surprising that some M.E. patients pass from a state of just being 'fed up' from time to time, into true clinical depression, withdrawal from family and friends, and even have suicidal feelings.

How psychiatrists view M.E.

Following publication of several research papers on M.E. during the mid-1980s, the media once again became interested in this controversial illness. When I discussed M.E. on Radio 4's *Medicine Now* programme, the BBC received well over a thousand letters requesting further information; and an article by Sue Finlay in the *Observer* brought in over 6000 letters – all from people who believed that they might have M.E. What had become an almost unknown illness was suddenly back in the public eye. As a result, I have no doubt that large numbers of people who were tired and unwell, and for whom the doctors could find no obvious cause for their ill health, became labelled as having M.E. Not surprisingly, the M.E. Association became one of the fastest growing medical charities in the U.K.

Although most psychiatrists had by now dismissed the idea that M.E. was hysteria, hypochondriasis or malingering, they remained unconvinced by the hypothesis of persisting viral infection affecting brain, muscle and immune system function. In March 1988 three such psychiatrists – Drs Anthony David, Simon Wessely and Anthony Pelosi – challenged this hypothesis in an article in the *British Medical Journal* titled 'Postviral fatigue syndrome: time for a new approach' (medical reference 6).

The psychiatrists' explanation, to quote from a letter to the *New England Journal of Medicine*, was that 'symptoms are perpetuated by a cycle of inactivity and a deterioration in the tolerance for exercise, compounded by a depressive illness'. To back up these opinions, they carefully looked at large groups of patients with chronic debilitating fatigue which had lasted for more than six months, but which were not necessarily related to a viral infection at the onset (i.e. M.E.). About 75 per cent of this group turned out to have a clear-cut 'hidden' psychiatric illness. In about half this was depression, but others had what is known as a somatisation disorder where a variety of physical symptoms are psychologically based. A small minority had anxiety or phobias. Only in about a quarter was there no obvious psychiatric disorder.

These findings received considerable publicity in both the medical journals and the media, both of whom used them to once again dismiss M.E. as being 'all in the mind'. Consequently, because of the absence of any evidence of active inflammation in the brain or spinal cord (encephalomyelitis), much of the medical establishment abandoned the term M.E. in favour of chronic fatigue syndrome (CFS) – the name now being used by the psychiatrists.

Now, I can fully accept some of these arguments. I would agree that CFS is a perfectly acceptable term to use when covering a wide variety of patients suffering from chronic fatigue, but I would still maintain that people with M.E. fall into a distinct sub-group with symptoms which are very different to those seen in depression.

This distinction is not only important from the point of view of future research into M.E., but it also affects how patients should be managed. I have no doubt that there are people (wrongly labelled as having M.E.) who fall into the vicious circle described by the psychiatrists of depression → fatigue and muscle pain → inactivity → exercise avoidance → more fatigue and pain → increasing unfitness → demoralisation and sick role behaviour → depression. Equally, there are a few patients with M.E. whose recovery is delayed by this sequence of events.

The appropriate management here may well be to break the vicious circle with antidepressant drugs, exercise regimes and cognitive behaviour therapy as advocated by the psychiatrists. However, I am not convinced that this is the best way to manage patients with genuine M.E. Antidepressants, as already mentioned, can help where depression occurs, but otherwise their value is extremely limited. Rest and exercise have to be carefully balanced; too much or too little of either is not advisable. And, although psychotherapy may occasionally have a role, it is not something I would routinely advocate.

The arguments put forward by the psychiatrists can be followed up in further detail by referring to the research papers listed on pages 354–6.

Recognising depression in M.E.

The big danger for anyone suffering from a depressive illness is not being able to recognise that it is occurring. Unfortunately, this fact may be all too obvious to family and friends, but not to the person whose mental health is steadily deteriorating. So, how can true clinical depression be separated from just feeling 'fed up' as a result of having M.E.? And which are the characteristic mood changes that can help to differentiate between the two?

There are a number of distinct features which are characteristic to all depressive illnesses. Two of them – fatigue and impaired memory/concentration – are well recognised features of M.E. However, the fatigue that is experienced in M.E. is dramatic in onset and overwhelming in nature. By comparison, the fatigue that is commonly seen in depressed patients is far less severe and stems from a lack of motivation to participate. As far as problems with concentration and intellectual functioning are concerned, I have already described the results of cognitive potential testing (page 64) which indicate that the brain malfunction in M.E. is not the same as seen in ordinary depression.

Other important features of M.E. which help to differentiate it from a primary depressive illness include:

- Rapid changes in mood throughout the day which are often related to distressing physical symptoms. Depressed patients tend to feel constantly 'low' in mood or worse at certain specific times of the day.
- Frustration at being unable to participate in work, hobbies or family pursuits which involve physical activity, but still being able to enjoy more passive pursuits. People with depression are said to experience anhedonia – the total and complete loss of interest in both forms of activity.
- Symptoms which are always exacerbated when patients push themselves beyond their limits of physical or mental

endurance. Depressed patients experience no such ill-effects from exercise, and often feel better as a result.

- A curious and highly characteristic phenomenon whereby physical or mental activity can both produce physical and mental fatigue. This is not something that is remarked upon by depressed patients.

- An 'encephalitic' component consisting of impaired intellectual functioning, clumsiness and unsteadiness which is not characteristic of straightforward depression. Here, there is a general 'slowing down' of all mental activity.

- The tendency to have grossly increased sleep requirements (hypersomnia) whereas the characteristic sleep disturbance in depression is early morning wakening.

Even so, there are some important mood changes which would strongly suggest that someone with M.E. was becoming depressed. A combination of three or more of the following, occurring as 'new' symptoms, for more than two weeks, would indicate the need for urgent professional help.

- Recent loss of appetite and/or weight.
- Change in sleep pattern to early morning wakening.
- Sudden loss of interest in sex.
- Apathy and complete withdrawal from social contacts and friends.
- Pessimism, hopelessness and a complete loss of self-confidence.
- Feelings of guilt.
- Inability to enjoy or sustain interest in passive activities.
- Suicidal ideas or plans – which must be taken seriously even as an isolated symptom.

Management of depression

One of the major problems with any type of depressive illness is the fact that it can create its own vicious circle. It's all too easy to spend vast amounts of time dwelling on your difficulties and negative thoughts – something that will only make you feel even more depressed. Although the vast majority of patients with true clinical depression gain considerable benefit from the type of drugs I describe later in this chapter, there are also some important self-help measures that can go a long way towards breaking the hold that depression so often creates. These include:

- Don't dwell too much on what's going on 'in your mind'. Take up some new interests which could temporarily take your thoughts away from being depressed.
- Think about taking some actions which would make you feel better about yourself. Don't neglect your appearance and leave the house untidy.
- A break from your usual daily routine can also be beneficial, or consider taking a short break away from home or a holiday – we all need something to look forward to.
- Don't bottle up your feelings: if you need to cry or get angry then do so, but preferably in the company of someone who understands your situation.
- Above all, don't be afraid to ask for help from friends, family and health professionals – the longer that a depressive state goes untreated the worse it becomes.

Drug treatments for depression

Doctors can now choose from a wide variety of effective antidepressant drugs. They all act by increasing levels of various chemicals in the brain (neurotransmitters) which are thought to be depleted in depression. The two most important neurotransmitters are called noradrenaline and 5 hydroxytryptamine (5HT). Interestingly, there is also some research which suggests that these drugs may act on the body's immune response by affecting Natural Killer cell function or histamine receptor activity.

Tricyclic antidepressants are the most frequently prescribed drugs for depression. Some of them are sedating (useful for anyone who has associated anxiety or difficulty with sleep), whereas others have a mild stimulating effect (more appropriate where someone has become withdrawn and lethargic). A few are combined with tranquillisers, but most doctors now feel that this is not helpful because it makes minor adjustments in the dosage very difficult.

A common problem with nearly all these drugs is that they have unpleasant side-effects (see table below) to which M.E. patients seem particularly susceptible. They tend to occur almost as soon as treatment is commenced, so it's not unknown for people to stop taking their antidepressant before any of the benefits have started to accrue. These side-effects can often be reduced by commencing treatment with a low dose which is then gradually increased over a few weeks to build up a tolerance. Taking the entire daily dose at night may also be helpful, but do check with your doctor first.

Side-effects also mean that tricyclic antidepressants must be used cautiously by anyone who has pre-existing heart disease, liver or thyroid problems, as well as conditions such as glaucoma, diabetes and prostate gland enlargement (elderly men). At the start of treatment they can also produce raised levels of liver enzymes, but these usually return to normal. Even so, they should be used with extreme care in anyone who started their illness with an infection in the liver (hepatitis); regular checks

---

Side-effects of Tricyclic Antidepressants

Gastrointestinal	dry mouth+
	weight gain+
	constipation+
	stomach upsets
	liver function disturbances
Heart	fall in blood pressure+
	palpitations
Nervous system	dizziness+
	nervousness
	tremor
	exacerbation of epilepsy
Miscellaneous	increased sweating
	allergic skin reactions
	poor diabetes control
	blurred vision
	urine retention
	impotence

+ = common ones

on liver function should be made. Tricyclics also need to be used with care during pregnancy.

Tricyclic antidepressants can also interact with other drugs, particularly alcohol; cimetidine (for stomach ulcers); and some blood pressure treatments.

Benefits from these drugs don't usually occur for several weeks. When they do start to work, one of the first effects is an improvement in sleep pattern. This is then followed by an increase in appetite, weight gain, and as mental activity once again quickens up, the depressed mood should start to lift.

Deciding on just how long to continue treatment with any antidepressant drug isn't always easy. It's quite likely that this will be necessary for several months and then for a short period after the depression has fully lifted. However, some doctors like to maintain treatment at a low dose for a much longer period of time as a precautionary measure. Unlike tranquillisers, there should not be any problems with unpleasant withdrawal symptoms.

New tricyclic antidepressants In the past few years a 'new wave' of tricyclic drugs has been developed which appear to have a faster onset of action and fewer side-effects (particularly on the heart) than the 'older' drugs. These new products include lofepramine (Gamanil), which is now being prescribed for quite a few patients with M.E. Although these drugs are considerably more expensive than the original tricyclics, their relative lack of side-effects may make them a more appropriate choice.

Tetracyclic antidepressants, like Bolvidon (mianserin), mainly act by raising the level of a chemical called noradrenaline. Although side-effects generally tend to be less troublesome, this particular drug can occasionally cause serious problems with the blood and liver, so regular blood counts are essential. Bolvidon tends to be sedating whereas Ludiomil (maprotiline), another tetracyclic, is not.

Monoamine Oxidase Inhibitors (MAOIs) tend to be reserved for patients who do not respond to first-time antidepressants or where there are special associated problems such as phobias or severe anxiety. These drugs all act by inhibiting the action of a specific enzyme in the brain called monoamine oxidase (MAO). The main reason why doctors seldom make use of MAOIs is because a long list of foods and drugs, which contain a chemical called tyramine, cannot be taken at the same time. This list includes cheese, Bovril, Oxo, Marmite, alcohol, pickled herrings, along with cough mixtures, nasal decongestant drops and some prescription drugs. They should also be avoided for two weeks after stopping treatment with a MAOI. So, if you are prescribed one of this group of drugs, do make sure you obtain a full written list of substances to avoid from either your doctor or pharmacist. However, some psychiatrists now feel that the side-effects associated with MAOIs have been over-emphasised, and that they are superior drugs in the treatment of depressive disorders where lack of energy is a prominent symptom. For this reason they are sometimes specifically recommended in the treatment of M.E.

Tryptophan, one of the essential amino acids, was found to be a useful mild antidepressant. It has now been withdrawn from use following the discovery that it could cause a potentially fatal condition known as the eosinophilia-myalgia syndrome.

5HT Re-uptake inhibitors are the latest addition to the already well-stocked antidepressant pharmacy. These drugs act by increasing the levels of a chemical called 5 hydroxytryptamine/ 5HT in a part of the brain known as the limbic system. At present there are just a handful of these new drugs available, which tend to be non-sedating, making them less useful where insomnia is also a problem. Whether or not 5HT drugs are more effective than the tricyclics remains uncertain, but they do seem to cause significantly fewer side-effects. The main problem seems to be that some users experience a sense of nausea and stomach fullness which leads to loss of both appetite and weight (which can occasionally be an advantage for patients with eating disorders). Other side-effects which are occasionally reported include a dry mouth, diarrhoea, delay in sexual ejaculation, tremor and increased sweating. As with tricyclic antidepressants, it may take several weeks before any positive benefits start to occur, but most of the side-effects also tend to decline in severity after a few weeks. There has also been a warning that 5HT reuptake inhibitors should not be used straight after a course of MAOI drugs. One 5HT drug, Prozac, has been the subject of concern in America where there have been reports of it making some patients suicidal or prone to violent behaviour. At the moment the U.K.'s Committee on Safety of Medicines are monitoring Prozac very carefully, but until the situation is clarified I would not recommend this drug for anyone who is susceptible to erratic mood swings (see medical reference 144).

New antidepressants, such as lofepramine and the 5HT reuptake inhibitors, may now turn out to be a much better choice of drug for patients with M.E. who require this type of treatment. Several trials are now under way to see if this is so.

Psychologically based treatments

Antidepressant drugs are undoubtedly a quick, easy and often very effective way of treating many types of depressive illness. However, they cannot be used in isolation, especially in the case of M.E. where several different factors may be contributing to the development of depression.

They won't have any effect on problems with the DSS, doctors or employers – all of which can become very depressing! Neither can they help to resolve a family or financial crisis. If these sorts of very practical difficulties exist and remain unresolved, there is no way that antidepressant drugs are going to be effective.

In addition to drugs, some doctors also make use of various kinds of 'talking treatments' or psychotherapy. With a GP this is unlikely to be anything deeper than simple problem-counselling, which gives the depressed patient an opportunity to talk through his or her difficulties, fears or frustrations. Other forms of counselling can be much more intense and prolonged, especially when they involve coming to terms with distressing events in the past which are still having a negative impact on your life. Building up a good relationship with a professional counsellor is essential if such an approach is going to be successful. If you want to find out more about this type of approach, MIND (see

Classification of antidepressant drugs

Type of Drug	Generic Name	Trade name	Comments
Original Tricyclics	amitriptyline	Lentizol	sedating
		Tryptizol	sedating
	butriptyline	Evadyne	non sedating
	clomipramine	Anafranil	non sedating and useful if phobias or obsessional features present
	desipramine	Pertofran	non sedating
	dothiepin	Prothiaden	sedating
	doxepin	Sinequan	sedating
	imipramine	Tofranil	non sedating
	iprindole	Prondol	non sedating
	nortriptyline	Allegron	non sedating
		Aventyl	non sedating
	protriptyline	Concordin	non sedating
	trimipramine	Surmontil	sedating
Combination Drugs		Limbritol	amitriptyline + tranquilliser
		Motipress	nortriptyline + phenothiazine★
		Motival	nortriptyline + fluphenazine
		Triptafen	amitriptyline + phenothiazine★
New Tricyclics	amoxapine	Asendis	rapid action, sedating, worrying side-effects, very costly
	lofepramine	Gamanil	non sedating
Tetracyclics	maprotiline	Ludiomil	non sedating
	mianserin	Bolvidon	sedating, blood counts
		Norval	advisable

Type of Drug	Generic Name	Trade name	Comments
Monoamine Oxidase Inhibitors (MAOIs)	isocarboxazid	Marplan	
	phenelzine	Nardil	for depression + phobias
	tranylcypromine	Parnate	side-effects+
	trifluoperazine + tranylcypromine	Parstelin	
5HT Reuptake Inhibitors	fluvoxamine	Faverin	
	fluoxetine	Prozac	may cause weight loss
	paroxetine	Seroxat	
	sertraline	Lustral	
Miscellaneous	trazodone	Molipaxin	sedating, less side effects than tricyclics
	flupenthixol	Fluanxol	avoid in severe depression or overactivity
	tryptophan		not in current use
	violoxazine	Vivalan	costly++ with a high incidence of nausea

*phenothiazines are tranquilliser drugs that I would not recommend in treating M.E.

page 335) publish a useful leaflet called *Talking Treatments*.

Psychiatrists may also suggest an approach known as cognitive behaviour therapy, which aims to correct negative thoughts and ideas which can become a very disabling part of depression. In the case of M.E. this type of approach is likely to be quite time-consuming, and will require a considerable degree of commitment from both therapist and patient. Between each appointment at the clinic the patient is given a list of tasks to do at home, as well as being asked to keep a careful record of their activity and severity of symptoms. In practice cognitive therapy aims to gradually increase activity – both mental and physical – at a steady pace, especially those activities which have been previously avoided because of pain or fatigue – the assumption being that symptoms in M.E. are perpetuated by psychological rather than physical factors.

The use of cognitive behaviour therapy in the management of M.E. has come in for a considerable amount of criticism. At the moment only one open trial has been conducted by psychiatrists working at the National Hospital in London (medical reference 117) involving fifty patients with some form of chronic fatigue. Their results have to be viewed with a considerable degree of caution because there was no control group or independent assessment of the outcome, along with a high rate of dropout or refusal to accept the treatment. Furthermore, it was impossible to distinguish between the benefits of antidepressant drugs and the purely behavioural approach to treatment.

In the UK the psychiatrists' view of M.E., and these type of psychologically based treatments have become very fashionable despite the lack of convincing results from clinical trials. Unfortunately, some doctors then go on and misinterpret what even the psychiatrists are recommending, and advise a far more aggressive exercise regime which can produce a dramatic deterioration in health. The way that many psychiatrists manage patients with M.E. is reviewed in a recent paper by Dr M Sharpe in the *British Medical Bulletin* (medical reference 126).

Relationship difficulties, which may be directly or indirectly attributed to the illness, can often be helped by talking them through with an experienced counsellor at the Marriage Guidance Council, which is now called Relate (see Useful Addresses). Equally, the M.E. Association's Listening Ear service has volunteers available who are willing to talk in confidence and give whatever support they can.

Unfortunately, for a small group of people with M.E., their depression becomes severe, a feeling of total worthlessness develops, even to the point of considering suicide as the only way out. At this point professional psychiatric help is essential, possibly necessitating a short spell in hospital during this 'crisis period'. If you are feeling this low and there seems to be nobody you can talk to, do phone the local Samaritans (in the phone book or see Useful Addresses) who can offer some immediate help and advice.

Doctors are also beginning to look at some more unusual ways of treating depression. Seasonal Affective Disorder is a newly recognised type of depression where symptoms gradually appear during the dark winter months. As with M.E., this disorder has been linked to an abnormality in the hypothalamus, and regular treatment using a source of artificial sunlight seems to be very effective. Perhaps this is something that M.E. patients who are depressed may soon be making use of?

Anxiety

Anxiety is a common and quite normal response to any stressful situation. Many public performers have palpitations as they go on stage and anyone's pulse rate will rapidly rise if, for example, they have a near miss in traffic. It's only when these sort of symptoms become commonplace and out of all proportion to whatever the individual feels worried about that a state of anxiety exists.

As already mentioned, differentiating some of the symptoms of anxiety from M.E. may not be easy, even for an experienced doctor, and in those patients who are naturally prone to anxiety there may be a combination of both.

Common symptoms of anxiety

Psychological:
  Irritability and restlessness; difficulty getting to sleep
  Poor concentration
  Increased sensitivity to noise
Physical:
  Overactive autonomic nerves
    palpitations, sweating, diarrhoea, frequently passing urine, impotence
  From overbreathing (hyperventilation)
    dizziness, paraesthesiae ('pins and needles'), fainting

From muscle spasm
  headaches, aches/tension in the neck or back

Some doctors are still far too keen on immediately treating any patient who has anxiety with a benzodiazepine tranquilliser such as diazepam (Valium). Such drugs act by dampening down nervous activity in the brain and in my experience at least half of all long-term M.E. patients have been given these sort of drugs to try at some stage in their illness.

On the whole these drugs should be avoided in M.E.; they have *no* effect whatsoever on the underlying disease process, and as they 'numb the mind' still further and exacerbate fatigue they may well make things worse. The only time to consider using them is for a very short period (i.e. days, not weeks or months) to deal with an acutely stressful event. Using them to blot out stress or anxiety is *not* a solution in M.E., and can lead to the problem of long-term dependence.

There are still far too many M.E. patients taking these drugs on a long-term basis, and in most cases this isn't helping them to recover from M.E. Once you've taken them for more than a few weeks, it is hard to stop, as many patients experience a withdrawal syndrome, very similar to the withdrawal problems seen with other drugs like alcohol, or even heroin. Many of the original symptoms of anxiety return as soon as there's no trace of the tranquilliser left in the body. As well, some of the withdrawal feelings can be very disturbing and frightening, such as increased sensitivity to noise, feelings of depersonalisation or being 'unreal', and occasionally hallucinations and delusions. Unfortunately these feelings can persist for weeks or months and be quite unbearable, so it is tempting for both doctor and patient to just restart the drug again.

Any M.E. patient who is taking long-term tranquillisers should seriously consider taking steps to 'come off', but as this withdrawal process isn't easy it must be done under medical supervision, and if your general practitioner isn't keen to help it may be necessary to ask for the advice of a psychiatrist. Self-help groups such as C.I.T.A. (see page 327 for address) can also provide counselling, and put you in touch with someone locally who has been through the withdrawal process. The dose must be reduced very slowly – over a period of four to twelve weeks, sometimes longer – to lessen any rebound anxiety taking place. Using one of the beta-blocking drugs during this withdrawal period can also help to reduce some of these unpleasant rebound anxiety symptoms.

If drug treatment is really thought to be necessary for a patient with anxiety – especially if there are a lot of symptoms connected with autonomic overactivity – one of the beta-blocking drugs may be a possible alternative approach to a benzodiazepine (such as Valium), but they must be prescribed at the lowest dose possible. Buspar (buspirone) is a new type of drug which is claimed to be just as effective as the benzodiazepines in relieving anxiety, but without impairing mental functioning or causing dependence. Exactly how it acts on the brain remains uncertain, but there do not appear to be any muscle relaxant or sleep inducing effects. Although the side-effects are claimed to be less than in conventional tranquillisers, Buspar can still produce headaches, dizziness, nausea, light-headedness, fatigue and nervousness. Also, like many of the antidepressant drugs, it usually takes several weeks before any benefits accrue. At present the role of Buspar in the management of anxiety associated with M.E. seems very limited. In view of the experiments conducted with this drug on hormonal control (see page 70) it would appear that people with M.E. may be more susceptible, so I would suggest that its use is still viewed with caution.

A much better approach to managing stress and anxiety is by self-help relaxation techniques, by which patients are able, themselves, to relax both body and mind – what one M.E. patient I know refers to as a 'dose of instant Valium'! You can discover how to do this from reading, learning from a cassette tape, or going to a relaxation class, but it does have to be carried out on a regular basis to be effective. Relaxation techniques can also be of help when getting to sleep is a problem.

A General Relaxation Technique

- Set aside a quiet period each day, preferably for about twenty minutes or so twice a day, when you know you're not going to be disturbed.

- Sit comfortably in your favourite chair, or lie down quietly on the bed. Take the phone off the hook as well, to prevent any interruptions.
- Close your eyes, relax, and take in slow deep breaths at a regular pace. Don't overbreathe though!
- Allow your mind to wander on to some pleasant thought, sound or experience – whatever you feel appropriate. Listening to some tranquil music at the same time can be very soothing.
- **For muscular tension** This can be particularly useful for dealing with areas of muscular tension in the neck, and shoulders, etc., when associated with stress. However, it's *not advisable* to follow this part of the method for muscles which are painful and weak purely as a result of M.E.

Learning to tense an area of muscle to the point of maximum tension and then having to relax it can be very beneficial. First, make a firm clenched fist with your hands, and notice the feeling of tension in the area. Then, let the fist suddenly relax and see how a warm feeling then follows – indicating that it's now become fully relaxed. This process can be repeated in other 'trouble spots' around the body where muscle spasm/tension seems to be a problem, using the same principle of artificially producing tension followed by sudden relaxation.

By the end of the session you should now be feeling totally relaxed, and your breathing should be slow and regular. Have a few minutes doing nothing and then get up again. If you're using these techniques to help you get off to sleep at night they can be carried out shortly before retiring.

Relaxation tape cassettes can be obtained from either the British Holistic Medical Association, Relaxation for Living or Lifeskills (see Useful Addresses). The latter organisation produce:

- *Relax – And Enjoy It!* – a comprehensive course in deep, quick relaxation techniques.
- *Control Your Tension* – teaches the skills of anxiety management, and is particularly useful where anxiety is associated with phobias.

Patients with anxiety problems may also find other alternative approaches such as yoga or meditation equally helpful (see Alternative Approaches to Management).

Panic attacks

For those M.E. patients who already experience anxiety, panic attacks can be a further incapacitating problem. These attacks are brought on by fear, which is out of all proportion to the stressful situation.

Fears of going into public places or crowds of people in the course of using public transport or shopping in a busy supermarket (agoraphobia) are common causes. In some severe cases an attack can be caused simply by the fear of going out of the house.

To appreciate what such an attack feels like imagine how it feels when you've just stepped off the kerb and nearly been knocked down by a bus – a panic attack produces exactly the same sort of symptoms, but not for just a few seconds. The incapacity can last for up to half an hour. During such an attack a victim will feel unreal and start to tremble and shake inside. This is invariably accompanied by palpitations, chest pains and shortness of breath – even a feeling of choking. This rapid overbreathing (hyperventilation) washes out the carbon dioxide from the blood and causes the sensation of pins and needles (paraesthesiae) in the skin. Other common accompanying symptoms may include dizziness, sweating or flushing. Once the attack is over the patient feels thoroughly exhausted and apprehensive. These symptoms are produced by the autonomic nervous system suddenly becoming overactive when a patient is confronted by what they fear most.

Interestingly, excessive amounts of lactate seem to trigger panic attacks in people who are susceptible, and this finding has been combined with a technique known as positron emission tomography (PET) to study blood flow to various parts of the brain during such an attack. The results show that anxiety is associated with *increased* blood flow to the temporal regions of the brain – the exact opposite to recent findings in some patients with M.E. (see page 112).

The solution of panic attacks requires expert professional help. The benzodiazepine tranquillisers are best avoided, as in anxiety, but antidepressant medication can be quite helpful. Drug treatment, however, won't succeed by itself, and patients have to learn to control their bodies, especially the overbreathing during an attack. The relaxation techniques already described to help anxiety may also be useful here, and a further approach known as behaviour therapy can also be tried.

Behaviour therapy involves the patient being gradually exposed to the sort of situations they fear. In the case of crowds and open spaces this may firstly involve just looking at pictures and thinking about the situations for short periods. This is then followed by short trips outside the house in the company of a friend or counsellor, until eventually the patient feels confident enough to confront what they fear most. This is a slow, time-consuming approach, which requires practical assistance from an experienced therapist, but when carried out can be very effective in reducing phobic anxiety. Further self-help can be obtained from Phobic Action (see Useful Addresses).

Hyperventilation

Hyperventilation, or chronic overbreathing, is frequently associated with anxiety and panic attacks, although it can also be caused by various other medical disorders including asthma, heart disease and chronic pain.

One group of specialists, at London's Charing Cross Hospital, have recently claimed that the majority of patients with M.E. have chronic hyperventilation, also known as 'effort syndrome' (see medical references 40 and 43). These claims have been widely reported in the media and have resulted in further adverse publicity for M.E., one particularly bad example being 'Yuppie flu is all in the mind' (*Sunday Times*, July 17th 1988).

The theory is that following an initial stressful event, such as a viral infection, the body reacts by chronically overbreathing (hyperventilating), even though both patient and doctor may be completely unaware that this is happening. The result is that too much carbon dioxide is washed out from the lungs alongside a rise in the level of stress hormone adrenaline. A vicious circle quickly develops with changes in the blood chemistry causing symptoms due to overexcitability of the nerves (palpitations, dizziness, pins and needles) and constriction of the blood vessels (cold extremities). Other common symptoms include shortness of breath, tremors, chest pains, muscle weakness and feelings of unreality.

Unfortunately, chronic borderline hyperventilation is not easy to diagnose, even using some of the most sophisticated lung function tests which are now available. One very simple test for hyperventilation is to lie down, place one hand on your stomach and the other on your chest. If you arc hyperventilating, the upper hand on the chest should be moving far quicker than the lower one. As far as M.E. is concerned, the findings from Charing Cross have not been confirmed by any other research groups, and Dr David McCluskey from Belfast, in a *British Medical Journal* paper (medical reference 138), concluded that 'patients with chronic fatigue syndrome do not hyperventilate'.

Where hyperventilation is confirmed, the principal treatment involves breathing exercises which are taught by a physiotherapist. Drugs have very little role in the management of this disorder, although some doctors use a controversial regime which involves initial sedation with large doses of tranquillisers such as Valium. This approach has come in for much criticism because of the serious risk of dependency.

My own view is that hyperventilation syndrome certainly exists and is probably under-diagnosed by doctors. I also suspect that it is the true cause of ill health for a *small number* of people who have been wrongly labelled as having M.E. However, hyperventilation is not the cause of M.E., and inappropriate treatment with drugs like Valium could end up causing far more harm than good.

If you require further advice or information on any aspect of mental health, I would suggest contacting either MIND or the education department at the Royal College of Psychiatrists (see Useful Addresses). They both provide useful leaflets; MIND acts as a pressure group on behalf of all people with mental health problems. I have also listed the titles of some helpful books on depression, anxiety and tranquilliser abuse in the reference section.

4. Alternative And Complementary Approaches To The Management Of M.E.

In view of conventional medicine's current inability to provide any really effective treatment for M.E., it is hardly surprising that many patients decide to opt for alternative approaches. Whilst remaining open-minded about alternative medicine, I feel that I can only recommend those therapies which seem to offer genuine benefit, and advise extreme caution about many of the others.

You may also find that your GP has strong opinions about alternative medicines. Some are well informed and supportive whereas others are hostile and negative. Whatever view your own doctor takes, it is always a good idea to discuss any specific treatment before going ahead, especially if it involves taking drugs, unusual supplements or having injections.

Many alternative practitioners now like to use the term 'complementary medicine' because they would prefer working with your own doctor rather than in isolation. Unfortunately, this type of co-operation is not always made easy when exaggerated and unsubstantiated claims are made by some alternative practitioners and 'pill pushing' manufacturers about 'breakthrough' treatments for M.E. There are no miracle cures for this illness.

It is important also to appreciate that so-called natural medicines are not always harmless as the scandal with germanium illustrated. This expensive mineral supplement was successfully targetted at patients with M.E. and AIDS during 1989 with claims that it could 'boost the immune system'. Germanium turned out to be potentially harmful and the Department of

Health had to withdraw it from sale following reports of serious kidney damage (see medical references 164 and 176).

Undoubtedly some M.E. sufferers do find alternative approaches helpful, but exactly why remains open to debate. It may, of course, be due to the fact that the therapy is beneficial. However, what could be just as important is the fact that, at last, you are doing something positive to improve your health. Alternative treatments aren't generally subjected to the same type of rigorously controlled trials as conventional drugs, so it is difficult to rule out a placebo effect as well. The fact that you are taking, and paying for, something which you've been told will help, can have a very positive effect. It is also quite likely that the sympathetic and optimistic approach of most alternative practitioners may be having an equal or even more powerful effect than their therapy.

So, if you're going to experiment with alternative medicine, what sort of questions should you be asking before going ahead?

- Is the therapist recommended, and does he/she have any worthwhile qualifications? This sort of information is not always easy for a lay person to evaluate as long as dubious diplomas are issued from unrecognised Colleges and Institutes.
- How much is a course of treatment going to cost? Some forms of therapy, especially from private medical clinics, can be very expensive. Bills of hundreds, even thousands, of pounds are not unknown.
- Does the treatment have any possible adverse effects? Particularly important in allergy treatments.
- How is the treatment supposed to help in M.E.? Has it been subjected to any form of objective and impartial trial? Very few have. Remember that there are many different views as to 'what is going wrong' in M.E. amongst alternative therapists.
- Will the therapist be informing your own GP about their findings and treatment?

It is obviously not possible to describe all the different types of alternative therapies currently being used by M.E. patients.

However, the following is an A–Z guide through some of the most popular.

Acupuncture

Acupuncture is a traditional Chinese technique which involves the insertion of very fine needles into specific points of the body – the acupuncture points.

The Chinese view of health and disease differs markedly to that of conventional western ideas. They feel that our bodies are in a state of flux between what they refer to as Yin (passivity) and Yang (activity). The healthy body is 'in balance', but the unhealthy body is 'out of balance' between these two vital forces. The aim of acupuncture is to restore balance, and so return the body to normal.

An essential part of the Chinese philosophy is that energy (Qi) flows through the body in channels, each channel corresponding to one of the vital organs such as the heart, brain, etc. If there is disease present in that part of the body then the energy flow in that specific channel is disrupted. These channels don't exist in terms of conventional anatomy. They can't be found at dissection like nerves or blood vessels, and this is why conventional medicine finds this theory hard to understand. By selecting sites where these channels of energy pass, and applying the acupuncture needle, the aim is to correct the dysfunction in energy flow.

The acupuncturist decides which parts of the body are unhealthy by first carrying out a clinical examination, not dissimilar to a normal doctor, but particular attention is paid to the pulse and the state of the tongue – considered to be key indicators of health by the Chinese.

Can acupuncture help M.E.? Conventional medicine accepts that part of the therapeutic effect of acupuncture involves the release of morphine-like substances (endorphins) in the body, which is why it can be so effective in pain relief and even anaesthesia. There is also the suggestion that acupuncture needles are capable of stimulating tiny nerve fibres which send messages back to the brain to control activity in other pain relief centres. Perhaps acupuncture might be a good alternative for any M.E. patient who requires an anaesthetic during an operation or pregnancy?

Anyone who has particular problems with localised bone or muscle pain, unrelieved by ordinary pain killers, might well consider making use of this approach.

Another effect of acupuncture is on the autonomic nerves (which cause vasomotor instability), and again patients experiencing such symptoms (e.g. palpitations) might find acupuncture worth trying. Acupressure at the wrist may also help in the control of sickness (see pages 92–3).

Acupuncture can't 'cure' something like M.E., but it could help with some symptoms. In China, acupuncture is a true form of complementary medicine, with acupuncturists working alongside colleagues in hospitals and clinics who work along traditional western lines. Acupuncture usually needs to be given in a course of treatments, if it's going to have any effect: you won't gain benefit from a one–off treatment. Benefits may not start to occur for several weeks or months, and further treatment may be necessary at a later date.

This therapy can now be obtained on the NHS, but with great difficulty. A few general practitioners have become interested and use it on their patients, but they are still few in number, and there's not much financial incentive for them to do it. A few of the NHS pain clinics also use acupuncture as part of a multidisciplinary approach. For most patients, though, it means going privately. For those who do, please make sure that you find a reputable practitioner because there is a risk of spreading HIV and hepatitis B viruses through the use of unsterilised needles. For how to find an acupuncturist see page 323.

Alexander technique

This aims to improve all aspects of general health by paying particular attention to posture and good breathing. The technique has to be learned by practical instruction from a teacher who has undertaken a three-year training course. An introductory lesson allows you to experience the process at first hand and to then ask any questions. For further details on how to find an Alexander therapist see page 324.

Allergies – are they a part of M.E.?

Allergies are included in this chapter on alternative approaches because it's quite wrong to infer that M.E. is an 'allergic disease', like asthma or hay fever. Some M.E. patients go on to develop secondary allergies as part of the disease process (and I've suffered from hay fever since developing M.E.). However, allergies are common in a normal population of adults, with up to 15 per cent having some form of allergy, and so the association with M.E. may be just pure coincidence. On the other hand there are now reports of some patients having raised levels of a specific antibody known as IgE which would support the link with allergies (see medical reference 85). The lowered levels of blood cortisol described earlier (page 156) could also result in an exaggeration of normal allergic responses.

The most likely explanation for M.E. patients developing allergies seems to be the effect of persisting virus and immune disturbances unmasking allergies in an already susceptible patient. It is worrying to find that some patients, who have no evidence of allergic symptoms, are spending vast amounts of money at private allergy clinics, trying to find what they are allergic to.

Of all the alternative approaches to the management of M.E. allergies are probably the most confusing. Allergy, in medical terms, is simply a way of describing an over-enthusiastic response by the immune system to factors which most people would regard as harmless. The allergic symptoms then occur whenever a sensitive (allergic) patient comes in contact with that substance – the allergen. A comprehensive list of all known allergens would be endless, but many of them are normal everyday constituents of our environment: pollens, furs, foods and drugs. Some truly allergic patients have allergies which change in the course of time. So, identifying which particular allergens are involved in any one individual isn't always easy.

Symptoms result from inflammatory responses taking place in different parts of the body. Inhaled allergens can cause asthma, chemicals on the skin can cause eczema and foods can produce varied symptoms: abdominal pain, changes in bowel habit, etc. When an allergic patient comes into contact with an allergen, the immune system responds by releasing chemicals like histamine which cause an immediate inflammatory response in the particular target tissue.

Both doctors and patients experience a considerable degree of confusion and misunderstanding over the distinction between allergy and sensitivity, and this might be particularly relevant with M.E. in relation to foods. Certainly, some people have a true allergic response to certain foods, most commonly milk and dairy products, wheat and nuts, but just because a certain food makes you feel unwell doesn't mean that you're allergic to it. Caffeine, for example, in coffee will quickly upset some people due to its direct effect on the nervous system causing palpitations, tremor and a headache. But this is a direct effect of the caffeine – there's no allergic response taking place.

Many patients seem to suffer from a variety of digestive (possibly malabsorption) problems once they've developed M.E., but if there is a persisting enterovirus in the lining membrane of the bowel this could well be causing a food sensitivity right there in the gut, as opposed to an allergic reaction in the body generally (see also page 90).

Whatever mechanisms are involved – allergic or increased sensitivity – the most reliable way of detecting a 'culprit' food is by an exclusion diet, followed by a challenge with the suspected food, but this must be done with the help of a doctor or dietician. This type of diet involves a strict regime of what we like to call 'non-allergic foods' for a week or so. This could consist of spring water, a source of protein such as lamb and a source of carbohydrate like rice. Foods can then be slowly introduced in groups (e.g. wheat products) to see if any one produces a recurrence of symptoms. If no significant improvement has occurred at the end of the strict exclusion, it would seem that food sensitivity or allergy is not the cause of the problem.

Allergy testing

Many patients are being led to believe that a whole range of allergies can be quickly and simply diagnosed by 'allergy tests', but this just isn't so. Conventional medicine tends to rely on the results of skin (provocation) tests and blood tests. These can be obtained on the NHS by referral to an allergy clinic at one of the larger district general hospitals.

Skin tests A small amount of very diluted allergen is pricked into the skin, and the inflammatory response – due to histamine release – measured. This type of testing is particularly useful for inhaled allergens causing asthma; for skin eczema; but only for a few food allergies (e.g. egg). For the majority of foods it's probably of little value as they don't tend to produce this type of response in such a short time.

Blood tests measure the levels of specific antibodies which allergic patients make in response to specific allergens. (This is known as the RAST test – standing for Radio Allego Sorbant Test.) These results again have to be carefully interpreted, as not all foods produce this type of response.

A wide variety of other allergy tests are now available, but conventional allergists regard the majority of them as being of dubious value; consequently, they are seldom available on the NHS. As medical adviser to the M.E. Association, I know that many desperate patients are spending hundreds, even thousands of pounds, searching for 'hidden allergies', using techniques which are reducing savings rather than suffering.

At one end of the spectrum are perfectly respectable private doctors and clinics. At the other are naive amateurs and charlatans with no recognised qualifications operating via adverts in various health magazines. Their advice ranges from the bizarre to the positively harmful.

Unfortunately, many people still believe, with some justification, that orthodox medicine regards allergy as a 'no go area'. Hence the current boom in private and alternative services of which your own GP probably has very little working knowledge. So, here is a brief guide to the most popular forms of allergy tests used by alternative practitioners.

Cytotoxic tests are available from several private laboratories. They rely on changes taking place in the shape of white blood cells when a blood sample is mixed with food extracts. Some conventional allergists accept that these type of changes can occur, but it seems that the current method of microscopic examination is far too unreliable. Cytotoxic tests produce too many false positives and negatives. *Not recommended*.

Hair analysis relies on detecting allergies from a sample of hair. There is no scientific evidence to back up such claims. *Not recommended*.

Kineseology is based on the supposition that muscle power falls when a patient and his allergy are placed in close proximity. *Unproven and extremely dubious*.

Pulse testing is amazingly simple – when an allergic individual eats a certain food the pulse will rise. *Unproven – not recommended*.

Radionics practitioners use a pendulum and do not require the presence of the patient. The patient and practitioner communicate by 'energy waves' which transfer all the necessary information. *Not recommended*.

Vega testing involves the use of electrical equipment rather like an ECG machine. It is said to be capable of diagnosing both food and chemical allergies based on the idea that there are changes in electrical resistance at acupuncture sites during illness. *Regarded with extreme scepticism by conventional allergists* (see medical reference 174).

Treatment of allergies

Once an allergy or sensitivity has been found the obvious solution is to try and avoid, wherever possible, the particular allergen.

Conventional medicine treats allergies with a variety of drugs. Antihistamines, sodium cromoglycate (which covers the histamine-containing cells and prevents its release) and the powerful anti-inflammatory steroids are all used depending on the type and severity of the symptoms. Steroids are not recommended for M.E. patients unless really necessary, as they dampen down immune responses.

Non-orthodox practitioners use a variety of approaches to manage allergic disease, and again their value is heavily criticised by some doctors.

The two methods which are most commonly used in the private allergy sector are enzyme potentiated desensitisation (EPD) and neutralisation therapy.

Enzyme Potentiated Desensitisation (EPD) This controversial method for treating allergies was developed by Dr Len McEwan, an allergist who originally worked at St Mary's Hospital in London. He is still the leading expert in this area and trains other doctors in how to administer EPD. Although this treatment is mainly used in the private allergy sector there are a few allergists working within the NHS who are open minded about its possible value.

The principal use of EPD is for treating food allergies, and the technique involves a mixture of multiple diluted food allergens combined with an enzyme (beta glucuronidase) which is supposed to increase the desensitising effect.

EPD can be given either by injection or by placing the allergen and enzyme mixture on to an area of skin on the arm. The treatment has to be administered several times during the first year, and boosters are then given at increasing intervals depending on the response.

The cost of a full course of EPD may well run into several hundred pounds. Unfortunately, a few patients also seem to have adverse reactions and cannot continue. So, in the absence of any published trials demonstrating clear benefits *I would not yet recommend the use of EPD.*

Neutralisation therapy This is another approach favoured by some doctors in the private allergy sector. A few conventional allergists feel that it may have some benefits, whereas others maintain that the investigation side produces too many false negatives and positives.

Allergies are first identified using a series of injections of food extracts which are placed just under the skin (intradermally). A series of weaker and weaker injections are given until the resulting reaction (a weal) is white, hard and raised as well as remaining the same size for ten minutes after the test dose. This is known as the neutralising dose – a precise concentration of allergen which should be able to 'switch off' the symptoms.

Neutralisation therapy then involves taking the food extracts either by drops straight under the tongue or by self-administered injections. As far as M.E. is concerned this technique remains purely speculative and *I would not recommend its use at the present time.*

The subject of allergies and M.E. creates a considerable amount of heated debate between those who support the theories and others who don't see allergies as having much to do with this illness. This is undoubtedly very confusing for patients, who can't follow the scientific arguments, and are baffled by what they ought to do. I've tried to present the facts as I see them. I don't accept that allergic reactions are a major part of M.E.; although there are some patients who have allergies (or sensitivities), and identification and correct management could help them feel a lot better.

Some useful books on allergy are listed on pages 363–4 as well as details about the British Allergy Foundation.

Aromatherapy

Here, small quantities of plant oils are massaged into the skin, inhaled or used in the bath. Aromatherapy is undoubtedly very soothing and relaxing, especially when using an oil such as lavender in the bath. Whether these oils have more beneficial therapeutic properties (as is often claimed) remains a matter of speculation.

Occasional allergic reactions have been reported from the use of some oils (e.g. lemongrass) which are far more concentrated than their original plant form. So, do look very carefully at the label and make sure the oil has been properly diluted.

Another concern is that some oils may also be absorbed through the skin and then enter the general circulation. For this reason the International Federation of Aromatherapists have drawn up the following guidelines:

- Avoid altogether because of possible toxicity – calmus, cassia, fennel, horseradish, mugwort, mustard, pennyroyal, rue, sassafras, savin, tansy, wintergreen, wormwood, sage, aniseed, hyssop.
- Avoid in pregnancy (may cause bleeding) – all the above plus basil, birch, clary sage, cypress, jasmine, juniper, marjoram, myrrh, peppermint, rosemary and thyme.
- Unsuitable for anyone with raised blood pressure – hyssop, rosemary, sage and thyme. Fennel, hyssop and wormwood can also trigger epileptic attacks.
- Avoid if you have sensitive skin (can cause an unpleasant irritant dermatitis) – basil, lemon, melissa, peppermint and thyme. These oils can also irritate when used in the bath. Also avoid bergamot, lemon, lime, orange and verbena in strong sunshine.

Some of the common oils which appear to be safe and may be worth trying include:

- Camomile – said to reduce tension and help sleep.
- Geranium – a cool calming oil useful for tension.
- Lavender – supposed to help stimulate the mind.
- Peppermint – said to relieve decongestion and headaches; also very cooling.
- Ylang Ylang – supposed to have a sedating effect.

Autoimmunotherapy

This is an unusual form of 'Own Blood Therapy' which originated in Germany. The technique involves removing a syringe full of blood from the vein which, after a short while, is injected back into the muscle. Treatments are given weekly for several weeks and the amount of blood used is steadily increased. Various homeopathic medicines may also be added during the process.

The theory behind autoimmunotherapy is that once outside the body the blood changes its composition. When it is reintroduced the body recognises that it is not quite the same and the result is a stimulation of the immune system. These scientific statements do not make sense to me and so *I would not recommend its use.*

Ayurveda

This is a traditional system of medicine which is very popular in India. It is now becoming fashionable here in the U.K. The treatment involves the use of herbal medicines and massage which is said to be less 'interfering' than orthodox medicine and allegedly results in far fewer side-effects. Anyone trying ayurveda should be careful to ask questions about the use of imported herbal medicines whose safety has recently been questioned (see later in this chapter).

Bach flower remedies

These were developed in the last century by a homeopathic doctor called Edward Bach. He claimed that extracts from certain flowers could reverse what were termed 'negative mental states' which led on to various types of physical illness. Bach flower remedies are alleged to work by a process of energy transfer – something that most orthodox medical opinion views with considerable scepticism.

Candida albicans

One aspect of M.E. that continues to create an enormous amount of controversy is the possible role of a yeast called candida. It's also an important reason why some doctors refuse to take M.E. seriously – they regard candida as yet another 'bogus illness'.

Having worked in the sexually transmitted disease clinic at London's Middlesex Hospital, I've spent more hours looking for this particular yeast under the microscope than any of the alternative practitioners advocating such a connection. I've also witnessed the whole spectrum of ill health that it can produce ranging from vaginal discharge through to life-threatening complications in patients with severe immunedeficiency. *My conclusion is that candida has no connection whatsoever with M.E.*

Unfortunately, large numbers of people with M.E. do believe that they have a significant candida problem and go to great lengths to treat it, using drugs, restrictive diets and probiotics. Some undoubtedly report improvement; in others there's no change, and a third group actually start to feel even worse with anti-candida treatment. These are results which are not that dissimilar to many of the other unproven treatments.

Reading the various other self-help guide books on the subject it's not hard to see why people become so convinced by the candida connection. The 'evidence' that more than 75 per cent of M.E. patients have candida is presented with such confidence – as though it was irrefutable. Unfortunately, it isn't – most of these 'facts' are based on supposition and pseudoscience. At the moment the case for candida leaks like a sieve. Perhaps the best way of trying to explore the arguments for and against candida is to look at how this yeast lives in our intestines, and what happens when the natural balance is upset.

Candida the alternative view

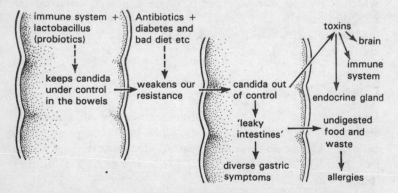

Firstly, there's no disagreement that everyone (healthy or unhealthy) has some candida living in their gut. The yeast is kept under control by the activity of 'good bacteria' (like lactobacillus) and the body's immune system. The presence of this small amount may actually be beneficial. As a result, it's not hard to grow (culture) candida in a stool sample, but this doesn't prove anything. Neither does looking for antibodies to candida – we all have this yeast as a life-long passenger, so it's not surprising that we make an immune response and produce antibodies.

From time to time certain factors allow candida to get out of control and this can lead to problems in various parts of the body. White patches in the mouth (common in babies and the elderly), vaginal discharge and skin or nail infections are all common examples; it's quite easy to confirm the presence of candida from any of these sites. People with severely disrupted immune systems (eg AIDS or those taking powerful steroid drugs) can develop far more serious candida infections in the lung or brain. There's nothing 'bogus' about these types of candida infections. The body's natural resistance to candida overgrowth can be weakened by a number of factors:

- Antibiotics – which kill off 'good bacteria', but the body's natural balance of gut organisms is usually quickly restored to normal after such drugs.
- Diabetes – which raises the level of blood sugar, the nutrient on which candida feeds.
- Immunosuppressive drugs and diseases like AIDS.
- The contraceptive pill is frequently cited as the fourth factor, but a review of all the current literature leads me to doubt such a connection. The contraceptive pill does not contain the type of steroids which significantly depress immune function. They do alter the body's sex hormones (oestrogen and progesterone) but whether this predisposes to candida is open to debate.

Orthodox and alternative medicine now part company. The latter's explanation is that candida turns into what is known as a hyphael form and starts to grow roots (just like a tree does) which penetrate the gut wall to produce a 'leaky intestine'. This in turn allows so-called candida toxins to enter the blood and affect the brain, immune system and hormone producing glands. Undigested food particles are also supposed to be able to seep through these tiny holes and set off allergic reactions. Lastly, waste products from yeast fermentation (acetaldehyde) are alleged to interfere with blood oxygenation.

This all sounds very impressive in theory, but where is the hard scientific evidence to support the hypothesis? I do not believe it exists and this is why:

- Claims that much of the candida overgrowth in M.E. occurs in the gullet/oesophagus and stomach could easily be verified by using a special type of X-ray (a barium swallow) or by having a look down the throat with an endoscope and taking a small sample of tissue (a biopsy). This type of oesophageal infection is a common complication of AIDS and can easily be confirmed by these sort of investigations. Nobody has, as yet, demonstrated the same findings in M.E.
- There is no reputable published material to show that candida behaves in the intestine by growing penetrating roots and producing a 'leaky' gut lining.
- Claims that candida toxins can have adverse effects on the brain or immune system are unsubstantiated. I recently asked one of the manufacturers of nystatin if they could do a world data search for toxins; they could not find a single reliable scientific reference on this connection. Incidentally, despite the enormous profit potential, the manufacturers of this drug have no desire to promote it to M.E. patients because they have still to be convinced about any such link.
- Acetaldehyde may well be produced in the intestine but it's doubtful if there are sufficient quantities to cause a significant lack of oxygen.
- Gastric symptoms, such as bloating and wind along with bowel disturbances, are far more feasible, but again remain unproven. If the gut really is 'leaking' then why don't far more serious problems arise? Why, for instance, doesn't the nystatin pass through these holes? After all, nystatin is a toxic drug which is only safe when not absorbed into the circulation.

Having examined all the arguments for and against candida, can it really do any harm embarking on a treatment regime? Possibly not, but I would still maintain that people with M.E. have quite enough restrictions placed on their lives without having to add limitations on diet, as well as spending money on supplements and probiotics. In addition, is it really such a good idea to be taking prolonged courses of antifungal drugs which some microbiologists now feel could result in the development of resistant strains – as has occurred with anti-biotics and bacteria? Although nystatin is thought to be per-fectly safe inside the intestine, there are drugs like Nizoral (ketoconazole) which can have serious toxic effects on the liver.

Finally, could it be that having some candida inside the gut is actually beneficial and forms a natural part of the environment there? My feeling is that the candida connection is another blind alley for desperate patients searching for a cure. By all means weigh up the arguments carefully, but remember – the case for candida is nowhere near as watertight as its advocates suggest.

If you want to read more about some of the research that has been published into this very controversial area please refer to the medical reference 169.

Treatment

Those who believe that it's essential to remove candida as part of an M.E. treatment regime rely on an approach which involves diet, conventional anti-fungal medication and other additional supplements.

Diet

The theory is that to help eradicate candida your diet will have to be free from both sugar and yeast, which denies the organism its essential nutrients. This sort of diet will involve cutting out foods like bread (which contains yeast), sugar and honey. Even your B vitamins have to be yeast free. Some practitioners also advocate a low carbohydrate diet to accompany this, but don't start this sort of dietary manipulation by yourself without prop-er supervision. One reason for the apparent success of this diet may have nothing whatsoever to do with its effect on candida. Instead, as Dr Robert Loblay, an expert on food allergies and intolerance, explained at the 1990 Cambridge Symposium, the reason may lie in the fact that this approach eliminates a number of common foods which contain chemicals such as natural salicylates and glutamine to which many people are undoubtedly sensitive.

Drugs

Anti-fungal medication, such as nystatin, needs to be prescribed by your general practitioner. Nystatin is the generic name, so it comes in a variety of preparations using different trade names – e.g. Nystan. It can be used as a cream or pessary for vaginal infections, drops and pastilles for thrush in the mouth, skin creams, tablets for bowel infections as well as powder. The powder form is taken between meals, and the dose is gradually altered according to the individual response.

Nystatin appears to be a perfectly safe drug, but like any medicine it should be used with caution during pregnancy.

One anti-fungal preparation, which M.E. patients use occasionally is ketoconazole (Nizoral). This drug is potentially *very toxic* to the liver, and I don't believe it should be used by anyone with M.E., unless there are very strong medical indications to do so.

A variety of other anti-fungal preparations are also used by the practitioners who carry out this form of therapy, some of them originating abroad.

Additional supplements

Lactobacillus acidophilus is a natural constituent of the bowel, and its presence helps to keep candida in check. It can be killed off by taking antibiotics, but restored by eating 'live' yogurt (from health food shops), or can be taken in capsule form.

Other additional supplements sometimes recommended include high doses of Vitamin C, as well as other vitamins and minerals. High-dose Vitamin C will produce diarrhoea, and it's claimed this will aid the removal of candida. This megadose therapy isn't without side-effects (see vitamins, pages 206–10) and shouldn't be stopped abruptly.

Anti-fungal candida treatment isn't a scientifically proven method of managing M.E. The exponents of this therapy don't claim it will cure M.E., but that it will help to make some people feel substantially better. Certainly, there are reports of patients apparently benefiting from this approach, although others say they feel worse. Some conventional doctors are looking at the relation between yeasts and specific bowel diseases, but this research is still in its early stages and it is too soon to draw any conclusions from it.

Chemical sensitivities

The controversial link between chemical sensitivities/allergies and M.E. continues to generate a great deal of publicity and is accepted without criticism by many patients. However, this is something that orthodox medical opinion, including my own, still views with considerable scepticism, because any such link is very difficult to prove. Whilst accepting that chemical sensitivity may be a problem (and occasionally a severe one) in a *small minority* of patients, I do not believe that everyone with M.E. needs to go to the lengths advocated by some practitioners, and remove almost every form of chemical from their home environment. Equally, you should be very careful about some of the very dubious investigative procedures and treatments which are now available in the alternative health sector. The possibility that some agricultural pesticides may be associated with an M.E.-like illness is discussed further on page 29.

Coenzyme Q10

This is one of the body's essential enzymes which is present in all human cells, particularly within the mitochondria, where it acts as an igniting force in energy production. Coenzyme Q10 may also have a role in neutralising harmful oxidants which lead to cell damage and degeneration. Inside the body this enzyme is manufactured in the liver, but it is also present in many foods including meat, fish and vegetable oils. Although there is no doubt about the theoretical value of Coenzyme Q10 *no reliable evidence* has been published to show that people with M.E. are either deficient in it or that commercially available supplements will boost energy production.

Dental amalgam removal

Although mercury is undoubtedly a toxic metal, there is still no good scientific evidence to support the view that the small amounts present in dental fillings are absorbed into the body to cause harm. Total replacement of such fillings is likely to be a very expensive procedure (up to £2000) and is *not something I would advise.*

Detoxification therapies

These involve various forms of 'colonic cleansing' which, in theory, help to eliminate a 'toxic load' from the large bowel. These types of approaches were very popular in the early 1900s and now seem to be the subject of renewed enthusiasm amongst alternative therapists. *Orthodox medicine considers them to be wholly unscientific,* and they should certainly be avoided by anyone who is already debilitated as a result of M.E.

Colonic irrigation involves regular visits to a colonic therapist (about £30 a time) who uses warm water to flush out debris from the bowel wall. Although adverse effects are rare it can upset the balance of electrolytes (body salts) and damage the gut lining in anyone who already suffers from any sort of bowel inflammation.

Fasting for days, or even longer, is another method of allegedly detoxifying the body. *This is one practice which I would definitely not recommend* – it could end up doing far more harm than good.

Dietary supplementation

Some practitioners advocate that M.E. patients should be encouraged to supplement their diets with a variety of trace elements, amino acids and vitamins. This type of approach is particularly popular in America for a variety of illnesses; once again the theories are quite attractive, although there is little evidence to back them up and win the acceptance of orthodox medicine.

The idea behind this approach is that there may be both faulty absorption of some of these essential substances, as well as an extra requirement to help in the repair process of essential cells which have been damaged by the persisting virus or immune dysfunction. A comprehensive list of all these substances would be endless, as differing practitioners recommend their own individual treatment regimes, often using a combination of therapies. However, amino acids and three trace elements which are quite frequently taken by M.E. patients do warrant some appraisal.

Patients who are interested in this type of approach, and want to follow it up can have tests done on various mineral levels in the body by: BIOLAB, The Stone House, 9 Weymouth Street, London W1N 3FF. Tel 071-636 5959. They are a private pathology laboratory who specialise in this type of work.

Amino acids are the essential building blocks which are required by the body to manufacture proteins. When food proteins, like fish or meat, have been digested, they are quickly broken down into their constituent amino acids. These are then removed from the circulation by cells in the brain, muscle, bone, skin etc. to build up their own proteins for either repair or growth.

Altogether there are about twenty different amino acids of which eight are known as 'essential' because they cannot be made inside the body – they have to come from our diet. Expensive preparations containing various amino acid supplements – both essential and non-essential – are now available. *Provided your protein intake is satisfactory, there seems little advantage in using these preparations.* However, if it can be shown that there are specific amino acid deficiencies in M.E. this sort of approach could be beneficial, and one small trial looking for possible deficiencies is now in progress.

Magnesium Deficiency of this vital element has been implicated in a number of disorders including premenstrual syndrome and high blood pressure. However, researchers remain uncertain about the precise role of magnesium in the body, although it does seem to be an important factor (like Coenzyme Q10) in catalysing energy production inside nerve and muscle cells.

In March 1991 *The Lancet* published a paper on the use of magnesium sulphate injections as a possible treatment for M.E. (medical reference 167). The paper created a great deal of press interest and, as a result, family doctors were inundated by requests to prescribe this new form of therapy.

The reaction from the medical profession was far more sceptical. Some doctors co-operated with requests for treatment whereas others were hostile and refused to experiment with such an unconventional approach to management.

The clinical trial involved 32 patients who were selected by general practitioners and by the Centre for the Study of Complementary Medicine in Southampton.

Firstly, the concentration of magnesium inside the patients' red blood cells was measured. (Only a very small amount of magnesium is present outside the cells, making ordinary blood tests an unreliable indicator of magnesium deficiency.) The results suggested that patients with M.E. were *slightly* deficient in magnesium. They were also asked to fill in a comprehensive health questionnaire so the response to magnesium could be objectively assessed.

The 32 patients were then divided into two separate groups so that a double-blind, placebo-controlled trial could be carried out. This means that neither doctor nor patient knew who was receiving active treatment (in this case injections of 1gm of 50 per cent magnesium sulphate) or a placebo-dummy injection (water).

The trial continued with six weekly injections after which everyone filled in their health questionnaire once again. This covered symptoms such as energy levels, emotional reactions and sleep pattern. Out of the 15 patients receiving magnesium 12 improved, of which 7 reported a significant improvement in energy levels. In the placebo group only 3 out of 17 reported any benefits.

So, although the numbers involved were very small, and the follow-up period surprisingly short (six weeks), the results were considered to be statistically significant. The paper passed the strict peer review (assessment by other doctors) necessary for acceptance in *The Lancet*.

So, why might magnesium be helping patients with M.E.? Magnesium is something that we all take in as part of a normal healthy diet. Foods such as green vegetables, cereal grains, chocolate and nuts are all good sources. So is 'hard' drinking water.

About 45 per cent of this daily intake is then absorbed in the small intestine. During times of deficiency inside the body this absorption can easily rise to 80 per cent. Once inside the body most magnesium is stored inside the bone and muscle.

The main action of magnesium is within the cells, particularly muscle and nervous tissue where it helps with numerous enzyme systems. As far as muscle is concerned, too much magnesium can seriously interfere with the way electrical impulses are transmitted from nerves to muscles. However, within the muscle cell itself it is stored in the mitochondria – the 'power house' of the cell – where it acts as a vital co-factor in energy production. So, there are some theoretical mechanisms why magnesium supplementation could be both beneficial and harmful.

According to most orthodox medical opinion, true magnesium deficiency is fairly unusual but it can occur in some types of gastrointestinal disease (where absorption is reduced), alcoholism (which increases its removal by the kidneys as do diuretic drugs) and some hormonal diseases (e.g. an overactive thyroid gland).

Incidentally, an underactive thyroid (hypothyroidism) can actually cause magnesium levels to rise. Whether or not magnesium deficiency is a significant factor in M.E. remains speculative despite these findings from Southampton.

Publication of the trial results was followed by a number of critical letters to *The Lancet* (see medical reference 167). One of the most important concerned the actual amount of magnesium contained in these injections. According to one of the pharmaceutical companies involved, this amounted to only about 100mgs which was then released over the following few hours. Given that our average dietary intake of magnesium is about 300–400 mg per day, it is difficult to see why an extra

15 mg per day on average should produce any major benefits.

It was also pointed out that measuring the red blood cell concentration of magnesium is not a reliable indicator for assessing magnesium deficiency inside the body. A more objective method is to assess the concentration in either muscle or monocytes (a type of white blood cell), or to carry out what is known as an intravenous magnesium loading test. In practice though, none of these tests are easily obtainable from the NHS so most people trying magnesium therapy will not know if they are actually deficient. It was also pointed out that the laboratory used to carry out some of the tests had been the subject of media investigations which had cast doubt on their accuracy.

Lastly, it should be noted that high doses of magnesium can cause serious side-effects, especially on the heart. So, it is a wise precaution to check that kidney function is satisfactory before these injections are given; I would not recommend that anyone with heart disease takes extra magnesium. These injections must be given into the muscle and *never* directly into a vein.

Given the way that the body absorbs and then distributes magnesium, it seems that small amounts taken by mouth are far less likely to have any beneficial effects.

The results of this small trial must be viewed with considerable caution, and further independent trials are now needed before any definite conclusions can be drawn. We also need to establish if significant magnesium deficiency is indeed a part of this illness. *Magnesium is not yet a proven therapy for M.E.*

Selenium This is another trace element which has recently been advocated as a possible treatment for M.E. Selenium is frequently combined in commercial preparations with vitamins A, C and E. In theory, this combination should act together to scavenge for harmful substances known as 'free radicals' which cause cell damage, ageing and possibly cancer. Selenium is also alleged to possess anti-inflammatory, antiviral and immune altering effects; concentrations are said to be reduced in some patients with rheumatoid arthritis.

Although it has been widely speculated that selenium may be able to modify the body's immune response to viral infections *there is still no reliable data to show that it has any beneficial effects in M.E.*, or that blood levels are reduced.

As with any other micronutrient, concern has been expressed about how important it is to leave a wide safety margin, and not to exceed the recommended dose of any selenium supplement. Toxicity does occur leading to hair loss, chronic eczema and damage to the sensory nerves (as with vitamin B6). According to the most recent government guidelines on vitamins and minerals a safe daily intake lies somewhere between 40 and 70 micrograms for a normal weight adult. Supplementation in excess of this should only be taken where a clear deficiency is shown to exist.

Zinc This trace element forms an essential part of our diet, and well over 200 enzymes are now known to require its presence to operate effectively.

At the moment there is no officially recommended daily intake of zinc in the U.K., but in America it is set at 15mg per day. Most people take in about 10mg a day in their diet, which is probably quite sufficient. Meat (30 per cent) and milk (25 per cent) are major sources of dietary zinc, but fruit and vegetables contain very little. Absorption from the gut is reduced by a high intake of dietary fibre and phytic acid which is found in soya beans. Even so, vegetarians do not seem to have any problems associated with zinc deficiency.

Orthodox medicine acknowledges that severe deficiency of zinc does occasionally occur, and this can result in inflamed skin lesions, increased susceptibility to infections and a general failure to thrive in children. Such deficiency is usually due to a malabsorption in the intestines, chronic alcoholism or loss during kidney dialysis.

The level of zinc in the blood is not thought to be an accurate indicator of zinc levels overall, as only a small amount is actually in the blood. Any chronic infection will probably reduce the level of zinc in the blood, but it seems that the total amount of zinc in the body doesn't fall significantly, so concluding that someone with M.E. has a mild zinc deficiency from a blood test isn't necessarily a logical conclusion.

Experimentally, zinc can interfere with virus multiplication.

Even so, there's no evidence that it stops the progression of the common cold (for which it's often recommended) or any other persisting viral infection. Some allergists believe that patients with food allergy or sensitivity have an abnormal ratio of copper to zinc status in the body, and that if this is corrected there can be a considerable improvement in food-related symptoms. Taking extra amounts of zinc may result in side-effects (eg stomach pains and decreased copper absorption); very high intakes can actually start to depress the immune system. Zinc also competes with iron for absorption within the gut; cases of anaemia associated with excessive supplementation have now been recorded.

At present, many of the claims made for zinc supplementation are unfounded, but taking a little extra probably does no harm. No M.E. patient should take any more than 50 mgm per day (Zincomed capsules contain this dose) if they decide to use this as part of their treatment. Zinc supplements should *not* be taken by any patient who has kidney problems.

Vitamins

Vitamins, when taken in normal recommended daily doses (RDAs), are extremely safe. However, many people with M.E. seem to be taking ever-increasing amounts of expensive vitamin supplements. In some cases the manufacturers have been giving the prescribing practitioners a substantial commission on sales – a practice which creates a very undesirable conflict of interest. *I am not convinced that large doses of vitamins are either necessary or desirable in this illness*.

The list of disorders (including M.E.) that large doses of vitamins are alleged to help is becoming endless. It seems that almost any 'sick cell' in the body can be restored to normal health by these pills. This trend towards high dose vitamin therapy is partly based on the ideas of the great Vitamin C enthusiast, Linus Pauling. He argued that many psychiatric illnesses (particularly schizophrenia) were due to deficiencies in transmitter chemicals within the brain (neurotransmitters) which could be solved by dietary supplementation. The same idea has now been applied to M.E. – taking large quantities of vitamins and minerals should help cells in the brain, muscle and immune system to recover. This all sounds fine in theory, but any alleged benefits are based on anecdotal reports rather than hard scientific fact.

All doctors acknowledge that vitamins are essential catalysts for the correct functioning of blood and nerve cells, the immune system and hormones; in fact almost any tissue in the body. However, these requirements are in *minute amounts* which any normal healthy diet should be supplying perfectly adequately. There is no scientific proof that people with M.E. are deficient in any of the major vitamins. Until such evidence exists, I would urge anyone with M.E. to carefully consider the pros and cons of megadosing on vitamins. The untoward effects of taking such large doses over a prolonged period of time is still far from certain and difficult to assess, as self-medication makes the reporting of adverse reactions very unlikely.

So, which vitamins do you need to be careful about and what are the dangers?

Vitamin A (Retinol) is currently being investigated as a possible anti-cancer substance; but there is no good evidence that M.E. patients are either deficient or would benefit from supplementation. The medical journals now contain well over 500 case reports of people being made ill by taking too much Vitamin A. In excess it can cause increased pressure in the brain and serious liver damage – deaths have even been reported. It seems that at levels as low as ten times the RDA, toxicity can occur.

Vitamin B Group Conventional teaching on vitamins used to be that it was only the fat soluble group (A, D, E and K) which caused harm as they could accumulate in body fat. The water soluble vitamins (B and C) are excreted in the urine when taken in excess, so nobody thought they could also accumulate. Research has now shown that life is not quite so simple, and although Vitamins B1, B2 and B12 appear to be quite safe, problems are arising in connection with Vitamin B6 (pyridoxine) and Vitamin C in high doses.

Vitamin B3 (niacin) is needed for the continuous release of energy from carbohydrates. The only people who really need to take supplements are alcoholics, people on a very poor diet and anyone on kidney dialysis. High doses of niacin (especially in the sustained release form) can cause severe liver damage and even death. There is no rationale for exceeding the RDA in the case of M.E.

Vitamin B6 (pyridoxine) is currently the vogue treatment for pre-menstrual tension (PMT), and it does undoubtedly seem to help some women with this condition. At doses of 150 mg per day (and possibly lower) it can damage sensory nerves causing pins and needles (paraesthesiae) and inco-ordination. What is worrying, and still far from certain, is at what level Vitamin B6 actually starts to produce nerve damage in the absence of symptoms. Dr Katharina Dalton, a world expert on hormone disturbances, has noted that adverse effects reoccurred at doses of 50 mg per day in patients who had previously stopped the high dose treatment and then resumed at this lower dose. (See medical references 163 and 168.)

Vitamin B12 is needed for healthy bone marrow and nerves. Deficiency leads to anaemia and nerve cell degeneration (pernicious anaemia). Deficiency occurs primarily due to lack of absorption, so it has to be given by injection. Oral preparations do no harm but their benefits are questionable. At present there is no evidence that M.E. patients have problems with B12 absorption. However, some doctors in both America and Australia are giving B12 injections in an attempt to saturate the body with this vitamin. Although there are anecdotal reports of success, the only placebo-controlled trial which involved vitamin B12 showed no significant benefits compared to a placebo (medical reference 149).

Vitamin C This is probably the most common vitamin to be megadosed by M.E. patients, due to claims that it can boost the immune system. Whether or not patients with M.E. need their immune systems boosting is a matter for debate. Even so, there is very little evidence that large doses can actually fulfil these claims in humans. If Vitamin C did have these properties, it would presumably have become a standard treatment for immunedeficiency conditions such as AIDS.

What worries doctors is the increasing number of adverse reactions being reported as claims for Vitamin C become more widespread. It is now known that excessive amounts can increase the levels of oestrogen in the body so converting a 'low dose' contraceptive pill into the 'high dose' equivalent. Vitamin C also increases the output of chemicals in the urine called oxalates which can result in kidney stone formation. Increased intake results in the body's natural removal mechanisms speeding up, so that any sudden cessation of treatment can produce a rebound scurvy – several cases of which have now appeared in the medical literature. Another disturbing effect of Vitamin C is the way it increases the absorption of iron. M.E. patients are not deficient in iron and it is undesirable to overload the system with this metal as it can cause serious liver damage. It has also been suggested that heavy metals like iron and aluminium may damage the nerve cells and be responsible for other neurological diseases such as dementia.

The harmful effects of excessive Vitamin C seem to be largely ignored whilst its benefits remain far from certain.

Vitamin D helps to maintain the level of calcium in the blood. Any excess will lead to kidney stones and further muscle weakness. The best way of maintaining an adequate calcium balance is from dairy produce, and calcium supplements if necessary.

Vitamin E This is another fat soluble vitamin which is also enjoying considerable popularity amongst M.E. patients. Many people are enthusing about Vitamin E's anti-oxidant role, meaning that it can mop up free oxygen molecules circulating around the body. There is certainly a theoretical benefit here, as these molecules do seem to be capable of damaging cells; and Vitamin E has been used experimentally on premature babies whose eyes have been damaged after being given too much oxygen at birth.

However, on the negative side, Vitamin E raises blood fats (triglycerides), can lower thyroid gland hormones; and it has been reported in a reputable medical journal as causing muscle weakness along with the release of muscle enzymes (creatine kinase), suggesting that excessive amounts may actually be damaging muscle cells.

The benefits of this vitamin in M.E. remain far from clear – I suggest any patient takes larger amounts with considerable caution.

So, vitamins need to be taken with the same type of caution that applies to any other medicine, especially if you're going to take more than the RDA. A daily multivitamin tablet isn't going to cause any harm and good value ones include Sanatogen Multivitamins and Boots Plurivite M. Specially formulated preparations from the health food industry often cost more and don't offer any significant advantages. In future I hope that alternative practitioners will give a great deal more thought (and publicity) to the possible disadvantages of high dose vitamin therapy. Apart from the dangers I have illustrated, all this is doing is making drug companies even richer and producing some of the most expensive urine in the world, as our bodies naturally remove what we don't require.

Further information on the benefits and side-effects of vitamins can be obtained by reading medical references 170 and 175.

Hair analysis

The value of hair analysis in the assessment of nutritional status and allergies is viewed with extreme scepticism by orthodox medicine. Nevertheless, several private clinics now claim to be able to detect deficiencies in vitamins and minerals such as zinc, magnesium and chromium from a sample of hair. The problem is that hair does not necessarily reflect the concentrations of minerals found in body tissues, and there are large individual variations in these levels according to age, sex and even which part of the scalp the sample is taken from. Even more dubious is the practice of diagnosing and treating allergies from samples of hair sent by post. *I do not believe that hair analysis has any value in either the diagnosis or treatment of M.E.*

Vitamins and minerals: the facts

	Recommended Daily Allowance★	Sources
Vitamin A: retinol	1000mcg	liver, green vegetables, carrots, oranges, eggs, cheese, milk.
Vitamin B1: thiamin	1.4mg	potatoes, bread, milk, vegetables, cereals.
Vitamin B2: riboflavin	1.6mg	liver, meat, milk, cheese.
Vitamin B3: niacin and nicotinic acid	18mg	liver, meat, bread, cereals.
Vitamin B6: pyridoxine	2mg	liver, cereals, pulses, poultry.
Vitamin B12: cobalamin	3mcg	meat, milk, cheese, eggs.
Vitamin B: biotin	0.15mg	liver, pork, cauliflower, cereals.
Vitamin B: folic acid	400mcg	green vegetables and fruit.
Vitamin C: ascorbic acid	60mg	fruit, vegetables, potatoes, tomatoes.
Vitamin D: calciferol	5mcg	sunlight, margarine, fish, eggs, butter.
Vitamin E:	10mg	vegetable oils, nuts, eggs, butter.
Minerals		
Calcium	800mg	milk, cheese, bread.
Iron	12mg	meat, liver, beans, bread, fruit, nuts.
Zinc	15mg	milk, liver, meat, wholegrains

★ European Community figures are quoted which are slightly higher than the RDA here in the U.K. Mcg and mg quoted throughout are per 100G.

Healing

The term healing covers a wide variety of different therapies, the theory being that patients can be healed by 'forces' which the healer possesses, and which can be passed on to the patient.

Many of these healers make strong religious claims in connection with their work, assuming, rightly or wrongly, that their powers are 'God given'. In practice the process of healing usually involves the laying on of hands, or some form of physical contact, although some healers claim to be able to transmit these healing powers by way of thought.

There seems to be an ever growing number of healers. Some of them are obviously frauds, so if you do decide to embark on healing do make careful enquiries first and try to find a genuine and respected healer. This 'mind over matter' approach can be of great value to some people, and obviously the chances of success are greatly increased if you believe in the healer and the principles of healing.

Patients who have strong religious beliefs (and even those who don't) may gain considerable benefit and comfort from Christian healing. Some churches now have specific 'healing services' as part of their worship, and your vicar will know of any which occur locally. Part of the service usually involves the priest giving an individual blessing along with the laying on of hands for those who require healing. Relatives are also very welcome to attend and to pray for recovery.

Some healers belong to the National Federation of Spiritual Healing (see page 331), but the best way of finding a healer would be by personal recommendation.

Herbal medicines

A recent survey in the *British Medical Journal* found that general practitioners understood less about herbal medicines than any other branch of alternative medicine. This is disquieting, because many of the drugs used by orthodox medicine are derived from plants, and some of the herbal medicines available for purchase have some disturbing side-effects if not used with care.

Herbalists are generally unqualified, although a few have taken some formal training. They will recommend and prepare herbal medicines for patients, but most people seem to use this branch of alternative medicine on a 'do-it-yourself' basis, by purchasing the remedies from health food stores – often without knowing a great deal about the product they're about to use. There is a vast range of herbal medicines available, and the current position with regard to licensing and control is far from satisfactory. Patients are taking substances of which the long-term effects, in some cases, have never been properly assessed. This is something that the Department of Health is currently investigating.

Although the majority are probably quite safe, some herbs are known to accumulate heavy metals and pesticide residues – which can be passed on to the patient. A few are known to cause cancer in animals (Comfrey and Sassafras) or produce severe liver damage in humans (Ragwort or 'bush tea'). Ginseng, which is quite popular among a few M.E. patients, is reported to cause high blood pressure, breast development in men (it can affect hormone levels) and 'nervous irritability'. Its benefits are far from certain. (See medical reference 160).

The *British Medical Journal* also recently reported on several cases of severe liver damage (hepatitis) which had been caused by products containing a herb known as valerian. At the time, valerian was said to be present in over eighty different herbal medicines which were being promoted for their sedating effects – two of those mentioned by the Journal were Kalms and Neurelax (see medical reference 177).

More worrying are some of the herbs used by hakims – the traditional Indian herbalists who still treat many members of the Asian community. These imported herbs have been found to contain toxic substances such as lead, mercury, arsenic and even strychnine. They should certainly be avoided. Further details on the adverse effects of herbal medicines are contained in medical references listed on page 366.

Even so there is no dispute that many of these herbs do have genuine and beneficial pharmacological effects, which is why Evening Primrose oil (Efamol) merits some serious consideration.

Evening Primrose oil has become an increasingly popular treatment for a whole range of conditions, ranging from premenstrual tension to rheumatoid arthritis, atopic eczema and multiple sclerosis.

Evening Primrose oil comes from seeds of the shrub *Oenothera biennis.* It's usually combined with Vitamin E, which helps to preserve the effectiveness of the oil once inside the cells. The oil is rich in two essential fatty acids. These are known as essential because our bodies can't manufacture them, and we have to take them in the diet. It's thought that these fatty acids play a part in chemical pathways that eventually have an effect on the body's immune system and inflammation responses.

There's no doubt that Evening Primrose oil has a number of firm supporters in orthodox medicine, and trials have recently been carried out to compare its effectiveness in relieving the pain in arthritis with traditional pain killers. The results seem to show it can be just as effective. There's also some good evidence that it can help quite a lot in skin conditions like eczema. In patients who are experiencing joint pain this drug might well be worth trying, especially as it doesn't have any nasty side-effects.

In 1990, the results of a properly controlled clinical trial using supplements of Efamol Marine (a mixture of gamma-linolenic acid and eicosapentaenoic acid) were published (see medical reference 162). After 15 weeks 84 per cent of those who received a high dose of Efamol reported improvement compared to only 22 per cent in the placebo group. Those receiving the Efamol also noted a significant decrease in their palpitations and heart rhythm disturbances. The authors of this study speculated that the high dose of Efamol might be reducing the production of lymphokines such as interleukin, as well as correcting any deficit in body stores of essential fatty acids resulting from a chronic viral infection. (The patients in this clinical trial took four capsules of Efamol Marine morning and evening. Each capsule contains about 35 mg of GLA and 17 mg of EPA.)

The oil usually comes in capsule form (250 mgm or 500 mgm). It is available from pharmacies and health food stores under a variety of trade names, and is quite expensive. It has recently been made available on NHS prescription, but only for the treatment of eczema and cyclical breast pain.

Although Evening Primrose oil appears to be perfectly safe it can occasionally cause nausea, diarrhoea and headaches. It should be avoided by anyone with epilepsy.

Eleutherococcus Senticosus (ES) This is a ginseng supplement which comes from Russia. There, it is claimed to promote resistance to infections, conserve stress hormones produced by the adrenal glands, and even help in the treatment of cancer.

At the moment no proper clinical trials have been published using M.E. patients to assess both the alleged benefits and possible side-effects. Reported adverse reactions include palpitations, high blood pressure, headaches and insomnia (see medical reference 160).

Homeopathy

Homeopathy was developed by Dr Samuel Hahnemann nearly 200 years ago. It's based on the principle that 'like cures like', and involves the use of very dilute preparations, which in a healthy person would cause specific symptoms, but could cure the same symptoms in someone who was ill. For example, because scarlet fever resembles belladonna poisoning, a very dilute dose of belladonna would be used to treat scarlet fever.

Homeopathic medicines are usually made from natural sources such as plants, minerals or animal products. The remedy is made by a process called potentisation, so that as the original solution (the 'Mother Tincture') is made more dilute, its effect is increased. Conventional medical thinking finds it difficult to understand how such a product could then be beneficial in purely scientific terms, as there's almost nothing left in the final preparation, now so diluted.

Homeopaths tend to take an holistic approach to patients and their illnesses, and will adjust the treatment to each individual case. There's no one homeopathic remedy for something like M.E. Homeopathic treatment depends on you and your individual symptoms. It's not a do-it-yourself type of alternative therapy.

Homeopathic preparations appear to be perfectly safe and free from side-effects. Many M.E. patients make use of them and some claim to benefit.

If homeopathy is the type of alternative treatment that you would like to follow up, there are now several consultants who are willing to see M.E. patients both privately and on the NHS. Everyone is entitled to be referred to one of the NHS homeopathic hospitals or clinics in Glasgow, Bristol, Liverpool, London and Tunbridge Wells. For further details on these clinics and a homeopathic pharmacy in London see page 333. Details of a paper on homeopathic approaches to M.E. can be found in medical reference number 173.

Hypnosis

Hypnosis can't and won't 'cure' M.E., but for patients who are experiencing considerable degrees of anxiety and apprehension about particular symptoms, or the condition in general, it may be of help for relaxation, and in coming to terms with M.E., instead of fighting against it. So, it may be appropriate and helpful with some of the emotional difficulties encountered with M.E., or occasionally with a specific symptom such as chronic pain.

Do remember, though, that *hypnosis in the wrong hands can do a great deal of harm*, especially if it's inappropriately used for psychiatric problems like severe depression. This is one form of alternative therapy which can do harm, and if you're considering using this approach I'd strongly suggest discussing it with your own doctor first. Any M.E. patient should consult a medically qualified hypnotherapist, and certainly not one out of the Yellow Pages. An increasing number of general practitioners are using hypnotherapy in their practices. One of the partners in your own practice may be interested (see also page 333).

Iridology

Iridologists believe that by carefully examining the colour and structure of the iris (the coloured part of the eye that surrounds the pupil) they can detect ill health in almost any part of the body. They use the iris rather like a clock face in which each small segment corresponds to a particular organ or specific anatomical part of the body. Like most orthodox doctors I find these diagnostic claims to be extremely suspect, and to date no objective clinical trial has managed to support the theory behind iridology. *I cannot recommend it.*

Kutapressin

This is a drug which is given by intramuscular injection several times a week. It is currently being used in America, but I am not aware of its availability in the U.K. The active ingredients are a mixture of chemicals derived from pig's liver and amino acids. Kutapressin was originally developed for the treatment of various skin disorders back in the 1940s, and came about as a by-product from the manufacture of vitamin B12.

Doctors who use Kutapressin in the treatment of M.E. claim that it helps to restore imbalances in the immune system, and that it also has separate anti-viral effects. Interestingly, as far back as 1939, Kutapressin was being used as a treatment for neurasthenia – a condition which some doctors feel was very similar to M.E. It is also said to be effective in treating shingles.

Although this drug is anecdotally supposed to improve fatigue and reduce muscle or joint pains (but not mental impairment) there are, as yet, no published trials to back up these claims. *I would be reluctant to recommend its use until such trials have been carried out.* Further information on Kutapressin is contained in the CFIDS Chronicle, Spring/Summer 1990, pages 25–30.

Meditation

Some M.E. patients gain benefit from the way meditation can relax the body and mind. Meditation can take any form you like, from the type of relaxation techniques described on pages 177–8 to Christian meditation, transcendental meditation or Zen meditation. Meditation seems particularly appropriate for patients whose stressful life continually exerts a powerful negative effect on their body's ability to recover.

Probably the best-known meditation technique is transcendental meditation (TM), which was originally brought to wide public attention by the Maharishi Mahesh in the 1960s. TM is based on principles commonly used in India, and which probably date back to well before the time of Buddha, over 2,500 years ago. It involves spending periods of about twenty minutes, twice each day, sitting in a perfectly relaxed state in a quiet room, with eyes closed and breathing easily. The aim a quiet room, with eyes closed and breathing easily. The aim is to use the mind to settle and slow down the body, creating 'inner stillness', using a special repetitive technique called a mantra. This can be a sound, or a repeated word or phrase, which is specially chosen to suit that individual. Once started TM needs to be continued on a regular daily basis, as the effect is cumulative – it's not a one-off form of therapy.

There's no doubt that this form of 'mind over matter' can reduce the heart rate and blood pressure, and it's possible that these purely physical effects may in turn be producing beneficial psychological ones as well.

TM is quite an easy technique to acquire after you've been instructed by a trained teacher. This will usually involve going through a series of introductory talks, followed by individual sessions on the actual learning process. After that you can continue on your own. TM isn't an approach that will suit everyone, but I do know of several patients who claim to have found it helpful.

Naturopathy

This therapy aims to use the body's natural internal healing powers as a basis for recovery from ill health, and makes little use of external treatments. Naturopaths tend to regard their role as helping the patient to heal themselves – so they tend to pay much more attention to the individual than the disease.

Dietary modification, with the use of fresh and unprocessed food, is one of the most important recommendations in change of lifestyle, but herbal medicines, manipulation and massage may also be included.

Part of the process of coming to terms with, and recovering from M.E., involves making changes in lifestyle, and if a naturopath fully understands the condition, they may be able to help to offer some good advice. For how to find a naturopath, see page 336.

Osteopathy and chiropractic

Probably the commonest reason for patients consulting osteopaths is back pain, which is often related to problems with the bony vertebrae themselves or the structures which surround and support them – the muscles and ligaments.

The osteopath becomes skilled in detecting positional changes in the vertebrae, and the way that they move in relation to one another. Like the chiropractor he aims to correct these abnormalities, and hence the symptoms which occur as a result, although the practical approach of the osteopath is somewhat gentler. Both osteopaths and chiropractors first carry out a careful clinical examination, and may also make use of X-rays to exclude any conditions which could be worsened by manipulative techniques.

Many M.E. patients have back pains along with muscle spasm and pain, and if this seems to be unrelieved by conventional medical approaches these are therapies which might be worth considering. If you do have any sort of back pain it's very advisable to discuss the use of manipulative therapy with your general practitioner before going ahead. Back pain in an elderly patient with M.E. could be due to osteoporosis, in which case manipulation wouldn't be a good idea. Many general practitioners now accept osteopathy as a valid form of treatment – in fact many of them use it themselves for their bad backs, and a few have even become qualified osteopaths. Osteopathy, however, is not available on the NHS.

Qualified osteopaths have to complete a comprehensive training, and then conform to professional standards. Unfortunately, as in other forms of alternative treatment there are unqualified people calling themselves osteopaths, who may end up doing more harm than good. For how to find an osteopath, see page 337.

Chiropractors use a variety of manipulative techniques based on the assumption that the cause of symptoms such as back pain or referred nerve pain (e.g. sciatica down the leg) results from what they term 'misalignments' or subluxations of the spinal column. They believe that by correcting these misalignments they can then restore the normal anatomy, and so relieve the symptoms, be they due to muscle spasm, bone misplacement or pressure on the nerves as they pass out of the spaces between the vertebrae.

As with osteopathy this is a form of alternative treatment that is becoming increasingly respectable amongst orthodox medical opinion; a recently published trial in the *British Medical Journal* did appear to confirm its beneficial effects.

Unfortunately anybody can set up in practice and call themselves a chiropractor, and just like osteopathy in the wrong hands this can have its dangers. Registered and trained chiropractors belong to a professional organisation, and there are a few medically qualified ones. For how to find a chiropractor, see page 326.

Oxygen therapy

Various forms of oxygen therapy are now becoming available. In theory it all sounds very impressive – increasing the amount of vital oxygen into the tissues ought to help muscle and brain function, rejuvenate 'sick cells', and boost the immune system etc., etc.

One form of oxygen therapy being used in the U.K. involves the injection of dilute amounts of hydrogen peroxide (bleach) into the muscle.

In America you can now pay out £50 a visit for 'Ozone Treatment' (three molecules of oxygen). This involves withdrawing a pint of blood, adding ozone till the blood turns bright red and then re-infusing it! In practice, playing around with the body's natural physiology is not nearly so easy or simple.

Some people with M.E. are now joining up with multiple sclerosis patients who use hyperbaric oxygen chambers – oxygen at very high pressures. Despite the widespread claims that this is an effective treatment for M.S. (and M.E.) there is no good published evidence from the neurologists to support this assumption.

Stabilised oxygen (SO) is yet another form of oxygen treatment whereby drops are placed into drinking water to allegedly enhance body oxygen levels.

I am not yet convinced by any of these claims about the benefits of oxygen therapies, and I suspect that most of them are of no value whatsoever.

Probiotics

These are concentrated cultures of 'good bacteria' (e.g. lacto-bacillus) which, supposedly, help to restore the imbalance of gut organisms following anything from stress to excessively prescribed antibiotics.

In theory the approach has some attraction but it is very unlikely that the minute quantities used in a capsule could significantly reverse such a disturbance. *There is no evidence that people with M.E. have any such disturbance in their gut organisms.*

The unsavoury activities of one probiotic manufacturer, who was promoting these faecal organisms to vulnerable M.E. patients, led to an investigation by the Department of Health in 1989 (see medical reference 165). Nevertheless, many people with M.E. believe that such a disturbance exists and regularly take probiotics as part of their anti-candida regime. I do not believe that probiotics in this form have any useful role to play in M.E., and would not recommend their use.

Reflexology

Reflexologists claim that by examining the soles of the feet they can detect all manner of ill health. Each part of the sole is divided into separate zones which represent a particular organ or a different anatomical part of the body. For instance, the big toe is supposed to represent the head, brain and pituitary gland. Then, once a diagnosis has been made, reflexology claims that by the use of massage, blocked energy channels can be cleared in the organ or limb to restore normal health. *I would not recommend this approach for diagnostic purposes in M.E.*

Relaxation techniques

For anyone under stress, relaxation techniques (teaching your body how to relax) are a far wiser idea than taking tranquillisers like Valium. One of the easiest, and cheapest do-it-yourself methods is to follow the instructions on tapes which are available from various organisations – including *Relaxation for Living* and *Lifeskills* – see Useful Addresses.

Royal Jelly

This is an expensive mixture of vitamins, minerals, amino acids and a 'mystery ingredient' which is alleged to have almost miraculous healing properties for an endless list of ailments including M.E. Although many alternative practitioners are now recommending this product the results from the M.E. Action treatment survey (see page 225) are not very impressive. Royal Jelly doesn't seem to have any adverse effects, but *its benefits in M.E. are unproven*. The cost can vary enormously, and expensive brands do not confer any extra benefits.

Signalysis therapy

This is one of the more unusual of the new alternative therapies currently being aimed at people with M.E. Signalysis involves taking a sample of blood which is then heated to a high temperature. It is claimed that by carefully examining the resulting crystals under a microscope that 'problems in any area or organ can usually be identified before changes in the body can be detected'. An individual 'therapy' is then prepared which is alleged to stimulate the body's immune response. *Signalysis is not an approach that has been accepted by orthodox medical opinion in the UK.*

Yoga

This is an approach that combines spiritual, mental and physical training. The movements involve light exercises which are designed to be carried out slowly, and then the particular position is maintained for several minutes. The aim of yoga is to develop both flexibility and relaxation.

Yoga does seem to produce genuine benefits in people with

back pain, anxiety, high blood pressure, asthma and PMT. I'm not sure about its possible value in M.E., although I do know of a few people who have found yoga useful. If you decide to try this technique do make sure that you find a teacher who fully understands about this illness and is able to advise on the most appropriate type of movements. The wrong type of yoga could end up doing far more harm than good.

Conclusion

As you can see there's a bewildering choice of therapies on offer from the alternative health sector. Some do seem to be of help, whereas others are extremely dubious and a complete waste of time and money. This is one area of health care where the consumer has to carefully make up his or her own mind on the evidence that is available. If you want to find out more about any particular therapy you could contact The Institute of Complementary Medicine (see Useful Addresses). A full list of references to papers on various aspects of alternative therapies appears in the reference section (pages 358–9). If you're unlucky enough to be ripped off or harmed by an alternative form of therapy, it's worth contacting Healthwatch (see Useful Addresses) who are actively campaigning for so-called 'natural medicines' to be subjected to the same controls of safety and efficiency that apply to ordinary drugs.

Appendix

In 1990, ME Action conducted a survey into treatments which had been used by nearly 500 of their members. With kind permission, the results are reproduced below. Perhaps one of the most interesting and disturbing points to emerge concerns cost – the average amount of money spent in the private or alternative health sector amounted to nearly £900, with one person spending over £16,000! However, only 8 per cent felt that they had wasted their money, and 53 per cent considered that it had been a combination of money well spent and wasted. The remainder did not feel strongly one way or another.

Analysing the results it seems that these therapies fall into three distinct groups. At the top of the list are those which seem to benefit the majority of users. In the middle are a much larger group where, I have to say, the results suggest a strong placebo response. Down at the bottom are a selection of treatments (e.g.

Therapy

	Useful %	No effect %	Harmful % therapy %	Trying this	No. of answers
Rest	94.5	5.2	0.3	88.9	618
Hydrotherapy (warm baths etc.)	79.6	11.1	9.3	15.5	108
Relaxation techniques	79.5	20.2	0.3	49.1	341
Diet	73.2	24.1	2.7	80.1	557
Massage	64.2	17.6	18.1	29.4	204
Natural anti-candida t'ment	55.4	38.3	6.4	42.9	298
Healing	54.4	44.0	1.6	26.2	182
Aromatherapy	50.9	45.4	3.7	23.5	163
Antidepressants	49.4	22.9	27.7	48.3	336
Vitamins and Minerals	49.2	48.0	2.8	87.2	606
Colonic Irrigation	47.5	45.9	6.6	8.8	61
Enemas	47.4	39.5	13.2	5.5	38
EPD Allergy Desensitisation	47.0	42.2	10.8	11.9	83
Anti-candida drug therapy	46.5	37.9	15.6	36.8	256
Evening Primrose Oil (EFA's)	45.8	50.2	4.0	72.8	506
Probiotics (Acidophilus etc.)	43.4	50.0	6.6	43.5	302
Reflexology	43.2	40.9	15.9	19.0	132
Oxygen sleep apnoea t'ment	42.9	57.1	0.0	1.0	7
Homeopathy	42.1	48.1	9.8	45.4	316
Desensitisation	42.0	44.0	14.0	7.2	50
Herbal Remedies	40.8	51.8	7.3	35.3	245
Gamma Globulin	40.0	41.7	18.3	8.6	60
Acupuncture/Acupressure	40.8	48.7	10.5	27.5	191
Sleep treatment Charing X	33.3	50.0	16.7	0.9	6
Dental Amalgam Removal	32.7	60.0	7.3	7.9	55
Amino Acids	26.6	62.6	10.8	20.0	139
Germanium	18.9	64.9	16.2	21.3	148
Royal Jelly	15.3	73.0	11.7	44.2	307
Graded exercise programme	37.0	13.4	49.6★	18.3	127
Tranquillisers	36.6	23.2	40.2★	16.1	112
Fasting	32.9	22.4	44.7★	12.2	85
Steroid drugs	14.3	20.4	65.3★	7.1	49
Antibiotics	11.3	16.7	72.1★	29.4	204

Reproduced by kind permission of M.E. ACTION

steroids, tranquillisers and antibiotics) which almost everyone would agree should be avoided in M.E.

Hopefully, in due course, some of these alternative therapies can be subjected to properly controlled clinical trials to see if they really are of any value.

Allergy, Conventional and Alternative Concepts is a highly critical report on many of these approaches, particularly those dealing with allergies. It is available from the Royal College of Physicians, 11 St Andrew's Place, London NW1 4LE.

Part 3
LEARNING TO LIVE
WITH M.E.

1. Three Case Histories

Looking after a young child who has M.E.
by Rachael Glover's mother

At eight years of age my daughter Rachael was an outgoing, active and very cheerful child, who enjoyed ballet lessons, gymnastics and long country walks. At the crack of dawn she'd be up, singing around the house, and generally driving us all to distraction with her 'get up and go'. She loved school, and couldn't wait to get there each morning. She even wanted to go at the weekends! Alas, I didn't realise how precious a time it was for us, and I now look back on those eight short years as being Rachael's childhood. For she was then struck down, quite dramatically, with what our GP thought was glandular fever.

Rachael had swollen glands, a temperature and an ulcerated sore throat. She was racked with pain all over her body, and this continued for several weeks. However, all the blood tests came back as normal, so we were told to get her back to school as soon as possible.

As time went on her symptoms didn't seem to improve, so I asked for a referral to the local hospital. The consultant agreed with our GP's opinion and felt she would be fully better within three months, and to continue going to school. She went back, but was too weary to take part in the general activities, preferring to sit in a quiet corner. The teachers were convinced that she'd become used to being at home, and wouldn't accept my doubts and fears concerning her non-recovery.

Rachael would only be in school for a couple of days before collapsing with the return of all her previous symptoms. Even when she did manage to go she was never totally well, and this continued for two years. Daily living was never ever to be the same again for any of the family. We attempted to go on one of our favourite walks one Sunday, when she appeared to be a little brighter, but after only 300 yards she collapsed and had to be carried home. So started the awful lethargy which has since dominated her life.

One day, looking through the family snapshots, trying to amuse her, I was shocked to realise the drastic change which had occurred. Gone were the lovely rosy cheeks and bright eyes, only to be replaced by a deathly pallor and dark circles under the eyes. I took her back to the hospital where she had every conceivable blood test they could do, but in the end the advice was that she should pull herself together, and stop thinking of herself as being an invalid.

We returned to our GP, and this time asked for a second opinion at Great Ormond Street children's hospital, in London. There we were told that, yes, Rachael was poorly, but they didn't actually know what was the cause. The consultant said he'd come across children like this before, and that after a time they always made a recovery, but he didn't know what ailed them. He continued to see Rachael on a regular basis, and fully backed us up with, for example, countless letters to the school, and most important of all gave us lots of moral support. However, other doctors and teachers involved with Rachael continued to maintain that there was nothing much wrong with her.

As so often happens when one has almost given up hope, I turned on the radio one evening and found myself listening to Dr Shepherd talking about M.E. It hit me that this was exactly what Rachael was suffering from. I duly got in touch with the M.E. Association, and was put in touch with another doctor who was experienced in M.E. After listening to our story, examining Rachael, and further blood tests, it turned out that Rachael had a positive test for enterovirus in the blood, strongly supporting the diagnosis of M.E. The medical advice was that there was no 'cure', but with rest – both physical and mental –

she would eventually get over it. We felt a great relief that, at last, we'd got a diagnosis of what was wrong.

By now Rachael was starting to require a wheelchair to go any distance, and by the time of her last Christmas at junior school it was necessary to push her to the local church for the carol concert.

There were times of despair and one particularly awful night she said: 'Mummy, it would be kinder to gas me, than to let me suffer like this any longer.' I was shocked and so very sad for her. We had a little weep together, but I felt so angry that my child was having to suffer for so long in this way.

In the midst of all this the school decided to threaten us with prosecution for Rachael's constant non-attendance. This resulted in a meeting with the Chief Education Officer to try and sort out the mounting difficulties concerning Rachael's education, or rather the lack of it. At last we seemed to have someone who was totally on our side. Soon after the meeting a letter arrived from the school, not quite an apology, but near enough, plus a pile of kind letters from all the children in Rachael's class.

It was arranged for us to have the services of a home tutor, and the authority decided that Rachael should be 'statemented'. We'd never heard of this procedure before, so I contacted the group leader of CASE (Campaign for the Advancement of State Education), as well as the Advisory Centre for Education (see page 324) and received a lengthy reply – all very much in favour of the statementing procedure. Statementing is basically a legal term connected with the English 1981 Education Act. It's a means of assessing the educational requirements of a sick or disabled child. It highlights the needs or support the child requires, be it a home tutor, flexible school hours, tutor support whilst in school lessons, provision of wheelchairs and ramps, etc. It outlines virtually everything the child needs within the school environment.

The process involves meetings between medical representatives, teachers, a child psychologist from the education department, along with the parents. Written evidence can also be submitted. If the parents disagree with the findings there are procedures available to have decisions changed. When it's been decided exactly what help is required a 'statement' is then

prepared. When everyone is fully satisfied with this final statement it's placed with the local authority, who must carry out
all the recommendations, and make any necessary funds available. If the school doesn't comply with any of the required
tasks the authority can make it do so. In essence, it's well
worth having, and so far it's certainly been of great help to us.

A home tutor was provisionally allocated to Rachael for
five hours a week. This was more than enough, as she was
rarely well enough for more. The teacher was fully aware of
the problems created by M.E., and on the days when Rachael
was well enough they'd read stories, and sometimes play a board
game. Unfortunately, they rarely managed to accomplish much
real work as Rachael's concentration was so low. However, it
was nice for Rachael to have this type of company and help
– a lady who could be trusted not to push her beyond her
limitations. It also gave me the first chance in many months
to have an hour or so to myself.

Children with M.E. do require a great deal of help and
support when trying to return to school. Your child, like
mine, may have been extremely bright and able prior to M.E.,
but now with concentration difficulties and muscle fatigue to
contend with, they may find themselves increasingly forced into
the situation where they need a statement in order to receive the
requisite help.

In September 1987 Rachael joined her new secondary school,
although she didn't actually make her first appearance until February 1988. The school was our choice, even before it became
obvious that she now had very specific needs. It's well known
in the area for its high standards of education, coupled with a
strong belief in caring for less fortunate pupils, who find the
staff helpful and sympathetic to their needs. The school has
ramps, a lift and other adaptations for pupils with disabilities.
At present there are six children who need these aids. Disabled
children are encouraged to take part in all aspects of school life
wherever possible, but if, like Rachel, rest is the name of the
game, they go to great lengths to make sure that they don't
overdo things.

By Christmas 1987, Rachael had been ill for four years.
She hadn't yet met her classmates, but the children sent her

a massive pile of beautifully written letters, jokes and stories. They said that the teacher and matron had often talked about her, so they felt they already knew Rachael, and looked forward to the day when she'd be well enough to join them. Girls had already volunteered to push her chair and be helpers. Needless to say this was all received with much joy, and she started to look forward to being well enough to be able to go next term.

As her health gradually improved I left it entirely up to Rachael to decide when to start her first day. In January she proudly hung up her new school uniform on the wardrobe door, and began to collect her pens and equipment together for the big day. We had a few false starts, but by mid-February she felt well enough to go for one lesson per day. I took her to school by car, and she was pushed in her wheelchair to meet the new classmates.

After that one short visit she was exhausted, and lay on the settee for the rest of the day. In the first week she only managed the one lesson, but after that she gradually built things up, until she was actually staying for school lunches with her new-found friends – always the same baked beans and chips, but who cares! – then home to rest. Suddenly she was a different girl, starting to feel a bit better day by day, and taking an interest in life again.

For me, this had been a very difficult time, having to stand back and watch her first few tentative steps, wanting to stop her from doing too much, but realising how important it was for her to learn for herself. It wasn't long before she'd actually accomplished three weeks of full-time schooling. There was nothing stopping her now. I'd hold my breath and clamp my lips firmly shut as she played in the garden with her friends, running to and fro. However, by bedtime one evening, the results of all this new activity were beginning to show. After a restless night she awoke once again with swollen glands, and feeling very low. I must say, though, she didn't get as unwell as I'd feared, and she didn't slip back too far. Recovering from M.E. can be two steps forward and one step back. Her level of activity – both physical and mental – was still obviously at a much reduced level, but a year earlier I had truly believed that my daughter had no future at all.

Her teachers have given her wonderful reports: 'keen, willing to work and a pleasure to teach' are all music to my ears. She still has to have a home tutor to sit with her for some lessons, as well as help from a welfare assistant during craft lessons. And instead of P.E., she spends time with the matron doing gentle exercises.

Rachael is now twelve-and-a-half years old, and is still painfully thin and frail. She gets tired very quickly, and has to rely heavily on her wheelchair to get around outside the house. The local school for the handicapped have a warm pool, and they've kindly agreed to let Rachael use it for half an hour each week. She just goes and lies in the water, and the physiotherapist gives her some gentle exercises in the pool. She is getting better, improving slowly day by day, and one day I'm sure that all of this will just be a painful memory.

I don't think that children of Rachael's age can ever come to terms with an illness of this magnitude – neither can many adults. She accepts that she has a strange disease, and is heartily sick and tired of it, but she still refuses to take any interest in it. The only time she'll put herself out to discuss M.E. is if she hears of another child going through black days with it, and then she tries to help them feel a bit better. She no longer plans ahead; she just says she'll see how she feels on the day before deciding what to do. She used to cry a lot, but now she tries to laugh things off by saying that it's 'only the bugs' which are bothering her. Until quite recently she didn't like to talk about her future aspirations, but now she talks about doing 'something with computers', so she's obviously feeling much more confident about the future.

The financial pressures on the family have been quite considerable during the course of Rachael's illness, especially at a time when I'd planned to return to full-time employment again. This I had to forego in order to be at home to look after Rachael. In view of her quite severe disability we applied for both an Attendance Allowance and a Mobility Allowance. Since then, like so many others, we've had to endure the full bureaucratic nightmare of the DSS system. The examining doctor for Rachael's Mobility Allowance wrote that she fulfilled the requirements, as the exertion required to walk exacerbated her illness. However, it then came as a shock to find this had been turned down by the authorities, who make the final decision. We decided to appeal, but the next doctor decided she was perfectly able to walk the required distance. The next stage is an appeal to the tribunal, but when you're physically and mentally worn down by caring for someone the last thing you want (or are capable of) is fighting for benefits. I've found a welfare rights worker, attached to the Benefits Unit of the town hall. They help prepare your case, and will even attend the tribunal with you.

As for the family, Rachael's illness has taken its toll on us all. Our youngest daughter, Emma, just eleven, has missed out more than anyone else on holidays, trips out, picnics, etc. Most of the time she's been uncomplaining, but just occasionally she would get bitterly upset and jealous about the disproportionate amount of attention Rachael was getting. Fortunately I'm now in a position to be able to spend more time with Emma, and am trying to mend the damage. But, just like Rachael, these precious years can never be replaced. It's not been quite the same for my sons, and Ben, who's now seventeen, is happy with his own friends away at college.

M.E. has taught us many things: first and foremost to take each day as it comes. If your child can't eat, sleep or whatever, don't worry – maybe they will tomorrow. When, as undoubtedly they will, your child begins to start taking the first tentative steps back to normal life, learn to stand back, as they've now got to find their own level of activity, and learn to have control over their own lives again.

Ignorance of this disease has only made Rachael's suffering worse, and I think the illness has lasted longer as a result. If only I'd known at the beginning what I know now, I think I could have handled things much more easily. Complete bed rest from the onset would, I believe, have significantly aided her recovery.

Believe, really believe, deep in your heart, that your own child can and will get better from M.E. It happens slowly but surely – just you wait and see.

Children and young people with M.E. – author's note

M.E. is not an illness that often affects children, although an increasing number of cases are being recognised – some as young as seven. There are also occasional outbreaks in schools and one recently occurred in Cambridgeshire.

As Rachael's case illustrates, children with M.E. present their own special problems. These include difficulties in obtaining the correct diagnosis, conflicting and sometimes harmful advice about management, and battles with education authorities over schooling.

Parents also face their own unique difficulties. Instead of receiving help and support from doctors and other caring agencies, they may have to pursue a series of battles on behalf of their sick child. They, too, can easily end up feeling isolated and bitter with the very professionals who are supposed to help.

Symptoms in children are generally similar to those seen in adults with fatigue and sometimes very severe muscle pain (myalgia) being the key features. Disturbances in sleep pattern can be pronounced with the child asleep during the day and then awake for most of the night. This sleep reversal is often accompanied by nightmares and irritability. Professor Behan has also noted that some boys develop difficulties in passing urine. Children with M.E. may lose a significant amount of weight early on, and occasionally this progresses on to true anorexia. After prolonged immobility in bed there is a real danger of muscle wasting and contractures occurring.

Diagnosis All too often these children are misdiagnosed as being hysterical, malingering or school refusers. The result is that the child is then dramatically forced back into full-time schooling and plenty of physical exercise (the 'in at the deep end' approach) which produces a rapid deterioration in both physical and emotional symptoms.

Some paediatricians and child psychiatrists still maintain that M.E. does not exist in children, or if it does it is nothing more than a short-lived period of postviral debility. Fortunately, a growing number are now accepting that, although rare, M.E. can present in this age group, and that for recovery to occur the doctor must take into account the physical, social and emotional factors that form a complex interrelationship in childhood M.E.

In the case of children I think it is essential that the diagnosis is confirmed by a paediatrician who understands the illness. He or she should then take an active role in co-ordinating all aspects of management.

Any good paediatrician will ensure that other treatable causes of chronic fatigue are excluded, including infectious diseases and blood disorders. In this respect I well remember the story of a child from Devon whose case was presented to a meeting on M.E. at the Great Ormond Street children's hospital. The boy had initially been diagnosed as having M.E., then, as having myasthenia gravis, before being properly assessed at this hospital. It turned out that he had a chronic infection called Lyme disease (see page 119) which was successfully treated with antibiotics.

One other advantage of having support from a paediatrician is when it comes to any problems with schools or refusal of DSS benefits. Remember, if you are not happy with a specialist's opinion, or if you are told that it cannot be M.E. because it does not occur in children, you can ask for a second opinion from another paediatrician.

Management Once again, the broad principles are not much different to those with adults, taking into account the fact that children have their own emotional, practical and education problems. Striking the right balance with rest and exercise, sleep, mental activity and good nutrition are probably the most important aspects of any recovery process. It's also important to remain optimistic about the chances of recovery whilst at the same time being realistic about the pace at which this will occur.

A period of bed rest may well be beneficial in the early stages, but following this, rest and exercise need to be carefully balanced. On the one hand there is a very real danger that prolonged immobility will result in further weakness, wasting and even contractures. On the other there is no doubt that when children do start to recover, there is a great temptation to suddenly start doing too much and precipitate a relapse. If children learn to pace themselves, both physically and mentally, they should be able to build on their progress, which in turn will have a very beneficial effect on self-confidence.

Children's appetites tend to decline rapidly when they are ill and this is especially so in M.E. Although it's never a good idea to make a great issue over meals or eating habits, I would recommend that their diet contains good quality carbohydrate, protein and an adequate fluid intake. If the diet really does become very 'faddy', then a mineral and vitamin supplement is advisable.

Drugs, I feel, should be prescribed as little as possible in the case of children; antidepressants have a very limited role in this group of patients.

It is also worth remembering that some of the DSS sickness and disability benefits mentioned later also apply to children; although obtaining them may involve yet another series of battles with the authorities.

Emotional and social For a child, any kind of unexplained illness that produces such a devastating effect on all aspects of their life is bound to be a frightening experience. So, just like adults, they need to be given some form of simple explanation about how it can sometimes take the body rather a long time to recover from an infection. They also need constant reassurance that although things may look very bleak at the moment there is a good chance that, given time, they will recover and start leading a normal life again.

The sudden loss of mobility, friendships and self-confidence can all mount up and have a severe effect on a child's emotional feelings. That's why it's important to make sure that close friends are still encouraged to keep in touch; that occasional trips outside the house are organised; and that some new non-active interests are encouraged. For some children a small pet might become a very welcome companion; others find keeping in touch with friends by phone or letter very useful.

Occasionally, these emotional and depressive aspects of the illness can end up having a very negative effect on recovery. Some children develop a clinging dependency on their parents, who in turn become over-protective and unduly cautious about altering the child's routine regarding exercise or return to school. Even though the physical side may be improving, the child becomes trapped by the psychological aspects of such a long-term illness. In this case the vicious circle needs to be broken in a firm but fair manner. If this is done correctly, the child can turn the corner and start to make a significant degree of recovery. They will require a great deal of encouragement to slowly start joining in all aspects of family life. This could involve coming downstairs for just a short period each day for a meal or to watch television, and then gradually increasing both physical and mental activity inside the home environment.

Unfortunately, at the other end of the spectrum, there are cases of very ill children in which the local authorities have decided to use a Place of Safety Order to separate the child from what they regard as 'over-involved' parents. This is then followed by compulsory admission to hospital where family visiting is deliberately limited and treatment may involve controversial forms of behaviour therapy and strenuous physiotherapy. The latter may turn out to be totally inappropriate and lead to a further deterioration in the child's condition.

Should this situation arise, I would suggest that a second opinion from a consultant with experience in M.E. should be requested. Secondly, legal advice from a solicitor who is well-acquainted with the law as it affects children should be sought urgently. The child may end up being made a ward of court.

Schooling and further education All too often children and young people with M.E. are being denied proper educational opportunities because of their illness. Those who are still too unwell to even make a small journey back to school may be denied home tuition because the authorities fear that it will encourage 'sick role behaviour' and cause a further delay in a return to school. Older children and teenagers may find that they have lost too much coursework to go back and complete A level courses; and some colleges and universities have been far from sympathetic when students have missed more than a couple of terms. Others, however, have bent over backwards to try and help by rescheduling exams and keeping a university place open for several years.

This is why it is so important to find a doctor who is

prepared to fully support the child and liaise on their behalf
with the school or college. There should then be no difficulties
with medical officers over suspected school refusals; and they
may well be able to persuade a college to hold open a place for
a further year.

Planning a return to school can be one of the most difficult
aspects of management in children. Ideally, this should involve
the family doctor, the education welfare officer, the teachers
and possibly a child psychologist if there has been a prolonged
absence. Careful advance planning needs to include transport
arrangements; avoidance of exam pressures; and, initially, being
very flexible about the actual amount of time spent in lessons. A
sudden return to full-time education is likely to be unrealistic.

Where the child still has significant physical disabilities (e.g.
uses a wheelchair), the statementing procedure (a statement of
special educational needs), described in Rachael's story, may be
very helpful.

If you are having problems with the educational authorities, it
is well worth contacting an educational welfare officer (EWO). If
this fails, write to the Chair of the Education Authority, sending
a copy to your M.P.

If home tuition is refused, you can write to the civil servant
responsible for home tuition at the Department of Education and
Science in London. Further detailed information on education
is contained in the M.E. Association's booklet 'Guidelines for
parents of children with M.E.'.

The good news is that children with M.E. do recover but
it may take a considerable amount of time; and you're likely
to receive much conflicting advice along the way. The M.E.
Association has also set up a working party with a mandate
to look into all the needs of children with M.E. Overall, the
attitude of doctors and officialdom does seem to be slowly
improving.

Medical papers which have been published on the subject
of childhood M.E. can be found on pages 347–8.

Pregnancy and M.E.
by Frances H. Woodward

I had been suffering from M.E. for two and a half years before we decided to have a baby. It was a very difficult decision to make because, at that time, my 'vertical hours' averaged only about five or six a day. My best time was, and still is, in the mornings. I would get up and potter around doing small jobs but by early afternoon I would start to fade away and for the rest of the time I was in bed. So my daily routine was not exactly congenial to having a baby.

One factor which encouraged us was that my condition was gradually improving. I'd had quite a dramatic start to my illness when, in March 1982, I had viral meningitis. I was in hospital for a week, and then in bed at home for several weeks. During the following months I suffered extreme fatigue: sometimes brushing my teeth was all I could manage before having to go back to bed. My doctor said that it was a slow recovery from meningitis, but I knew there was something else wrong with me. I was experiencing more and more symptoms: muscle pain, back and neck pains, head pressure, difficulty in walking and extreme fatigue. After almost a year I was eventually sent to a neurologist and he diagnosed benign myalgic encephalomyelitis. I couldn't believe there was an illness with such a long name and thought I would never remember it! I was, in fact, greatly relieved that what I was feeling had a name.

I immediately joined the M.E. Association and discovered the importance of rest and sleep. Instead of trying to push myself to do things, I established a new daily routine. I would get up in the mornings, at first for only one or two hours and then return to bed. Gradually, over the next year or so, I increased those vertical hours to five or six.

My husband and I had always wanted children and were anxious that this debilitating disease might prevent it. My GP and the specialist had suggested it would not be a good idea. However, in May 1984, we asked the advice of Dr Smith, the M.E. Association Medical Advisor. His advice was what we wanted to hear. If we really wanted children then life without them may make us unhappy and discontent. It was better to go ahead, being fully aware of the problems and with the provision of plenty of help.

When my pregnancy was confirmed, in January 1985, I really became very anxious about whether our decision had been wise. I wrote to Dr Smith for reassurance and also to another M.E. patient who had had a baby. Her letter boosted my morale as she was coping well and was, in fact, expecting her second child.

My first visit to the hospital was interesting because, at that time, little was known about M.E. The nurses and midwives were all interested to know how the disease affected me, were sympathetic in their manner and admired our decision to battle against the odds and have a baby. The gynaecologist had little experience of M.E. but suspected that I would cope all right with the first stage of labour but might have a problem in the second stage and be incapable of pushing. As I was thirty-seven, he recommended an amniocentesis which I had at sixteen weeks. My stomach was sore and uncomfortable for a week afterwards and I found it difficult to stand upright. Presumably this was because with M.E. the muscles are particularly tender and take longer to recover. Anyway, three weeks later the results came through as clear, so all was well.

I think having M.E. prepared me quite well for the aches and pains of pregnancy. In fact, the slight and temporary discomfort seemed mild compared to the long-term and severe pain and fatigue of M.E. I was used to resting and pacing myself – other people have to learn to do that while pregnant. Gradually, however, over the nine months, my M.E. symptoms eased. The acute pains I suffered in my neck, head, back and arms seemed to be duller but the major relief I had was the fading of that awful 'ill' feeling. My head cleared, and although I still get pressure in my head, that mental numbness which was constantly with me disappeared. I felt almost part of the real world; almost a real person instead of a zombie!

I must explain here that all during my pregnancy I was having acupuncture. I had started a course of treatment about three months before I became pregnant, in an anxious attempt to do something positive to help myself. It is difficult to judge which made me feel better – pregnancy or acupuncture – but I am inclined to attribute the growing feeling of well being to pregnancy and the more specific relief of things such as heart palpitations and nerve pains to acupuncture. These two problems were very severe before I started acupuncture and were starting to decline before I became pregnant. Even though I am no longer having acupuncture, they have never returned with such severity.

During the later weeks of pregnancy we discussed with the consultant the possibility of a Caesarean if labour became too much for me. General anaesthetic can worsen M.E. symptoms so it was decided that an epidural Caesarean would be our best option.

I thoroughly enjoyed my pregnancy. Not only was I relieved of some of my symptoms but I developed a sense of purpose. Previously I had felt worthless, now I had something to live for.

In August 1985, our daughter Anna was born. As the consultant predicted, I could cope with the first stage of labour, but by the second stage I was completely exhausted. I had no urge to push and no strength to push either. It was decided to use forceps. Anna was very solid (8½ lb) and needed tremendous tugging to get her into the world – an experience I would not want to endure again!

The nurses on the ward were marvellous. I had been in labour for seventeen hours and was totally exhausted. I could not walk for about twenty-four hours and during that time they brought me bed pans and gave me bed baths. When Anna cried a nurse would give her to me to feed and then return her to her cot to save me the effort. My arms were too weak to hold her so I fed her lying down. At night the babies were taken to the nursery and mothers were woken to go and feed their babies there. I did not have to do that. A nurse would bring Anna to me, return to change sides and then return again to take her back to the nursery. This was such a help to me, and whenever I expressed my appreciation they merely said that's what they were there for. I was touched by their kindness and regard for my problems. One sister even stayed on duty late one night in order to show my husband how to change a nappy and bath the baby. She had realised that he would be doing much of the caring when we got home, and took it upon herself to teach him. We really appreciated her concern.

I stayed in hospital for six days after the birth before I felt strong enough to go home. My husband took the first week off work and then my mother came for a week so it was a little while before I had to cope on my own.

We had decided that my limited energy should be concentrated on Anna and looking after her. We employed a cleaner to do the housework and a child minder to have Anna for two afternoons or whenever I needed a rest. We installed such labour saving devices as a microwave, a tumble drier and a dishwasher. I used disposable nappies to save time and effort. I could not have coped with carrying a nappy bucket, let alone washing and drying them. I find hanging clothes on the line difficult and still only put them out if it's a perfect day. There's nothing worse than having the effort of bringing clothes in, because of rain, before your arms have recovered from putting them out. If I am having a bad day or there is a hint of rain I use the tumble drier.

I found breast feeding worked well for me. Those who prefer to bottle feed have the advantage that other people can help – especially at night. However, I enjoyed breast feeding and found it very relaxing. My arms were weak and my back prone to spasm, so I lay down to feed Anna, which was restful for me and cosy and comfortable for us both.

To save my arms I would lift Anna and then sit down so her weight was supported on my lap. If she needed cuddling at length I would wear a baby carrier. I bought a second-hand carry cot which was left permanently in the car, so that I only had Anna to carry in and out – not a carry cot as well. To save my back and leg muscles I had two sets of changing equipment, one upstairs and one downstairs, with the mat at table height to save bending. I only ever tried to do one task a day, apart from caring for Anna. I would see a friend, or do a little shopping, or go to the clinic, all on different days.

My husband helped with the more strenuous daily tasks. He would empty the nappy bucket (used for disposables), put out or bring in washing, do ironing, empty the dishwasher, push the shopping trolley and often cook the meal. His main daily task was bathing Anna. I found it impossible to bend forward and hold her, so bath time was his time.

Motherhood with M.E. would be virtually impossible without a sensitive and willing partner. My husband has been indispensable in the caring for Anna. As well as all the daily tasks he helps with, every Saturday and Sunday afternoon he takes over completely while I go to bed and rest.

Although having a baby is hard work and often very tiring, the rewards far outweigh the difficulties. Anna has brought joy to our lives. She has given me an aim in life and stopped me focusing my attention on myself. When I'm in pain or feeling down, her smile uplifts me and a cuddle makes it all worthwhile.

We are so glad that we risked the consequences of having a baby. Not all people with M.E. have experienced the relief of symptoms during pregnancy, but I'm sure they will all agree that life with a baby is a reward to be treasured.

Pregnancy and M.E. – author's note

I now know of several women, like Frances, who have decided to start a family in the course of their illness. However, this is a decision which must never be taken without a great deal of thought and careful advance planning.

For many women the onset or continuation of M.E. into their mid-thirties means that they face the inevitable problem of steadily decreasing fertility. In purely practical terms they may soon lose the option of ever becoming pregnant. Even so, I would not advise anyone with M.E. to contemplate pregnancy until their condition has significantly improved or remained stable for at least a year. If time is on your side then it is far better to wait till you are well on the road to recovery.

Ideally, any pregnancy should also be planned to avoid giving birth during the late autumn and winter months when infections are far more common, and the cold weather is making you feel less well. For anyone who does decide to go ahead and become pregnant, two important questions will inevitably pass through your mind.

Firstly, what effect does pregnancy have on M.E.? In my experience about 75 per cent of women notice an improvement in their general health, sometimes quite significantly. This type of improvement also occurs in several other conditions, including rheumatoid arthritis, where there is also an immune component. The precise reasons are uncertain but are probably connected with changes in the levels of the various sex hormones, as well as the partial suppression of the immune system which helps to prevent the fetus being rejected. However, I must emphasise that a significant minority of women will find that pregnancy causes an actual *deterioration* in their M.E., so it should never be viewed as a way of trying to get better.

The real practical problems tend to arise at the end of the nine months and during labour. So, you must inform the midwives and doctors about M.E. (although they will probably know very little about the subject) because labour is likely to be very exhausting and you may need additional help.

Once you are back home again, looking after a newborn baby will become very demanding – both physically and mentally. Arranging family and social support to help you cope must be planned well in advance. It's also important to remember that otherwise healthy women commonly experience fatigue and emotional changes during this period which are once again related to changes in the hormone levels. These problems may be even more pronounced in someone with M.E.; especially if they have had any form of depressive illness in the past.

As far as the baby is concerned, breast feeding has many advantages, including the fact that it's an excellent way of transferring vital antibodies. On the other hand, bottle feeding will provide your partner with the opportunity to become actively involved as well as taking some of the strain away from night time feeding.

The second important question is whether a mother's M.E. presents any risks to the unborn child. As far as miscarriage is concerned, we know that 10–20 per cent of all pregnancies end this way; but there is no published evidence to suggest that this is any higher in M.E. There is, however, a *theoretical possibility* that a persisting enteroviral infection could be passed to the fetus. At the moment the degree of any such risk is very difficult to assess. I know of several women with M.E. who, like Frances, have all gone on to produce perfectly healthy babies. I am also aware of a couple of cases where the baby has failed to thrive and no obvious cause has been found. Here, the possibility of transmission of a virus during early development cannot be discounted. This is obviously an area where accurate data needs to be collected from all women who become pregnant during the course of their illness.

Any final decision on pregnancy is bound to be influenced by a number of factors – your social circumstances, your age, and above all, your current state of health. Before going ahead with such a major decision I would strongly advise discussing this with your family doctor, as well as another woman with M.E. who has been through pregnancy and knows all the benefits and problems at first hand.

M.E. and the single person
by 'Sue'

Perhaps the first thing to say is that coping with M.E., whatever your circumstances – alone, with a partner, with children or other dependants – is made a good deal easier once a diagnosis has been made, especially if one's nearest and dearest can then understand what is happening and are able to be supportive. It cannot be stressed enough, to anyone reading this who may have M.E., or who knows someone who may have it: seek out a consultant and get a diagnosis. To anyone with M.E. it makes a world of difference just knowing what the matter is. It means that your self-esteem doesn't take such a knock, and that you don't go making things worse. No more feeling 'I should be able to do this so easily. Why can't I?', and no more pushing beyond personal limits. One can then take account of the illness in practical planning from day to day. So much of the secret of dealing with M.E. is illness management – but first you have to know the beast you're dealing with.

I write as someone who has had the syndrome for the best part of twenty-five years. It started in my teens, and I am forty now. I have only known what is wrong with me for three of those years. My illness has followed a chronic relapsing/remitting course, with about five prolonged, major outbreaks and never quite feeling 'well' in between-times. For years, I've alternated between saying to myself, 'Oh, this is just how I am. Not much stamina. Always tired. Often ill,' and asking, 'Do other people ever feel like this, and so often? Surely there must be something fundamentally wrong with me?' Now I know!

For part of my twenty-five 'M.E. years' I was married. So, in writing about coping with M.E. now, as a person who lives on her own, I can also look back and compare lifestyles. Such comparisons are difficult, however, because the major difference between previous years and now is not between being married and being single, but between not knowing and knowing what is wrong. My basic message would be that coping with M.E. has its good and bad, its difficult and easier bits, irrespective of your personal situation. The great divide lies between before and after diagnosis.

Once that diagnosis has been made, the next hurdle is acceptance, and learning to live within your limitations. Glibly said. At first, and perhaps for some time, there will be trial and error. You have to find out what you can do, and when to stop, to prevent a relapse. One way in which living alone can be a real boon, is that it's so much easier to leave tasks half-done, to be flexible, and alter a set routine, if you don't have a family to look after, or anyone else to take daily account of. Conversely, of course, there is no one there to help either. Shopping, cooking, cleaning, washing and all the other household chores have to be managed, spaced out between periods of rest. Forward-planning has to be done with military precision.

If someone with M.E. lives alone there are several things that make life a bit easier. First, friends can be persuaded to form a rota to do basic tasks. If that is difficult to organise, or if a sufferer prefers to seek out voluntary help on a less personal basis, then most towns have a Council for Voluntary Service, and some have a university or a polytechnic where students may have formed a 'caring group'. Or use your local church if you have one. A phone call to any one of these places can produce a team of helpers. The key is not to be afraid to ask for help, not to be deterred by apparent rebuffs, and to keep on asking until you do succeed.

For shopping, be on the look-out for firms that will deliver, and large stores that operate special bus services often door-to-door. Some health-food stores in particular offer delivery services. Ask around, and don't hesitate to make your special needs clear. You may find – especially with a health-food store – that many customers have problems with carrying their supplies, and just one query can trigger the start of a delivery service. Also, find out if your area operates a dial-a-ride system for the disabled. Contact the Disability Unit of the council, the Passenger Transport Authority and/or social services. If there is nothing – ask for one! It can help, not just with shopping, but with any trips that you have to make.

To take the best advantage of bulk-shopping a small freezer is invaluable for single people. I find it is also useful for 'bulk cooking' if and when I feel like it (and a food processor is also a boon). And I always make sure that, along with a well-stocked freezer, plenty of fresh fruit and vegetables, and all the healthy, yeast-free foods, I also have convenience foods and a range of items that are easy to prepare. Then I am ready for the bad days, because I know that however careful I am, there will be relapses.

If, like me, you have a lot of muscle problems, or arthritis, or heart problems; or if you just have the whole syndrome badly, and are more often 'flat out' than not, then do not hesitate to apply for a home help too. I have one who just does the vacuum-cleaning. The rest I can manage without too much damage, but vacuuming takes me ages, is very painful, and finishes me off afterwards, for days. In other words: choose carefully what you can do without ill effect, and follow up all channels of possible help for what you can't do. Contact with the home help section of your nearest social services office is also likely to produce an initial visit from a social worker, along with the home help organiser. This can be a helpful contact to have in reserve for if the going gets really rough and extra help (meals-on-wheels, household aids and so on) is needed.

Once you have your basic routine and regular sources of help all sorted out, it is also good to work out, *in advance*, ways of coping with times of crisis – when you feel so ill you think you're dying, and can't do a thing for yourself. If you can, get yourself an emergency 'back-up team', using the kinds of resources and techniques described above: friends, various volunteers, home help, social services. Make it clear to these people in advance what your requirements will be if you do have a long period of bad relapse: meals cooked, washing done, all the shopping and so on. Divide out the tasks, so that people are prepared to take on whatever they can best cope with. Get it all sorted out when you are having a reasonably good patch, and so have your 'emergency services' at the ready for when you are most decidedly not. Just the knowledge that you have such a team of people to call on can be a great security blanket. Likewise, being on the telephone is a great comfort, especially with an extension by the bed. If you can't afford the luxury of a telephone, investigate whether your local council offers financial help with a phone for those in special need.

If you feel too ill to remain at home during a relapse, a referral from your GP to a local consultant and a hospital admission for short-term bed rest and nursing can be invaluable. If that can't be achieved, then another possibility to consider is going on a 'retreat', if necessary using the Ambulance Service to get there and back! Some religious orders offer board and lodging irrespective of one's beliefs or denomination. It can be a good way of obtaining rest and being looked after, if friends or relations can't produce a short-term place to stay, and if there is no hospital bed in time of crisis. Ideally, however, a good back-up team will make it possible to remain at home even during the worst of a relapse.

For M.E. patients living alone, perhaps the worst problems actually start when both the routine mechanics of life and crisis management have been sorted out. All too often the illness leaves one with just enough energy to cope with basic survival, and no more. But what of work, social life and hobbies? What indeed!

My current bout of M.E. has been my worst ever: really quite bad for about six years, though I am now, slowly, getting better. I have had to stop work (I get Invalidity Benefit) and have now reconciled myself to not being able to do my old job again. It is too hectic, too physically, emotionally and mentally demanding. Work has always been a major part of my life and a large chunk of my identity, and not being able to continue has been a considerable loss. And yet, changing my perspective in this regard, looking at new ways in which I can value myself and enjoy being alive, without such a work-centred existence has been a very productive experience. Many M.E. patients have a 'work-centred' outlook – we are often busy, energetic kinds of people.

Those of us who live on our own are perhaps even more likely to put a lot into our work. However, if stopped in our tracks by M.E. we are also the lucky ones, because we have an opportunity to try to reorientate ourselves without the added worry of letting our families down. We can apply for benefit, and, after a period of adjustment, can come to enjoy a more balanced lifestyle. Perhaps, eventually, we can find a less demanding job, if well enough. I am not saying that giving up on work is an easy process. It requires a lot of effort to change a lifetime's habit. But it can be a process that offers its own rewards – and professional help is obtainable if necessary to assist in making the adjustment. (Ask your GP for a referral to a psychologist; seek out local counselling services, again via your GP; or, if that fails, your local Community Health Council.)

If one can continue at work, then it is essential to be quite up-front about what is going on. If people know about the M.E. many will understand, make allowances and be supportive. Job-sharing, going temporarily part-time, working from home, can all be discussed as possible solutions to the difficulties presented by the illness. But first, before they can help, people have to know what it is they are dealing with.

And then what of the rest of life? For those of us who have the illness badly that has to be very restricted too. Often the M.E. patient who is a little less ill, and so able to carry on working, is too exhausted to do anything else. There is no energy left for friends, going out: all the things that normally get taken for granted, and that make it good to be alive. And, all too easily, friendships fall away, people lose touch, and the person living on his/her own becomes increasingly isolated. So, what to do?

Once again, it helps to be well-organised and not backward in announcing one's needs loud and clear. I try to take the initiative most of the time in organising visits to and from friends, and other social events, so that I have control of when I do things, and can plan surrounding time accordingly. I discourage chance visits because I find I have to keep a strict control on the energy I put out each day. One unexpected caller can drain resources, easily overload a day, and set me back, for several days. However, I find that it is sometimes essential to remind myself that having control over my contact with others is how I want it to be. The temptation can be to 'bleat' if people, out of consideration for my needs, do not take the initiative to contact me! One can't have it both ways!

Despite all the problems, the illness can have a positive effect on social life. It doesn't just illustrate who friends really are, but also forces one to reassess the bases of friendships – what one values friends for and vice versa. Friends can play an important part, too, in broadening out one's life beyond the confines of M.E. This is particularly essential for those living alone. Often,·I think, this is an easier role for friends to play than asking them to be a sympathetic ear about the illness itself. For anyone on their own it is perhaps particularly difficult to share the various facets of the illness with others, because so few people see us at our worst. Most, therefore, will not know what the whole syndrome is really like. (At our worst we are often stuck behind closed doors, and usually alone.) So, for anyone alone, perhaps the best people to turn to to discuss the illness are others in similar circumstances. The 'Singles' Group run by those members of the M.E. Association who are living alone can be of particular help here.

Useful though friends and acquaintances can be, the bedrock of being able to deal with the illness successfully has to lie inside yourself. It is necessary, if possible, to develop a sense of self-value and enjoyment of your own company, of small details, the daily minutiae of life, that can be savoured on your own: having a few plants and watching them grow; a beautiful picture to look at; a tree outside, and so on. I suppose it is a bit like holding an individual glass bead up to the light, turning and turning it, and watching how the light changes, rather than trying to string whole necklaces together, one after the other. It *is* possible to arrive at a whole new perspective on life and how to relish it; learning how to live totally in the present, moment by moment; giving all that one has (however much or little) to whatever one is doing. To live fully and completely in the present is an opportunity that doesn't come at all in most people's lives and is a real gift. For those of us who are on our own this 'gift' can also be fairly easy to obtain. Once we have our basic routine established, together with appropriate back-up for times of crisis, we can afford, within that framework, to savour the freedom that being ill can bestow, get the most out of little things, without the pressure of also having to respond to others' needs on a day-to-day basis. It is remembering this that most sustains me at all those other times, when I feel very alone, berate the restrictions of being ill, and wish there was someone there to talk to, get me a meal or sympathise over the pain.

What also keeps me going is 'breaking out' occasionally. A person alone lacks people to sound-off to about the illness. A lot of the time he or she simply has to keep going because there is no one else there to take over. Occasionally having a good cry does wonders for pent-up frustration, grief, anger and loss – and to get these emotions out can only be good for enhancing the prospects of long-term recovery. Likewise, giving yourself a treat can help – even if that treat is detrimental in the short term and causes a temporary flare-up of symptoms. Sometimes it is good simply to 'live' and take the consequences of any flare-up that comes after. In such ways it is possible to overcome some of the feelings of loss, sadness and frustration caused by M.E.

So far I have talked of loss in conjunction with not being able to work, and not being able to pursue an active social life. There is one other important area to look at: the effect M.E. has on a person's ability to sustain a close, sexual relationship.

Some of us 'aloners' may have a sexual relationship with a partner, although we may not actually share a house. The amount of energy and effort needed if two people are to sustain a close, loving sexual relationship whilst living apart can become, at worst, prohibitive and, at best, a great source of stress, if one partner develops M.E. And for those M.E. patients who are prevented from developing any close sexual relationship at all because of the restrictions of the illness, or whose relationship has ended because of it, there is another whole area of grief, loss and loneliness to come to terms with. I feel the only way to do this, is again to try to use the experience of the illness to re-evaulate both one's own sense of self, and the range of ways in which one is able to relate to and value other people. Our society tends to emphasise the importance, above all else, of having a sexual relationship but in reality, there are lots of ways of loving other people that can be equally satisfying. If one can accept this, then one opens oneself to what is on offer, rather than using up energy in hankering after the unobtainable. Obviously this is easier said than done, and there will still be moments of acute sadness, not to mention sexual frustration, but these can at least be tempered, by masturbation on the purely physical level, and by the quality of life that can come from being completely open and responsive to all kinds of relationships with other people, and all kinds of experiences.

But what if none of this is possible? What if your M.E. is so bad that you simply cannot manage to live alone at all, never mind about such luxuries as work or relationships? What happens then?

Any solution to this will mean giving up a measure of independence, which is difficult for anyone accustomed to living alone. If your parents are fit, and able to care for you, you can then return 'home'. Alternatively, other relatives or friends may offer somewhere to live. In such situations a 'granny flat' can be a good compromise, offering carers and M.E. patients alike a measure of freedom, privacy and independence, whilst also affording regular care for the sufferer and mutual company/privacy for all. In such circumstances, maximum use still needs to be made of additional outside help, to ensure that neither carers nor sufferers are over-burdened, the former by practical tasks and resentments, the latter by guilt and claustrophobia.

Another solution for anyone unable to look after her/himself is some form of sheltered accommodation. This, however, is difficult to come by. Supply is vastly outstripped by demand. It is only those of us who have the illness very badly who are likely to qualify for a place, either in a council-run complex, a Housing Association development or in accommodation provided by one of several voluntary organisations working in this field. It should be stressed, however, that the nature of M.E. makes it difficult for a person to obtain sheltered accommodation in all but the very worst cases. Most of us do get better, even if the illness lasts a long time; most of us do have good periods in among the relapses. In this hard-pressed world of cut-backs, such fluctuations in our illness put M.E. patients at the end of a very long queue when it comes to obtaining sheltered housing. However, if the M.E. is really bad, and a person has nowhere to go, then a fight should be made to get an adequate placement, with help from the local housing manager, GP, consultant or social worker.

As a final point, however, it should be stressed that, even with quite bad illness, by enlisting the type of help described above, it should be possible for anyone with M.E. not just to manage on his or her own, but also to get real enjoyment out of life, minute by minute.

2. Relationships

One of the most distressing aspects of M.E. is the way it interferes with all aspects of one's personal and social life.

It can be very difficult at times maintaining your friendships, but don't ever lose the ones who are kind and understanding. There will be some who just can't comprehend what you're going through, and who will make the most stupid and insensitive suggestions about what you might try and do to get better. You're bound to find that existing friends are going to take varying attitudes towards you and your illness. The more they understand about M.E. and the way it affects you, the more likely it is that they'll remain the sort of friends you still want to see – so do explain M.E. to them.

Most patients will find that a whole range of sporting and social activities, which previously made life so enjoyable, now have to be abandoned or curtailed. For many people this inability to participate in any form of sporting activity is a severe blow, as outside work, sports and hobbies are a very important way of meeting people and maintaining friendships. Some M.E. patients try to maintain their involvement by becoming spectators instead. It may also be possible to keep in touch by performing some sort of administrative function for the club or organisation.

This reduction of interests and social life is something which partners and carers also find difficult, and so for their sake it helps to try to have some form of 'non-active' social life together from time to time. It could just be a visit to the cinema or theatre, or a quiet meal out at a restaurant. If you really can't face the thought of going out, why not make an event out of an evening at home, perhaps by hiring a good video and getting a take-away meal?

Don't ever forget about those people who are closest to

you – your partner, your children and your best friends. These relationships are going to come under great strain from time to time, but these are the sort of people you're going to rely on for a great deal of support.

Caring for someone who has M.E.

The person who is closest to someone with M.E. – be it spouse, parent or child – has a very difficult job.

Suddenly, the carer finds that their family member is not the person they once were. They cannot cope, physically, as they once did, and there may be psychological problems as well such as loss of confidence and self-esteem, exaggerated mood swings and depression. Just as the patient is coming to terms with all sorts of problems, so may all those around him or her be experiencing similar difficulties in learning how to cope.

Caring isn't just providing physical help. Most people with M.E. won't need the extra sort of physical care with lifting and bathing that someone with multiple sclerosis, for example, might require. Caring involves a great deal of emotional help as well.

Neither of you can predict the eventual outcome of the disease, and this can make forward planning very difficult. M.E. patients do stand a good chance of getting better and returning to normal health and a normal way of life. Unfortunately, this can take a long time, and it's all too easy to give up hope when they've had M.E. for several years, and to become convinced that he or she is never going to get better.

A key part of the carer's role is not only to understand what the patient is putting up with, but to give hope and encouragement that recovery will take place, and keep the person in a positive frame of mind that he or she will get better. Part of this positive approach is to encourage them to look after their personal appearance, to maintain their friendships and social contacts, and pursue their work, hobbies and interests – provided they are not exceeding their capabilities, and are having the proper amount of rest.

It helps to talk about the illness. Join the M.E. Association – where at a local group meeting you'll be able to meet other people who are close to someone who's living with M.E.

M.E. patients will obviously have differing physical and emotional needs when it comes to receiving help from other people. Many will be the sort of individuals who haven't been used to asking for this type of assistance in the past, so it's not easy to be specific about what to do for them. Here are suggested guidelines to be followed with a wide degree of flexibility, according to each individual's needs and personality.

A four-point plan to help carers and relatives

1 Find out all you can about M.E.

One of the first practical steps that any relative or carer must take is to find out as much as possible about this illness, and the way it's affecting the patient.

Above all, this means listening and learning from the patient about how M.E. is affecting his or her life, which may mean encouraging them to express feelings about both physical and emotional difficulties – something which some people may find very hard to do, and which they haven't been used to doing in the past.

It's a good idea for both of you to go along together, on at least one occasion, to a consultation with the patient's general practitioner or consultant – any reasonable doctor shouldn't object to this. It's quite likely that there are questions which the patient may not want to ask – here the doctor may be willing to see the carer separately, but some would regard it as unethical to talk about a patient's illness without their permission. Do find out all you can about how the doctor feels the individual illness should best be managed, any drugs that are being prescribed, what sort of things cause a relapse, and whether there are any reasons for the patient to be seen by a specialist who's 'expert' in M.E.

It's a very natural reaction for some relatives, when an illness like M.E. has been diagnosed, to start spending vast amounts of money and time chasing an elusive 'cure'. They write to experts all over the world, and request second opinions from anyone involved with the condition. Others take a completely opposite view and almost deny that any problem exists, or that it will go away if ignored. Some are even so successful in this type of approach that they don't realise that they're doing it! If the patient wants to try out some 'alternative' remedies or change their diet, don't denigrate such an approach. It may help, and many patients undoubtedly feel better simply by the fact that they are now taking some management decisions about their illness.

Read all you can about the illness; it's not hard to find up-to-date medical information on M.E., and the M.E. Association can often help if you're having difficulties. Once you've got the basic facts straight in your head about how M.E. behaves as an illness, it should be a lot easier for both of you to start making the sort of essential changes in lifestyle, without which progressive recovery is unlikely.

2 Involve the whole family

Where an M.E. patient is part of a family group it's often a very good idea for all the members to get together for a sort of family conference, so that everyone can appreciate how the illness is going to affect both the patient and their family life.

It's an opportunity for everyone to make their feelings – positive and negative – known about any particular difficulties or anxieties, as well as reallocating some of the household and family duties. Hopefully, everyone can be flexible, and decide on practical ways of getting around any current problems. This is far better than members of the patient's family quietly grumbling away behind their back, and no solutions being found.

Getting children to understand the effects of M.E. on one of their parents can be a particularly difficult task. Try to explain the disease to them as honestly as possible, so they can understand, why mum or dad can't do the sort of activities with, or for them, that other parents do.

Children find it very difficult to cope with a parent who has M.E. Like everyone else, some will be extremely supportive and even start to take on an adult role in the way they help about the house. Unfortunately, others will be the exact opposite, being completely unhelpful, and even isolating themselves from the parent and their illness.

At the age of five or six many children will want to know why mum or dad doesn't go out to work like his friends' parents, and why he or she can't come out and help with the game of football or go on a weekend camping trip. Some children will even make up fictitious occupations for you in order to avoid teasing and embarrassment at school – children can be very cruel to each other at times.

There aren't easy solutions to problems with the children, but talking to other families who are coping with M.E. might be very helpful and give you some ideas as to how some of your own problems might be tackled.

3 Get organised – find out about help that's available

Find out about all the extra sources of help and advice which are available, and might be appropriate to your particular needs and circumstances. Practical help for the disabled, and advice on social security benefits are covered comprehensively elsewhere (see pages 290–316).

Don't forget that besides friends and family, other people such as your neighbours, may be only too willing to give a bit of help – if only they were to be asked. If you are receiving help from people not closely associated with you, it's a great help to them if you carefully explain the nature of the illness and how it affects the patient. People can be quite afraid of illnesses (and people with illnesses) which they don't understand, so it's important that you or the patient puts them fully in the picture. They may be quite happy to offer a bit of practical help, such as doing a bit of regular shopping each week, and you or your partner might also be able to do something for them in return, such as looking after a pet when they go on holiday.

With the loss of mobility that M.E. imposes, many M.E. patients will find that new friendships now come from neighbours and people living close to them, when previously they may have only known one or two people who lived in the same street.

There is a new umbrella organisation, the Carers National Association (see page 325), which now exists specifically for people who are caring or helping to look after people with disability. They act as a source of further information on a whole range of practical problems anyone acting as a carer may face. They also organise local groups where you could meet other people who are having to cope with similar feelings and experiences that you may have with M.E. It's not the sort of help that everyone requires, but it's there should you need it.

4 Self-help for the carer

It's all too easy, when caring for somebody else, to start putting your own interests and life into second place. After all, you're trying to perform a kind of balancing act between your own needs, the rest of the family, and caring for your partner. It can become easy to start neglecting your own health, both physical and emotional, and it's no use falling ill as well, when you've become the central pillar to family life. If you find yourself getting depressed, do go and seek help from your general practitioner, or try to arrange for a counselling session. And if you've got any physical symptoms, don't neglect them – do go and get them sorted out.

You'll also have a lot of personal feelings about the way M.E. is affecting both your lives; some will be positive, but many will be negative and upsetting. You'll probably start to get fed up at times (just like the patient) about the restrictions M.E. is placing on your life. You may start to feel despondent when your partner doesn't seem to be making any real progress, or some new treatment isn't having any effect.

All this is a very natural reaction. There aren't any *easy* solutions, but whatever feelings you do have about either the patient, or the M.E., try not to bottle them up. If you don't find it easy to discuss them with your partner, it can help a lot to talk to a close friend or relative, or the partner of another M.E. patient whom you may have met at a local group meeting. Such a third party may even be able to intervene and help defuse a family crisis by tactfully putting your point of view about a particular issue.

Unfortunately, there may be times when the relationship comes under great stress, even crisis. If you find it very difficult dealing with frustrations or putting your feelings into words, try writing them down. It's something of a last resort, but just occasionally it can be very effective to relieve the pressure.

A variety of pressures may build up: health, personal and financial worries. It can be very helpful to talk things over with someone completely detached from the family. This might be a social worker, a sympathetic general practitioner or even a professional or volunteer counsellor. (The British Association for Counselling trains such people – see page 326.)

Although you may find that for much of the time you're having to put your interests, and even your work, into second place it's terribly important not to abandon them altogether.

It's unusual for any M.E. patient to actually require full-time physical help throughout the day, so giving up work for that reason isn't usually necessary. However, when a wife with small children develops M.E. (especially if they're of pre-school age) the husband may well have to make some very major decisions regarding his own employment, especially if he spends a large amount of time away from home. Alternatively, if the bread-winner has had to give up work due to M.E., it may be the carer who's now got to consider going out to work, for pure-ly financial reasons and on top of all the other responsibilities. Making the correct decisions in such circumstances is not easy, so do try and talk to other people who've had to make similar decisions before finally making up your mind.

If you're already working and happy in what you're doing, and there are no practical problems at home, there are good reasons for you to continue. It gives you respite from each other, and the opportunity to continue with outside friendships and social life. Also, do try not to give up hobbies and interests, even though there may be practical difficulties, or activities which you can no longer do together any more.

Don't feel guilty about going out on your own once or twice a week to an evening class, or a game of sport with some friends, even though your partner isn't well enough to come. It is important, at the same time, to try and develop some new interests and hobbies which you can do together. This might be swimming, a gentle walk in the countryside, or a trip out to a meal or the cinema if your partner feels well enough.

Sexual relationships and M.E.

Sexual feelings are a natural and essential part of any caring relationship, especially in the age group affected by M.E. In fact, sex may be one of the few pleasurable physical activities that patients still feel they can enjoy.

It's hardly surprising that many M.E. patients experience sexual problems at some time during their illness, with, probably, both physical and emotional factors interacting. Those who are going through a bad patch may withdraw emotionally from those around them. When this happens, the partner may feel rejected, so he or she loses interest in sexual activity as well. Some M.E. patients may also develop a negative body image, no longer seeing themselves attractive to their partner, and in such cases experienced psychosexual counselling can be very helpful.

Patients who have become anxious or depressed because of the illness, especially when they are taking some of the prescribed drugs, will find this often causes a further dampening down of sexual feelings. Normal sexual arousal stimulates nerves which help open up the tiny blood vessels in the penis to allow an erection to take place. Any anxiety will dampen down this nervous activity, and if the male partner fails on one occasion to achieve an erection, subsequent anxiety about a repetition may prevent him achieving an erection on the next occasion. Male impotence isn't a part of the physical disease process in M.E. When it does occur, emotional factors are probably much more significant. I've also become aware that some men with M.E. go on to develop a variety of other sexual problems, particularly in maintaining an erection. If your GP seems unable to help I would recommend asking for a referral to a urology specialist who is interested in this type of sexual problem.

For some patients, the physical problems associated with M.E. may make sex no longer an appealing activity. Pain in the muscles and joints may severely limit capabilities, and of course, sexual intercourse does involve the expenditure of a large amount of energy in a very short space of time. Intimacy doesn't have to end in intercourse, so foreplay, caressing and touching can be equally satisfying, as an alternative to 'active sex', if the energy just isn't there. Do also remember that sex doesn't have to necessarily always take place at night when you or your partner are feeling tired and ready to go to sleep.

If pain in the muscles, joints or back is a significant factor in reducing sexual pleasure, try taking a warm bath before going to bed, and consider taking an aspirin or other anti-inflammatory drug a couple of hours before. Back pain can be eased by placing a pillow under the lower back of the partner in the passive position. Don't be afraid to explore new positions which you may find more comfortable. Get a 'guide book' if you're not quite sure what to do! A man with M.E. will use much less energy if he lies underneath, and the wife becomes the active partner. Alternatively, lying side-by-side may be more comfortable.

Sex can also be therapeutic. Arthritis sufferers sometimes report pain relief following orgasm, which is thought to be due to the release from the brain of chemicals known as endorphins, which are like the body's self-produced morphine.

If you are experiencing sexual difficulties, do get help. Some GPs are excellent, as in other aspects of M.E., but others don't have a clue when it comes to sexual problems, and are just as embarrassed as their patients. If your GP doesn't seem the right person to approach, then the local family planning clinic or marriage guidance council will point you in the right direction. The British Association for Counselling have counsellors available and SPOD (Sexual and Personal Relationships of People with a Disability) can also provide advice and help (see page 341).

As far as contraception is concerned having M.E. is *not* a contra-indication to using either the standard contraceptive pill or the progesterone only pill. In fact, for many women with M.E., using the most reliable form of contraceptive is extremely important because pregnancy is not something that I would recommend in the early stages of the illness; later on it requires very careful consideration (see also pages 239–45). Equally, dealing with the problems of an unwanted pregnancy may well cause a further relapse. One method of female contraception that I would not particularly recommend is the intra-uterine contraceptive device (IUCD) because of its associated increased risk of infection. If you've completed your family then the ideal method of contraception may well be for the male partner to have a vasectomy – something which can be done quickly and easily using a local anaesthetic. However, it should be noted that concerns have recently been expressed as to whether vasectomy could occasionally be a factor in the development of M.E.

3. M.E. And Your Job

One of the most urgent problems facing many people with M.E. is trying to adjust financially to the limitations imposed by the illness.

Where the patient has been the main breadwinner, and is also quite young, with rapidly rising financial and promotional expectations from work, the loss of income can be abrupt and severe. A large mortgage might have been taken out on a new house, or other costly financial planning entered into, and now these commitments may be impossible to keep going. Even the most fortunate individuals (in Britain) are unlikely to receive more than six months' full sick pay and an equal period of half pay. After that, the total family income may rapidly diminish to a combination of state sickness benefits, and whatever other members of the family are bringing in. And, where a wife is at home looking after small children, this may mean no other source of earned income.

A financial crisis may then ensue, forcing sudden decisions to cut back on spending. It's far preferable to try and avoid this by talking to one's bank manager or building society before such a crisis occurs, to put them into the picture, and hopefully make some arrangements to ease the burden in the short term.

This chapter is designed to give practical help and advice on the sorts of problem which occur, and the options to consider in trying to solve them.

Returning to work

For those who have been diagnosed early on in the illness, a period of sick leave with complete rest, followed by gradual convalescence is the aim. Then perhaps a staged return to work, which will have to be flexible, and avoid excessive amounts of stress or overwork on any one day. Other patients who are diagnosed late, when the condition seems to have stabilised and possibly become chronic, may have much more difficult decisions to take. The choice may have to be between making a major readjustment in occupation or leaving the current type of occupation, if the physical and mental stresses are too much.

Unfortunately, the financial and psychological consequences of giving up work may also have their own negative effects on recovery in M.E. – unemployment can also damage your health. So, like all the other routes to recovery it's a question of trying to strike the right balance between the advantages and disadvantages, and at the same time keeping within your limitations.

It may not be easy to find such a person to talk to, but I always think it can be of immense help in these circumstances to listen to someone else in the same occupation as yourself who has M.E. and find out what they did. An M.E. self-help organisation may be able to put you in touch with someone.

Here is a quote from a recent article in the *Journal of the Society for Occupational Medicine*, by Dr Mike Peel, who was an Occupational Physician with British Airways. This is an account of the problems in returning to work which some of his patients with M.E. have faced, and is to be recommended to any other occupational health physicians.

The most important impression is that they are all very active, fit and dedicated workers: the last ones likely to exaggerate symptoms. Managers have expressed relief that a trusted colleague is genuinely ill and not hysterical. It is probable that the attitude of fighting on despite illness is a critical factor, in that they continued working long hours and taking regular exercise long after their bodies told them to stop.

J. Soc. Occup. Med. (1988) 38, 44–5

Problems at work

In the early stages of the illness, often before a firm diagnosis has been made, employers tend to be fairly sympathetic about sick leave but this approach tends to rapidly evaporate as the months pass by, and your absence becomes a steadily increasing inconvenience. There comes a time when the employer begins to wonder if you're ever going to return to work. Just how long can this persisting virus go on? Unfortunately, neither you nor your doctor can provide them with the answers they require, and their impatience gets worse.

You may attempt to go back to work, even though you know you're almost certainly not well enough to do so. This attempt fails, and you end up feeling even more demoralised. The company then decides it's looking extremely unlikely that you're going to return in the near future, and the next thing you hear is that somebody else has been promoted into your position: there's no job to go back to even if you are well!

It's a popular misconception that you can't lose your job due to ill health – unfortunately this isn't so. After a prolonged period away from work your employer may be able to argue that this is a valid reason for dismissal.

The first important step, if you feel you're about to enter this situation, is to get in touch with your trade union or professional body, and talk to one of their industrial relations advisors. It's essential to take expert advice here, as the law is complicated, and these people should be fully up-to-date with the legislation, and be able to refer you on for appropriate legal advice if necessary. If you don't belong to such organisations the local Citizens Advice Bureau (in Britain) should be able to give you some help.

Secondly, do keep in touch with work (probably the personnel officer) and let them know what's happening about your progress, or lack of it – they may even be able to help financially. Admittedly, some employers are excellent when it comes to problems related to ill health, but others just don't want to know, and hope you'll quietly go away.

It's also worthwhile making an appointment with the company doctor, if you have an occupational health service, to keep him informed. If he's interested and sympathetic towards M.E., he may be able to offer help in the future, and his opinion will be important if it comes to taking early retirement on the grounds of ill health.

If you are claiming sick pay under an occupational sick pay scheme, dismissal shouldn't be a way of stopping such benefits, but again, check the law with your trade union.

Dismissal on grounds of ill health – going to law

If it comes to the point of actually being dismissed because you've got M.E., there may be an internal company appeal procedure to which you or your trade union could present your case. Your employer may argue that your contract of employment has been terminated, because in the legal jargon, it has been 'frustrated'. (This means that your employer now considers that you are unable to perform your contractual duties due to continuing ill health with M.E.)

If you are dismissed, and all appeals to the company have failed, you may still have a case which could be taken to an industrial tribunal – but you *must* do this within three months of dismissal. The industrial tribunal will have to decide if your employer was acting in a 'fair and reasonable manner' when they decided to terminate employment. You may think that it's very unfair to be dismissed through no actual fault of your own, and a tribunal may agree with you if you can successfully argue points such as:

- You were never in any way consulted about your illness and possible return to work by the employer.
- The employer never went to the bother of obtaining relevant medical reports on your state of health from either your doctor or their own occupational health physician.

The tribunal also has to take into account the fact that your ill health could be endangering other employees, and in the case of M.E., this could well be relevant where a manual worker is operating dangerous machinery, or somebody driving public transport.

Anyone with M.E. who has registered as being disabled

for the purposes of employment may find this gives some added protection against dismissal.

The law regarding employment and dismissal on grounds of ill health is very complex, so do get expert advice before you make any irretrievable decisions.

Further information on sickness and unfair dismissal is contained in the *Disability Rights Handbook* (see Useful Addresses). Two useful legal precedents involving failure of the employer to adequately consult with the employee and their doctor are:

• Polkey v A E Dayton Services Ltd [1987] 3WLR 1153, HL.
• Wright v Eclipse Blinds Ltd [1990] 411 1RL1B 11, EAT.

Retirement on grounds of ill health

If you've been in a company pension or superannuation scheme and you decide to retire due to ill health, then some form of pension may now be payable. Unfortunately, a common problem is that the qualifying criterion for obtaining a pension, at a very early age, is 'permanent ill health' (i.e. you're not going to ever work again due to the illness). As the outcome in any individual case of M.E. is so unpredictable, especially in the first few years of the illness, no medical specialist is likely to firmly give the opinion that you're inevitably going to remain in a state of 'permanent ill health'. Consequently, the pension or award may then be frozen until it becomes clear that you are very likely to remain permanently disabled by M.E. – and this may be several years. Problems with insurance companies are covered in more detail on pages 138–40.

Occupations commonly affected by M.E.

Although M.E. undoubtedly affects people across the entire social spectrum and in all types of occupation, there does seem to be a bias towards those who are employed in the health care professions and teaching. I believe that there are a number of factors which may help to explain this curious vulnerability. The most important lies in the fact that both groups are working in an atmosphere of above-average physical and mental stress; they also face considerable pressure not to go 'off sick' when they are ill because it is often extremely difficult finding colleagues who are willing to cover their absence. In addition, teachers and health workers are frequently in close contact with other people's infections.

As far as the medical and nursing professions are concerned, there is now a good chance that permanent disablement with M.E. will be regarded as a work-related illness – provided that there is good evidence that the initial infection was contracted from a patient.

A recent survey, carried out by the M.E. Association, suggested that the situation was nowhere near as satisfactory for teachers with M.E. The average age at which they first became ill was 41, and of those off work nearly 45 per cent did not expect to return to classroom duties. This is not only a tremendous loss to the country in terms of professional experience; there is also the very large economic cost in terms of pensions and sickness benefits.

Once again, stress in the classroom was frequently cited as a major factor, not only in precipitating M.E., but also in perpetuating their ill health. The lack of part-time or flexible working opportunities appeared to be a major obstacle in planning a graded return to work.

At the moment the National Union of Teachers is actively campaigning to have M.E. recognised as an industrial disease for teachers. This is very important because it seems that several teachers with M.E. have been forced into unwise decisions over their contracts without taking competent professional advice. Others, under pressure, have just opted out and resigned. So, if you are a teacher in this position, do consult with the NUT, and also try to speak to another colleague who has had to make similar decisions, preferably one who has been employed by a sympathetic local authority.

The high incidence of M.E. in the teaching profession has also been confirmed in a recent survey by Dr Darrel Ho-Yen into the occupation of 275 patients in Scotland (see medical reference 50). Teachers and students accounted for 22 per cent of the total; 16 per cent were retired; 13 per cent were housewives; 11 per cent worked in various service industries; 9 per cent were clerical staff; 9 per cent were skilled workers;

8 per cent unskilled; 7 per cent worked in hospitals, and the remaining 5 per cent were in various professions (lawyers, civil servants, etc.). These figures should finally dispel the myth that M.E. is almost solely confined to middle class *Observer* reading professionals!

Other occupational groups who appear to be unduly susceptible include staff in mental subnormality institutions, and water and sewage workers – all of whom are exposed to an above-average incidence of infective illnesses.

Self-employment and M.E.

One further practical possibility worth exploring is that of becoming self-employed and carrying on some form of work from home. This has some distinct attractions, as it can be very flexible, carried out at times when you're fit enough, and temporarily abandoned when you're unwell.

Obviously, this is only an option for those who feel able, and want to continue with some form of work. I fully accept that for many M.E. patients, what I'm suggesting just isn't going to be possible now, but it may be later on when you start to make progress. It's also important to appreciate that if you do continue to claim invalidity benefit, there may come a time when the DSS will review your position. And, if they feel that despite being unable to perform your normal occupation, there is some 'suitable alternative work' you could do, this could be used as a reason to stop benefit.

Whatever you do decide to do about work, try not to make any hasty decisions – take time to consider all the options available, and take account of what other members of the family feel is right. And, don't ever resign from your job because of M.E. until you've first taken expert advice – you may end up disqualifying yourself from financial assistance.

There are no simple answers to the very common question: 'What do I do about my job?' It very much depends on the stage of the illness, what you do for a living, and the attitude of your employers and possibly the company doctor.

Help from the government

In theory, anyone who is disabled should be covered by legal protection against dismissal and redundancy, as well as being entitled to maternity leave, sick pay and time off work for public duties, etc. The 1986 Wages Act also means that disabled people should not be employed on less favourable terms than able-bodied employees. In practice, though, the situation regarding employment rights for many disabled people remains far from satisfactory.

In the past few years the government has brought in a number of measures to try and improve work prospects for the disabled. One of the most important is the fact that employers with 20 or more employees now have a duty to make sure that they have at least 3 per cent of their workforce made up of people with disabilities. And, under the 1985 Companies Act, those companies with more than 250 employees are now required to produce details in their annual reports on their policy regarding recruitment, training and the career development of disabled employees. Some of the other recent government initiatives include:

Registering as disabled This is not the same as registering your disablement with the Social Services (see pages 290–94), although you can do both if you wish to. Registration of disability for employment purposes is purely voluntary, but it can help in obtaining extra financial benefits and added protection at work. To become registered you need to be in a situation where it is highly likely that you will remain disabled for the next twelve months, and have some prospect of obtaining work, or actually be in work. Once registered, you'll be given a 'Green Card' which can also act as a passport to other benefits. This will include cover under the Disabled Persons Employment Act if you are threatened with dismissal from work. If this does happen, you should contact your trade union/professional body and the Disablement Resettlement Officer without delay.

Disablement Resettlement Officers (DRO) are available for consultation at most large Job Centres, and you can make your own appointment to see one – there's no need to be referred.

Their role is to deal with applications for registration from people with disabilities, and to advise on employment prospects and suitability for work in relation to specific disabilities. My personal experience is that most people with M.E. who have sought advice from a DRO have found it helpful.

Job Introduction Scheme is available to any disabled person who, in the opinion of the DRO, is in need of a period of adjustment to help them demonstrate their work capabilities to a new employer. You don't have to be registered as disabled to take part in this scheme. The Employment Service pays about £50 per week to a company that agrees to take anyone on for the 6-week trial period.

Enterprise Allowance Scheme is designed to help disabled and unemployed people become self-employed. To qualify you must be able to invest £1000 in whatever business you are planning to set up. If accepted, you'll then receive a taxable allowance of between £20 and £90 per week which can last for between 26 and 66 weeks. This scheme is run by the Training and Enterprise Council.

Employment Aids The Employment Service can provide certain work aids (e.g. typewriters, special chairs) on permanent loan to registered disabled people to keep them in employment. There are also some capital grants available (of up to £6000) to employers who may need to adapt the workplace in order to employ a disabled person.

Fares-To-Work Scheme can help anyone who is registered as disabled but is unable to use public transport for all or part of their journey to work. This could, for example, include taxi fares up to 75 per cent of the total cost.

The Disability Working Allowance (DWA) is a 'new' benefit introduced in April 1992 which is designed to supplement the income of disabled people on low wages who are working at least 16 hours per week. For further details on this benefit please refer to pages 310–11.

VAT concessions Anyone who is substantially disabled may be eligible for various VAT exemptions on capital expenditure – see VAT leaflet 701/7/86, Aids for Handicapped Persons, which should be available from your local VAT office.

Some other options with employment

You may feel that if you've had to give up your job because of M.E. there's nothing else you can now do, but it is important to explore other possibilities.

It may be possible to arrange some part-time work in your previous type of occupation, or do some 'flexitime' to fit in with the times of day when you seem to function most productively. Another employer might be able to offer you a similar type of job, but at a less demanding pace, and probably at a less demanding salary. However, for many patients these sorts of option may not exist, or be practical, and then there's no choice but to rely on financial support from the various state sickness benefits.

Being at home all day, no longer making any decisions and missing out on the social life and friendships that are all part of 'being at work' is a very demoralising aspect of M.E., which often exacerbates the feelings of isolation and loss of self-esteem. In this situation it may be worth considering making an application to the Open University. They are particularly keen to encourage students with disabilities on to their courses, and have a special tutor who can give further advice (see page 336).

It obviously depends on how unwell you are, what stage the illness is at, and how variable the symptoms are, but giving up work for good is one of the most difficult decisions to make in M.E., so *do* look at the other possibilities – state of health permitting. It may also be worth making contact with an organisation called Opportunities For People With Disabilities (see page 336) who liaise with employers who are sympathetic to the needs of disabled employees.

4. Running Your Home

The disabling physical symptoms of M.E. mean that many patients share the same sort of practical difficulties that other chronically disabled groups have in trying to lead a normal life. You're not alone in experiencing the sort of frustrations imposed by M.E. These may range from the pure physical inability to summon up sufficient strength to carry out a routine task like mowing the lawn, to difficulties with gripping or manipulating everyday objects used in the kitchen.

The combination of muscular fatigue and unsteadiness also produces great difficulty in coping with tasks that involve prolonged standing and concentrating. This not only prevents many patients following their normal occupations but it also makes many of the domestic tasks involved in running a home equally difficult.

To make life easier there are a number of practical aids available either free, on loan, or to buy, which will help to make many physical and manipulative tasks less fatiguing. There are also various professionals and agencies who can give invaluable help when it comes to learning to cope with disability (see 294–6). It's perfectly natural to feel reluctant to label yourself as being 'disabled'. You don't have to use the term if you don't want to, but if you are having practical difficulties do make use of the resources which are available.

Before approaching anyone for help it's a good idea to make a comprehensive written list of the sort of practical problems with which you require help. This might be something as simple as obtaining a device which can open tight tops on the marmalade jar, to how you can obtain expert assistance and financial help in making major adaptations to the home for a very disabled M.E. patient. Don't be afraid to go round asking questions.

The people involved are usually very approachable and only too willing to help.

If adapting your home involves making a claim for a benefit or grant don't be put off because you're not sure about your eligibility: as long as you provide the officials with honest information it can't do any harm. If you are then refused, but still think you have a good case, do make an appeal, as the success rate in challenging the bureaucracy over disabled benefits is quite high. In the meantime, there are many ways you can conserve your energy and make life easier.

In the home

Here are some practical suggestions, room by room.

Kitchens

- Keep commonly used foods and kitchen utensils together in an easily accessible place – preferably at chest height, to avoid repeated reaching up and bending down.
- Use level work surfaces for heavy objects: they can be pushed around instead of lifted.
- Raise the washing-up bowl in the sink so you're not stooping over, and let the washing-up dry by itself.
- If you can afford it, consider purchasing a dish-washing machine.
- Again, if you can afford it, consider other types of electrical apparatus which can make life easier: a microwave, a freezer to store some essential foods in, or an electric tin opener.
- There are numerous aids which make a whole range of domestic duties and cooking much easier, e.g. specially adapted cutlery and cooking utensils, plugs with small handles so they're easier to pull out of the socket, etc. Visit one of the disabled living centres (see pages 294–5), and see what's on display that might help you.
- With modern adjustable ironing boards it's easy to iron while seated, and with coat hangers to hand, plus an airer to put all the ready ironed items on to, you need not move from start to finish. Obviously, try to keep ironing to a minimum, and get the rest of the family well trained in how to do this

vital task! You may even be lucky enough to find someone locally who charges a small fee to do the weekly ironing.

- When cooking consider preparing double quantities and then freeze the remainder for a later date.

Living rooms

- If you have difficulty getting out of a low chair or sofa due to weakness in the hip muscles, consider getting a comfortable high chair, or one with a raised seat.
- A sofa bed may be a very useful additional piece of furniture if you're frequently confined to bed for 'relapses', and don't like spending your time upstairs confined to the bedroom.
- A remote control for the television set.

Stairs

- These can be a major problem for anyone who has been severely weakened by M.E., and may mean that a patient is confined to either the downstairs or upstairs for long periods. Chair lifts, although expensive, are a very useful device in such circumstances, but do take expert advice before spending large amounts of money: visit a disabled living centre for further practical help.
- If you do tend to live downstairs during a relapse, and sleep down there, it may be worth considering installing a downstairs toilet and shower.

Bathroom

- A hand rail, fixed to the wall by the bath, will help getting in and out.
- Buy a non-slip bath mat.
- Sitting in a shower can be less tiring than taking a bath. Use a special board across the bath top to sit on, but make sure it's stable and won't slip. (The Red Cross may loan you one.)
- Washing hair in the bath is a lot easier than bending over the sink.
- If your 'carer' is often having to lift you in and out of the bath, consider installing some form of hoist device.

Bedrooms

- Cut down on the bed-making by making use of fitted sheets

and duvets. The amount of warmth provided by a duvet is shown by its tog value. In a well-heated house a 10.5–12 tog duvet should be fine for all-year use. If M.E. makes you feel particularly cold then an extra-warm tog 13.5 might be better. If you really cannot tolerate the cold winter months it's now possible to purchase 15 tog duvets!

- Remember that all the household bedding doesn't necessarily have to be changed on the same day.
- A comfy upright chair for use when you're recovering from a period of bed rest.
- A lightweight vacuum cleaner saves lifting a heavy one up the stairs each time. If you use an extra long flex you can do an entire floor from just one plug.
- An extra telephone socket or a portable phone can be a great help, especially when you're not well and there's nobody else at home.

Out and about – shopping

- Local voluntary groups may be able to provide an able-bodied volunteer to help with a weekly shop, or a driver to take you there. Some schools also have volunteer sections.
- Find out about any local dial-a-ride services or other schemes to improve mobility. Shopmobility schemes now operate in nearly 30 cities in England and Wales. They are usually administered by the local authority – see Useful Addresses for a full list. The schemes provide battery operated scooters and wheelchairs to help people who have limited mobility to use all the shopping facilities in a city centre. Shopmobility is particularly helpful if car access is very restricted and where the large shops are grouped together in pedestrianised zones. Anyone with mobility problems can make use of this facility – you don't have to be registered as disabled or possess an Orange Parking Badge to qualify. Neither do you have to be resident in that particular town. Although there is no charge made for using the scheme a small deposit will be required. Shopmobility is usually open from 9.30 a.m. to 5 p.m. from Monday to Saturday. It's a good idea to book in advance, and car parking spaces are sometimes provided. Staff are also

available to demonstrate the use of wheelchairs and scooters. Remember, you will need some form of identification such as a driving licence.

- Consider alternatives to going out to the shops. Shopping from home can be done via mail order; some shops will still deliver groceries; and the milkman now carries an increasingly diverse range of produce.
- Ask a friend or neighbour to buy certain goods on a regular basis when they go to the supermarket.
- Find out about supermarkets and department stores which have special shopping hours reserved for the disabled; some also have priority parking facilities. An increasing number of shops are also willing to provide extra help for their disabled customers. Boots, for instance, now have trained staff who are willing to fit the wires into a plug correctly – something that might be very useful in the absence of legislation requiring the manufacturers to do it.
- Get the able-bodied members of the family (or friends) to buy certain items in bulk, as long as you have the storage space.
- Make sure that you've always got a stock of essential items of food, so that in a relapse when you can't get out for several days, there is something to eat.

The most useful source of information on all forms of practical aids for disabled people is an occupational therapist, who can also give useful advice regarding more major adaptations within the home. If you think that an occupational therapist might be able to help then contact your GP or local social services department. A list of useful publications describing aids and appliances for the disabled can be found in the reference section on pages 365–6.

5. Increasing Your Mobility

Problems with mobility are a major cause of social isolation for the disabled, as well as creating extra difficulties in obtaining employment, so do take advantage of any of the help that's available and appropriate to your own individual needs.

Pure financial help may be forthcoming from the DSS with a Disabled Living Allowance but this isn't easy to qualify for. The Department of Employment can also help with fares to work (see page 310).

Walking aids

A walking stick will help to provide extra support, relieve muscle and joint pains, and increase mobility.

Make sure that the stick you buy is the correct length for your body – you shouldn't end up leaning towards the stick (too short) or away from it (too long). If the stick has a metal or wooden tip it can easily slip in wet weather. A soft rubber tip is the best way to increase the friction and grip, and just like the tyres on a car these rubber tips need to be changed when worn. Pyramid sticks have either three or four legs and may be helpful if you require a considerable amount of support. If you're out and about quite a bit, it might be worth buying a shooting stick which has a fold-up seat on the top.

For those who are severely disabled the Zimmer type of walking frame may be necessary – a physiotherapist will give you appropriate advice.

Wheelchairs

Only a very few M.E. patients are ever likely to have to make use of a wheelchair, and this may be something which is used on a temporary rather than permanent basis to aid mobility during an arduous day's activities.

Wheelchairs can be obtained from a variety of sources.

1 From the NHS Artificial Limb and Appliance Centre Your doctor will have to complete a special assessment form in order to get one from this source. The best way of obtaining the model most suited to your individual needs is to make arrangements to visit a 'wheelchair clinic' at one of these centres, so your requirements can be assessed by an expert. You can also be visited at home for this assessment. Alternatively, a local physiotherapist or occupational therapist can help with the choice of the most appropriate model – and the NHS has over 140 available!

Wheelchairs from the NHS are given on free loan. All the models which are available from the NHS are described in the 'Handbook of Wheelchairs' (MM408) which is available from the NHS store, Manchester Road, Heywood, Lancashire.

2 Purchased privately There are perfectly reputable private suppliers of wheelchairs, but do take advice first before spending large sums of money.

3 The British Red Cross is very willing to make short-term loans to those who just require extra help for a short period, e.g. when going on holiday. They also produce a useful leaflet, 'People in Wheelchairs – Hints for Helpers'.

The exact type of wheelchair you eventually choose will depend on a number of factors. Are you going to use it indoors and out? Do you want to self-propel it or be pushed? Do you want to spend a lot of money on an electric model? Most people will require a chair that's suitable for both indoor and outdoor use, which will also fold up to fit in a car, and which is comfortable.

Features which increase the comfort and ride include pneumatic tyres (which, along with the brakes, need regular checking), a good cushion and a plywood base. You can also add various accessories such as trays, and cushioned backrests.

Some decide to purchase an electric wheelchair, but they do have their disadvantages – they're fairly heavy, can't be folded up, require quite a lot of space, and are fairly expensive. Indoor electric wheelchairs can be provided by the NHS, but the outdoor type have to be purchased privately.

Although the cost may be high, with a Disability Living Allowance you may be able to get help through the Motability scheme (see later in this chapter). Local authority housing departments may help with ramps and widening of doorways in the home, but you may need back-up from your general practitioner, occupational therapist and local councillor.

So, if you do decide that a wheelchair might help to increase your mobility, either permanently or just occasionally, do go and talk to some other users about their experiences and opinions on the types available, and seek the help of the professionals who can offer expert advice.

RADAR (see Useful Addresses) publish a very useful book called *Choosing a Wheelchair*. This is a wide ranging guide which includes up-to-date information on the various models which are available for both adults and children. It also contains further advice on how to obtain a wheelchair from the NHS or commercial suppliers, what features to look for, as well as the various sources of funding, insurance policies and loan schemes that are now available.

You and your car

Car insurance Anyone with M.E. who continues to drive a car ought to inform the motor licence authorities about their present medical condition. This may then involve a medical assessment on your continued 'fitness to drive'. Whether or not M.E. patients should be driving depends on each individual case, but some patients who are still driving probably should not be.

Many insurance companies also want to know about any physical or mental problems which could 'in any way impair your ability to drive', so check the small print, as you may be invalidating your policy. If in doubt most insurance companies have a medical advisor at their head office you could write to. If you do act accordingly, the insurance company will in all probability want to know what the licence authority have decided.

Help from motoring organisations For those who continue to drive (in the U.K.) there are two motoring organisations specialising in the problems faced by disabled drivers (see page 329). Both the Disabled Drivers' Association and the Disabled Drivers' Motor Club can give advice on car adaptations, and membership may also help with financial concessions on car ferries, motor insurance and RAC membership.

The AA has also launched a telephone information line to help disabled motorists. This service is open to both members and non-members, and provides help and advice on all aspects of mobility. AA helpline's number is 0800 (freephone) 262050, and the service is open daily. Both the AA and the RAC now operate a priority car breakdown service for disabled drivers, which gives a small financial discount to their normal rates. The AA RADAR Group membership costs £62.35 per year and covers the disabled person in any car. It is limited to profoundly deaf motorists and anyone who has been granted an Orange Badge. Details from the AA telephone number above. The RAC Response scheme costs £79 in the first year, and then £69 per year after that. It covers the disabled person and a spouse, in any car being used. Again, it is restricted to Orange Badge holders. Telephone 0800 (freephone) 400432 for more details.

MAVIS (Mobility Advice and Vehicle Information Service) This is an organisation set up by the Department of Transport to help disabled people choose a car and any adaptations which are most appropriate to their individual needs. Information is free but they may make a charge for other types of help (see Useful Addresses).

Mobility Information Service This is a voluntary organisation offering a wide range of information on cars and adaptations. It has a great deal of expertise in the field of mobility for the disabled. They have a number of leaflets on choosing, buying and converting a car. Personal assessment may also be possible within a 100-mile radius of Shrewsbury (see Useful Addresses).

Motability is a voluntary organisation, sponsored by the Government which aims to help people with disabilities use their Disability Living Allowance (mobility component) to buy or hire a car. The scheme offers both hire and hire purchase agreements. Using the hire purchase facility it is possible to buy an electric wheelchair or a good used car as well as a brand new one. Full details of Motability can be obtained from their head office (see Useful Addresses).

The Orange Badge parking scheme This entitles recipients with 'severe mobility problems' to various parking concessions, and is administered by the local authority's social services department. The scheme covers both disabled drivers and suitably disabled passengers, so non-drivers can also apply.

To quality you must already be receiving a Disabled Living Allowance (usually at the higher rates of the mobility component) from the DSS, or in legal jargon have a 'permanent and substantial disability to walk, or a very considerable difficulty in walking', something that tends to be open to wide individual interpretation.

To apply phone your local social services department and ask them to send an application form. If a DSS benefit does not give you automatic entitlement it's quite likely that you will then receive a request to see your GP who will carry out an assessment of your degree of physical disability. This will probably involve payment of a small fee.

If your request is refused there is no right of appeal, although your local councillor may be able to exert some pressure. All I can suggest is that you try again in about six months' time if you feel that you have a strong case.

One other useful advantage that comes with an Orange

Badge is that similar concessions are often available when travelling abroad.

RADAR also produce a comprehensive guide entitled 'Motoring and Mobility for Disabled People'.

The Department of Transport (see Useful Addresses) publishes an excellent free guide called *Door to Door* which provides information on all kinds of mobility problems.

Exemption from Road Tax This is a very useful financial benefit for anyone claiming a Disability Living Allowance mobility component; but the car must be used 'solely by or for the purposes of the disabled person', in legal jargon. In other words a wife with M.E. claiming Disability Living Allowance could not claim tax exemption on her husband's car if he is using it all day to go to work in! If you do receive the new Disability Living Allowance mobility component and think you might qualify, ask the local DSS to send you a Vehicle Excise Duty (VED) exemption form. This allowance can sometimes be claimed by a passenger who is receiving a care component of the Disability Living Allowance.

Public transport

For many M.E. patients who've had to stop driving their cars, or never even driven, increasing reliance on what often seems to be a declining standard of public transport becomes a necessity. Fortunately, the administrators of public transport have in recent years become more aware of the needs of their disabled travellers – particularly British Rail and the airlines – and some real progress is, at last, being made.

There is also some genuine financial help available with fares on most public transport, but the level of disability to qualify varies considerably.

Local voluntary organisations are now producing a range of access guides to toilets, shops and public buildings, and RADAR (see page 338) has started a scheme of specially designed toilets for the disabled. For a small fee you can get a special key (from

RADAR) which gives automatic access to these conveniences.

British Rail charges a small fee for their disabled person's railcard which gives reduced fares for both the holder and a companion. Anyone who receives a Disability Living Allowance from the DSS should qualify. This also now applies to those receiving the Severely Disabled Allowance, after I pointed out to British Rail that if you're deemed to be 'severely disabled' you ought to be sufficiently disabled to receive a 'disabled railcard'.

If you are severely affected by M.E., particularly if you are using a wheelchair, and want extra help during your journeys do let British Rail know (in good time and to the right department) as staff can be very helpful. They produce a comprehensive leaflet, 'British Rail and Disabled Travellers', which details all the ways they will help the disabled, and whom to contact for what.

Bus travel Many local authorities give financial help by issuing concessionary fares to people who've registered as disabled. Phone the local treasurer's department for further details.

'Dial-a-ride' schemes Some towns now operate 'dial-a-ride' schemes for disabled people, who are unable to make use of public transport. This can be of immense value for shopping trips, or just being able to get out once in a while for a social occasion. The service usually operates on a door-to-door basis. The Citizens Advice Bureau will know if there's one near you.

In London this scheme is administered by London DART (Dial-a-ride and Taxicard) – a central body which campaigns on transport funding for disabled people. London dial-a-ride is organised from six regional offices in the capital, but the joining criteria varies from region to region. However, a doctor's certificate or being registered as disabled should be sufficient. Telephone 071-482 2325 for further details.

The London Taxicard This unique scheme is administered by London Regional Transport, and funded by the individual boroughs, some of which are now sharply reducing their contributions. So, availability will depend on where you happen to live in the capital. Unfortunately, outside London few such schemes exist for the disabled.

To apply for a London Taxicard you need an application form which requires a doctor's signature. Once accepted onto the scheme you only pay the first £1-25 in a £9 taxi fare. After £9 the normal rate applies. For further details telephone 071-918 3588.

Shopmobility (see page 340) provides a range of battery operated wheelchairs and scooters on free loan for the day in the shopping centres of some large towns.

The DSS will provide cash help with fares to hospital for some people claiming low income benefits. Ask the hospital fares office or the local DSS for leaflet H11 and the AG5 and AG1 claim forms. Anyone on Income Support or Family Credit should qualify automatically, and close relatives in similar financial circumstances may also be able to make a claim.

Taking a holiday

Just like everyone else, people with M.E., along with their carers and relatives, need to enjoy a good holiday. However, the effort involved in getting away can be very tiring. But once you've got to the destination, a pleasant holiday in the right climate, with good accommodation and food can produce a considerable improvement.

The first thing to do is plan well ahead, and discuss with the whole family what sort of holiday seems most suitable, and where you're going to – home or abroad. Obviously, a holiday in the U.K. may be easier to get to if you're intending to go by car, and you're having to help with the driving. Alternatively, many pleasant parts of France can easily be reached using the car ferries, although this may mean the frustrations of having to hang about at odd hours, and climbing awkward stairs from the car decks. If you can't cope with stairs get in touch with the ferry operator beforehand, and they should let you use the lift. Some families have invested in caravans – obviously there must be another very fit member of the party, but this is an option worth considering.

Most of the large tour operators now welcome people with disabilities. Thomson advise them to contact their client services department (tel 071–387 9321) well before booking a holiday abroad to find out if the hotel, resort or country you intend to visit is going to be suitable. Others seem likely to follow suit.

If you're particularly disabled by M.E., and especially if you have to use a wheelchair, there are many hotels which make a point of having special rooms with appropriate access and washing facilities. Again, if you have special dietary needs some hotels will be very helpful. The Disabled Drivers' Association can give further help with the sort of problems you may encounter travelling abroad.

Useful publications include *Holidays and Travel Abroad* and *Holidays in the British Isles*, both of which are obtainable from RADAR. These books contain a mass of information on accommodation, transport and the addresses of helpful organisations specialising in holidays for disabled travellers. *The AA Guide for the Disabled Traveller* is available from AA shops. It is free to members but costs £3.50 for non-members. This book gives details of 600 hotels and self-catering establishments and 500 places of interest (including many National Trust properties) which cater for the disabled. Incidentally, the National Trust have specially adapted cottages in England which can be rented and they, too, publish a leaflet about facilities for the disabled at their properties (see Useful Addresses).

Some M.E. patients make the mistake of believing that a holiday in the hot sun will improve their condition. Unfortunately this is very rarely so, and the heat often makes M.E. worse. I personally find a warm, but *not* hot, rural part of France, with clean air and good food very beneficial, avoiding the very hot summer months.

If you are going abroad do make sure that you have adequate health insurance, and check the policy carefully to make sure about exclusions for 'pre-existing medical conditions'. There are still plenty of companies who will happily provide cover for M.E. patients, but you may have to shop around. Going abroad should be all right, providing you don't travel 'against your doctor's advice'. And don't forget to fill in form E111 (available from the post office) for you and your family if the holiday is being taken anywhere in the European Community.

This form acts as a passport to the use of these countries' state health services.

Compulsory vaccinations are seldom required for most popular European holiday resorts, and the chances of picking up nasty infections are fairly remote, provided you keep to simple rules of hygiene. (For further advice, see page 154.) If you get travel sickness, cinnariazine (Stugeron) is a useful drug. If you're abroad it's worth having a note of any important drugs you take already translated into the foreign tongue, just in case you lose them. The same applies for any other important medical conditions apart from M.E. The chances of finding a doctor abroad who's even heard of M.E. are going to be fairly remote.

If you want to find out anything more about the various vaccinations and potential health hazards in different foreign countries I can thoroughly recommend Dr Richard Dawood's book *Traveller's Health* which is published by Oxford University Press.

Airline travel

Aeroplane travel can be quite an exhausting experience, with crowded departure lounges, long walks with luggage to the planes and the inevitable delays. If you use a wheelchair, and let the flight operator know in good time they can be immensely helpful. One friend of mine with M.E. – an occasional wheelchair user – always uses his for transit through airports. Your travel agent should be able to give you some idea on conditions in foreign airports (and hotels) if you're considering travelling abroad.

The Air Transport Users Committee (tel 071–242 3882) produces a leaflet called 'Care in the Air' for anyone with disabilities who are intending to fly abroad.

British Airways produce a useful leaflet ('Travel Wise' – for incapacitated passengers) which is available from BA Customer Services, Comet House, Heathrow Airport. This gives details about their Frequent Traveller's Card (FREMEC) for disabled passengers, and how to arrange for escorted help through arrivals/departures and getting on to the aircraft. If you're flying it may be a good idea to go to the airport the day before and stay at a hotel for the night.

Always try and do as much of your packing and attend to anything else that needs doing in the home several days before you're going away. Ideally, this should then leave you with a forty-eight-hour gap before you depart, in which you can rest as much as possible.

Last, don't forget about the needs of your partner or the rest of the family. If they're having to do most of the organising or driving, why not suggest an overnight stop to break the journey? Or even consider using the motorail – both here and abroad.

6. Additional Help and Benefits Available in Britain

Registering as disabled

One of the first things you can consider doing to get additional help, is to register yourself as disabled, with your local authority. This is not the same as being registered as disabled for employment purposes – you can, in fact, do both if you wish to. After contacting the social services department, this will then involve an appointment with either a social worker or occupational therapist to assess your disability. They can come and do this at your own home if you wish.

Registering is quite voluntary, but it can help you obtain certain benefits which the local authority administers (concessionary bus fares or an orange parking badge, etc.). It also gives your local authority some idea of the number of disabled people in their locality, what their needs are, and to what extent they're meeting those needs. The actual benefits aren't great, but the more people who do register, the more pressure 'the disabled' as a group can put on both central and local government to take notice of their problems. So, by registering, you're not only helping yourself.

Financial benefits may also include help with VAT and some social security benefits.

Local authorities can help with advice (and sometimes finance) on adaptations to the home. They are also responsible for administering Housing Benefit (see later) and rebates connected with the Community Charge (Council Tax as from April 1993).

Financial help for alterations is very limited, but anyone who is a tenant in council property should qualify if they have a good case for, say, a wheelchair ramp.

Social workers know about all the services that a local authority can and should provide; if you're not happy with the response from the council's officials phone the local social services department and ask to speak to the relevant social worker.

You can also approach your local councillor or Citizens Advice Bureau if you're not satisfied by their response.

Local authorities also administer home helps, Meals on Wheels, transport concessions and orange parking badges.

Home helps are very sought after, but often not available! The home help organiser at your local social services office will be able to give you further information. If you are able to obtain this help you'll probably have to pay part of the cost, unless you're on a very low income. Due to demand often exceeding supply you'll probably only qualify for local authority help if you're living alone (or with a relative who isn't very fit) and quite constantly disabled by your M.E., so unable to do most household tasks. Here a doctor's letter will be of help. What they actually do in the home should be suited to your particular needs, but it can include helping with cooking, cleaning and shopping.

If you can't get help from the local authority you can always try to find someone by advertising in the local shop or newspaper, or ask around to see if a neighbour has a home help who might be prepared to work a few extra hours each week.

Meals on Wheels This service operates in most parts of the country, but again tends to be overstretched, so has to be limited to those in real need, who aren't well enough to be up and about to shop and cook a hot meal every day. The service operates on weekdays only, and a small charge is made. The quality of the food is usually very good. Contact your local social services for further information.

One alternative is to make use of restaurants who are providing home delivery of pizzas, etc. It is costly, but it does mean you can have a hot meal if you can't face cooking yourself. If you've got a freezer, and are living alone, check out the already prepared meals for one, which can be kept in store.

Social workers offer a wide variety of practical help and advice. They don't just spend their time dealing with problems. They may be able to put you in touch with an appropriate agency or help you steer the correct path through the minefield of DSS benefits.

Many social workers are experienced in listening to people who have a multitude of difficulties – financial, social, emotional, medical, etc. – and don't see any way out of their predicament. If you feel you've got to this stage, it's often very useful to sit down and talk about your anxieties with someone like a social worker, who's detached from the situation, yet has helped many others in similar circumstances. They should know all about the local authority services which are available, and may possibly 'negotiate' with the relevant department on your behalf. They also tend to have good contacts with local community and volunteer groups.

Some social workers are now attached on a part-time basis to general practitioner health centres, but the best way to contact one is to phone the local social services department and ask for an appointment, or a home visit if necessary.

District Nurses are nurses (sometimes with non-qualified helpers) who have undertaken extra training to become expert in the problems of nursing patients at home. For an M.E. patient who is spending long periods in bed they can offer practical advice to the carer on how to lift correctly, as well as assisting with bathing and dressing if there's nobody else to help someone living alone. They can also advise on what other sources of help may be locally available, and provide aids such as sheepskin mattresses to help prevent bed sores, hoists for the bathroom, bath seats, etc. The best way to make contact is via your general practitioner.

Physiotherapists don't just work in hospitals; they also work with patients out in the community. Active physiotherapy isn't usually part of M.E. rehabilitation and can even be harmful, but a physiotherapist who knows about M.E. and what isn't good for M.E. patients could be of great help. If you're on prolonged bed rest a physiotherapist could come in and show you how to carry out passive exercises on the arm and limb muscles, to stop them becoming too weak. Physiotherapists can also help with advice on wheelchairs, and what sort of walking aids may be available, e.g. Zimmer frames.

Ask your general practitioner if there is a community physio-therapist available.

Occupational Therapists work in both hospitals and out in the community, where they're employed by the local author-ity. You can contact your local occupational therapist directly (without a doctor's letter) at the local social services department. They will then probably come and visit you at home to assess and advise you on ways in which your daily living can be made easier. Occupational therapists are quite used to advising clients about aids to help with washing, bathing, dressing, etc., as well as equipment for the kitchen and the possibility of making more major alterations to the home.

If you're going to start making life easier in the way your home is run, you'll have to accept that a whole range of domestic duties aren't going to be carried out as often, or perhaps as efficiently, as they used to be. If you find standing and carrying out tasks particularly difficult, try to sit down whenever possible. It's obviously not so easy to do the cooking, washing-up or ironing from a seated position, but it may be the only practical way to complete the task. Here, an occupational therapist can help with advice on lowering of work surfaces and suitable high seating.

Home visits can also be made by a chiropodist, dentist and optician. Your local Family Health Services Authority (FHSA) should know if this is possible. A Citizens Advice Bureau worker will try to visit you at home if you are house-bound when it is not possible to give advice over the phone or by letter. Some local authority libraries make arrangements for home visiting as well.

Prescription charges M.E. is not an illness which entitles you to exemption from NHS prescription charges. If you regularly need two or more items every month it may be worth buying a four-monthly or yearly 'season ticket' which gives you unlimited free prescriptions for a set charge. Apply on form FP95 (EC95 in Scotland) which is available from the post office or social security department.

Free prescriptions are available to anyone who is:
- under 16 or under 19 if in full-time education
- aged 60 or over (women) or 65 (men)
- pregnant or is looking after a child under one year old
- claiming Income Support, Family Credit or living on a very low income
- also suffering from diabetes, myxoedema, hypoparathyroidism, Addison's disease, myasthenia gravis, epilepsy or who has a permanent colostomy or ileostomy.

Forms P11 and AB11 explain in detail about free prescriptions.

Public Services British Gas, British Telecom and the Electricity Boards have all become much more aware of the needs of disabled customers, and may be able to help with special adaptations to their equipment (e.g. easier knobs on a gas cooker) or, in the case of British Gas, offer free safety checks if you are registered as disabled. If you cannot manage to handle a large printed phonebook, register for free use of Directory Enquiries by calling 0800 (freephone) 919195 for an application form from British Telecom.

Further sources of practical help

The Disabled Living Foundation This is probably the most important, and now has over twenty disabled living centres throughout the country. (Full list on page 330.)

The Foundation now has well over 10,000 different technical aids for the disabled on its database, and many of these can be seen on display at the living centres. At these centres patients, carers and health care professionals can find out what's available, and where they can buy or hire such equipment. The centres don't actually sell anything on display. Occupational therapists and physiotherapists are on hand to give advice on aids for any individual problem. This can be for any aspect of daily living, indoors or outdoors, ranging from those designed to help with bathing and dressing, to highly sophisticated electronic aids for the severely disabled. There's no charge made to visit the centre, and they're usually open weekdays from 9.30 to 5.00.

You don't require a doctor's referral, although the staff do like you to phone or write beforehand to arrange a fixed appointment, so they can give individual attention. If you've got a severe disability associated with M.E. it's useful to have a doctor's letter as well, giving some information on your medical state.

Disablement Information and Advice Line (DIAL) Provides locally based information on how to obtain aids. There are numerous local centres, listed in the phone book (see pages 328–9).

Royal Association for Disability and Rehabilitation (RADAR) can offer advice on a whole range of issues affecting the disabled, and they publish a number of useful books (see page 338).

British Red Cross Local branches (see phone book) can make short-term loans of aids such as wheelchairs and commodes. They publish a helpful booklet, *Home-made Aids for Handicapped People*.

Centre for Accessible Environments will give free advice if you are considering extending or making some major alterations to the home. They are in contact with the sort of architects who are interested and experienced in this type of work (see page 325).

The DSS publish a leaflet 'Equipment for the Disabled' (Code HB2), which is available from DSS supplies (see page 327).

Equipment for the Disabled publish a series of illustrated booklets on a wide range of disability problems, and act as a reference source for aids and equipment (see pages 330–31).

Volunteer Bureaux exist in many areas and aim to put

anyone with disabilities in touch with willing, able-bodied helpers, who are prepared to help with a very wide variety of tasks. Your Citizens Advice Bureau will know if there are local groups operating, and they sometimes have a list of volunteers available and jobs to be done printed in the local weekly paper. If you've got a specific task which needs doing, e.g. some gardening, decorating or help with getting to the shops each week, get in touch with your local bureau organiser. They may have someone willing to help (see Useful Addresses).

Care Attendant Schemes are being increasingly organised by both local authorities and voluntary organisations. They will provide paid helpers who try to help disabled people with a wide range of tasks on a fairly flexible basis. The type of care provided can be on a personal basis, e.g. helping with washing or dressing, or more general tasks in the home. Such help is probably only available for M.E. patients who are quite badly affected, and either living alone or being looked after by a carer who also isn't in the best of health. This sort of service doesn't occur everywhere, but your local social services department or Citizens Advice Bureau will know if it does.

Crossroads Care Attendant Schemes aim to relieve some of the stresses which inevitably result from looking after a disabled person in their own home. They have been set up to complement, but not replace, existing statutory services and to work closely with them in the home. One particular area where Crossroads tries to offer practical help is when a carer also falls ill and there is a danger that the whole system of care will break down necessitating admission to hospital or residential care. Crossroads Care Schemes are now operating in well over 100 different towns in the U.K. They are all locally administered but form part of the national organisation. For further details on your nearest Crossroads branch contact their headquarters address (see page 327).

The DSS: sickness and other benefits available

You may find that you need to make use of state social

security benefits which are available if you're out of work. You contribute taxes throughout your lifetime, so now there shouldn't be any feeling of guilt in claiming benefits if necessary. Unfortunately, even though M.E. is a genuine illness, some examining medical officers still aren't up to date with the facts on M.E., and don't always see it that way.

On the positive side, there's no doubt that there has been a significant change in the way the DSS views M.E. as an illness, and the disability it causes. Claims for benefit are being considered in a more sympathetic manner, and patients should no longer have to get their doctors to write some form of psychiatric diagnosis on the sick note in order to get the benefit. And, in the House of Commons (*Hansard*, 13 November 1991, col. 582W) Mr Stephen Dorrell MP stated that 'the Government and NHS recognise M.E. as a debilitating and distressing condition'.

The different benefits, and rules governing your eligibility, are often complex, and sometimes misunderstood by the people who administer them. If you are in any doubt about your eligibility, do make a written claim and see what happens – it can't do any harm, providing you're not being dishonest in the information you provide. If your application is refused, don't give up, and make an appeal if this is possible – after all, you're not only fighting for yourself, but for other M.E. patients in the same position as well.

If it becomes necessary to appeal against a DSS decision, some lawyers aren't very well informed or helpful, and it's often better to 'do-it-yourself' with the help of a disabled rights organisation or trade union.

Some of the best impartial advice can be obtained from the various disability rights organisations such as the Disability Alliance, local Citizens Advice Bureaux and Welfare Rights Centres set up by local authorities. There are some very useful handbooks published by these organisations – see page 365.

Some practical advice on dealing with the DSS (and other parts of officialdom)

- Always try to find out who you are talking to, either

on the phone, or at an interview.

- Preferably do things by letter, and *always keep your own, dated copy of any correspondence.* If you're sending important documents keep a photocopy of them in case they get lost, and post them by recorded delivery. If you deal with the office by phone, always make a note in your diary about what was said, and by whom.
- If you want to discuss something at the office, phone to make an appointment, and if you're not happy about tackling officials by yourself, take a friend or relative along as well. There shouldn't be any objection if you explain your disability.
- Make a written note of what you want to ask before you go, and then record the official's replies.
- If you're not happy with the answers, ask to speak to a supervisor of the relevant department, or write a letter to the manager.
- If you're getting nowhere with a claim, a letter to your MP (at the House of Commons, London SW1) will be passed on to the local DSS office with a request for a swift reply. As a last resort write to the Minister for Social Security at Alexander Fleming House, Elephant and Castle, London SE1 6BY. If this doesn't work a letter to Her Majesty the Queen can be extremely effective in making officialdom move!

Guide to individual benefits

DSS benefits for the sick and disabled fall into three broad categories:

1   Those which help replace income for anyone who is no longer able to work:
   Statutory Sick Pay
   Invalidity Benefit
   Severe Disablement Allowance – if you've no national insurance contributions.
2   Benefits providing extra help for the severely disabled are:
   Disability Living Allowance (replaced Attendance and Mobility Allowance in April 1992)
   Disability Working Allowance

Where to go for help on individual benefits

Benefit problem	Who can help	Address or phone number
General Social Security advice and problems with DSS benefits	DSS	Freephone BELL – the Benefit Enquiry Line for Disabled People. 0800–882200 9.00–4.30 Monday–Friday
		Or phone your local Social Security Office – in the phone book under Social Security
DSS leaflets and claim forms		Either BELL (who can help you fill one in), your local DSS office or Post Office. Leaflets are available by post from: DSS Leaflets Unit PO Box 21 Stanmore Middlesex HA7 1AY
Housing Benefit & Community Charge Benefit	Your local council	
Income Support	Unemployment Benefit office	
Hospital travel costs	The hospital where you are being treated	See page 337
Further help	Welfare Rights Officer at your local council	
	Disability Alliance	See page 329
	Disability Rights Handbook	See page 365
	Citizens Advice Bureau – free local advice	

Invalid Care Allowance
Home Responsibilities Protection
Independent Living Fund
3   Benefits to help anyone on a low income:
Income Support
Family Credit
Housing Benefit
Social Fund
Community Charge Benefit

Statutory sick pay

At the onset of any illness, providing you're at work, you'll receive Statutory Sick Pay (SSP) from your employer, which may then be 'topped up' to a percentage of normal pay, depending on how long you've been employed.

Invalidity benefit

For people who have been incapable of work for the past twenty-eight weeks, and previously claiming Statutory Sick Pay (SSP) from their employer, or a non-contributory sickness benefit. It's still possible to claim Invalidity Benefit, if you haven't been claiming SSP. This may apply to some self-employed, and unemployed as well as widows/widowers. Payment can continue till 65 (women) and 70 (men).

The total, non-taxable, weekly payment is made up of three separate parts:

a) Invalidity Pension which gives a payment for the claimant, plus allowances for dependants. If a wife or husband earns (after expenses) more than a certain amount per week, his or her extra allowance, and children's allowances will be appropriately reduced.
b) Invalidity Allowance is only paid if you start claiming more than five years before pension age, and is paid according to how old you are at the start of the claim.
c) Additional Earnings Related Pension is based on your earnings after 6 April 1978, and is paid to anyone who

claims after 6 April 1979. However, the DSS have decided that nobody can now receive *both* the Invalidity Allowance and the Additional Earnings Related in full. Further details can be found in DSS leaflet NI 16A.

Invalidity Benefit can affect other social security benefits being claimed by either yourself or your dependants.

Invalidity Benefit is probably the most frequent benefit claimed by M.E. patients. You have to keep sending in sickness certificates (Med 3s) signed by your general practitioner indicating that the doctor considers that you are unfit for work. When the condition has become prolonged the general practitioner may date the certificate 'till further notice', but many GPs still like to keep an eye on their patients, and so limit it to six months or a year.

The decision to award the benefit is made by the DSS adjudication officer – a non-medically qualified civil servant – at the local benefit office. These unnamed officials will usually accept your GP's opinion, but after a while your claim will be referred on to one of their own doctors for an opinion.

Therapeutic earnings Anyone claiming Invalidity Benefit is also allowed to have some 'therapeutic earnings' (up to £39 per week in 1991), plus a few connected expenses. You must first get written approval from your GP that the type of activity won't have any adverse effect on recovery, and then send it to the DSS for their approval. The sort of work you might do is something quiet and non-demanding like writing, or occasionally doing your normal type of work, but for a very limited period. But you've got to be very careful that the DSS don't then use this activity as an excuse to say that you're fit to start looking for a full-time job again.

Invalidity Benefit cut-off The major problem that many M.E. patients experience in long-term sickness revolves around the DSS definition of being 'unfit for work'. They accept that you can be off sick from your normal occupation for a certain period of time, but after that they'll only continue to pay benefit, on an indefinite basis, if they're certain that there is no other work – full-time or part-time – from which you could reasonably earn a living. For example, in the case of M.E., they might well accept that a manual worker could no longer cope with this sort of work from the physical point of view, but he could cope with something less demanding. In my case they decided I couldn't be expected to cope with making important life and death decisions when my brain wasn't functioning, but that I could do something like collecting tickets at the car park, or even be a night watchman!

The process of reviewing fitness for work is complicated. To try and explain the steps which are taken it's helpful to refer to a flow diagram.

1 The first stage is when a form arrives through the post instructing you that such a review is about to take place. This can be because either the DSS or your GP wants a second opinion on your eligibility to benefit.

2 The examination will take place at a local DSS centre. If you (and your GP) can persuade the DSS that travelling would be very difficult and harmful in your present state of health, the examining doctor might be persuaded to do the assessment at home.

The RMO is employed by the DSS and sends an *opinion* to the local benefit office. While you're there it's worth asking if the RMO has received a report from your GP. In some cases it may not have arrived, but they're unlikely to tell you what it says if they do have a copy. It's worth noting that the examining doctor has, on average, only 24 minutes to deal with each patient, and this includes filling in the medical report!

3 The RMO has to decide if you are 'fit for work'. If it seems to him that you can't return to your normal occupation, he then has to decide if there is *any* possible work you could do. The fact that the type of work may not actually be available in your locality is of very minor consideration. Could you do it if it were available? Remember, the RMO's report is only a *recommendation*, not an arbitrary decision, although the way this information is conveyed, on Forms BF130 or BF114a, makes this far from clear. If this happens to you – reading the impersonal, stereotyped form from the DSS telling you that your benefit has

HOW THE SYSTEM WORKS

1. SUMMONS to attend DSS medical (form RM3)

↓

2. EXAMINATION by RMO —— Agrees 'UNFIT' —► Benefit continues

↓

FIT (?)

↓

3. RMO RECOMMENDS that you are 'capable of work' which can either be:

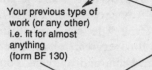

Your previous type of work (or any other) i.e. fit for almost anything (form BF 130)

Suitable alternative employment i.e. some form of 'light work' (form BF 114A)

↓

4. RETURN IMMEDIATELY to see your GP with the relevant form and request a fresh sick note. This shows that your GP has reviewed the situation and still agrees you should be off sick

If you do not go and see your GP the DSS adjudicating officer (AO) will now decide on your fitness for work

↓   *danger!*

FRESH NOTE given by your GP. Send this back to the DSS in the usual manner

your GP gives you a CLOSED NOTE

Benefit will now STOP and you will lose the right to any appeal

↓

The DSS should now arrange a further medical opinion from another RMO —— Agrees 'UNFIT' —►Benefit continues

2nd OPINION : still FIT FOR WORK

↓

5. DSS Adjudicating Officer (AO) makes his decision

Agrees 'UNFIT'

↓

Benefit continues

Decides you are 'FIT FOR WORK' INFORMS you on form BS25. BENEFIT WILL NOW STOP

↓

6. CLAIM UNEMPLOYMENT BENEFIT
Your GP can still issue sick notes if he disagrees.
APPEAL within three months to the Social Security Appeal Tribunal (SSAT) —► WIN APPEAL —► Benefit restored and backdated

↓

LOSE APPEAL

↓

7. FINAL APPEAL TO SOCIAL SECURITY COMMISSIONER

been stopped or your claim has been rejected – it's only natural to feel very angry, and even quite shocked.

Try not to get too upset, as the additional stress will only make your M.E. symptoms even worse. Sit down and calmly think things through, preferably with the help of a friend or relative for moral support, and plan what you're going to do next. Read up all the information you can get on the relevant benefit and the appeals procedures, and go and talk to someone at the local Citizens Advice Bureau. It's very tempting to start firing off a series of angry letters – by all means write them, but don't post them for forty-eight hours, as your feelings may have calmed down and changed by then. You don't want to be taking any actions in the heat of the moment which you might regret later.

When this sort of thing has happened to me, my natural reaction has been to phone the DSS, and to try to speak to the official who's made the decision. Unfortunately, this is easier said than done, as these bureaucrats are usually well protected from members of the general public!

Where a medical decision has been taken, a form may be signed by a named divisional medical officer. These doctors aren't used to members of the public phoning them up, but if you really feel aggrieved and confident enough to do so it's well worth a try, and you may get through to the top. Again try to contain your anger, and put forward your case in a reasoned and constructive manner – you may be lucky and end up receiving some sympathetic help and advice. It's worth remembering that many of these officials and doctors don't always agree with some of the decisions they have to take when making assessments on benefit claims, and they're only too aware of defending the indefensible!

4   If you disagree with an RMO recommendation you should immediately go and see your general practitioner and discuss the situation. Take the form with you as the doctor may not have heard from the DSS. If your GP takes your side, and disagrees with the opinion – accepting you are still unfit for work – you should ask for a fresh sickness certificate, even if your old one hasn't yet expired. Unfortunately, some GPs are still afraid of upsetting the DSS Regional Medical Officers (RMOs), who

carry out these assessments, and don't always give their patients the support they deserve. Others, however, are excellent, and don't have any qualms about fully supporting your case, and if necessary disagreeing with a colleague's opinion.

Your GP doesn't have to agree with the RMO – if he now issues you with a closed note (saying you are now 'fit for work') your benefit will stop, and you lose any chance of taking the case to appeal.

If the DSS now receives your fresh certificate, they should then arrange a second medical opinion by another of their RMOs.

5 With the above medical recommendation(s) the DSS Adjudicating Officer (AO) will now make a *decision* on the claim. The AO is a lay person, not a doctor.

6 If the AO decides to agree with the RMO the benefit will stop. However, you can now make an appeal to the Social Security Appeals Tribunal (SSAT) which consists of a lawyer and two independent people. In the meantime you do no harm by signing on as unemployed in order to get some financial help, but there's nothing to stop you sending in sickness certificates – providing your GP will still issue them. You must now prepare for the appeal by:

(a) Obtaining written support on your incapacity to work from both your GP and consultant – if you have one. The DSS is unlikely to have obtained a consultant's report, and if this supports your claim it can be very persuasive with the tribunal.

(b) Get as much advice as possible on how to appeal from the local Citizens Advice Bureau (they might be able to send someone along with you for support), your trade union, or a disability rights organisation – e.g. the Disability Alliance.

(c) Write down a list of your symptoms and how they incapacitate you during the day, especially in ways which would affect your capacity to work – e.g. you can't be reliable as your symptoms vary so much from one day to the next.

7 If you lose this SSAT appeal you still have one last chance, by appealing to the Social Security Commissioner (see p. 339).

Severe disablement allowance (SDA)

For anyone who has been unable to work for twenty-eight weeks or more, but doesn't qualify for state sickness benefit or Invalidity Benefit, due to insufficient national insurance contributions. You must be aged 16–60 (women), or 16–65 (men), as well as being both incapable of work, *and* be assessed as being 75 per cent or more disabled.

Assessing a percentage disability for say loss of a limb is relatively straightforward, but with M.E., where the disability is fluctuating and hard to assess objectively, it's quite likely that different doctors will come to differing conclusions. You'll almost certainly have to go for a medical examination, and if your general practitioner or consultant is prepared to support your case, it's important to make sure they send in some written evidence to this effect, clearly stating the nature of the disabilities M.E. is causing. The assessment should take into account both your physical and mental disabilities associated with M.E., and how they are preventing you carrying out 'normal living', with particular reference to employment prospects.

In the case of M.E. the disabilities which are particularly relevant are:

- Limited energy, which affects your ability to walk or carry out physical tasks.
- Brain malfunction, affecting your mental abilities.

It's important to get these facts clear in your mind before you go to the examination, so you can present them to the examining doctors when they question you about how M.E. affects your life.

SDA is a very complex benefit in its qualifying criteria, and so before making an application I'd recommend anyone to read more about it in the *Disability Rights Handbook*. More specific information is contained in – *The SDA – Handbook for Adjudicating Medical Authorities*, from the DSS leaflets unit (see page 327).

If you apply and are then refused you do have a right to appeal – within three months – to a Medical Appeal Tribunal. From talking to M.E. patients who've been refused on their first attempt, my advice is to appeal, and if still unsuccessful to try again at a later date. Unfortunately, one doctor's view of disability isn't always the same as his colleagues'.

SDA provides a weekly payment which is tax-free and not means-tested. There are extra additions for any adult or child dependants. Anyone already receiving a Disability Living Allowance should be able to claim SDA automatically. As with Invalidity Benefit you can also have 'therapeutic earnings' (see page 310). Further details on DSS leaflet NI 252.

Disability living allowance (DLA)

In April 1992 the DSS amalgamated the old mobility and attendance allowances to create this new benefit. In theory, anyone claiming either of the two previous allowances should have been automatically transferred to DLA. There is no doubt that the implementation of a major new benefit is going to have teething problems, especially in the case of M.E. where the guidelines issued to DSS officials are far from satisfactory. So, *the criteria listed below may well change* in the course of time, and if you are considering applying for this benefit, it is well worth asking the DSS for up-to-date information regarding your individual circumstances.

The DLA consists of a care component payable at one of three separate rates and a mobility component which is payable at one of two rates.

The criteria for the top and middle rates of the care component are very similar to those which applied to people claiming higher and lower rates of attendance allowance. As far as M.E. is concerned, this means requiring a great deal of help and attention with what the DSS refers to as 'bodily functions'. By this, they mean assistance from other people with walking, dressing, washing, eating and going to the toilet, etc. Anyone who thinks they may be eligible should read more about the DLA criteria in the Disability Rights Handbook.

The highest rate of DLA can be paid to anyone who satisfies *both* one of the day-time *and* one of the night-time attention or supervision rules. The middle care rate is payable if you satisfy *either* a day-time or night-time attention or supervision rule. The lowest rate can be claimed by anyone under 65 who on account of physical or mental disability:

(i)   requires in connection with his or her bodily functions attention from another person for a significant portion of the day (whether during a single period or a number of periods); or

(ii)   cannot prepare a cooked main meal for himself/herself even if he/she has the ingredients. (Children under 16 cannot qualify under this test.)

The DLA mobility component is payable at one of two rates to people aged 5 or over who claim before their 66th birthday. Here the highest rate is payable to anyone who satisfies the previous rules for mobility allowance. These are:

(a)   Being completely unable to walk. This means that you cannot take a single step, and very few M.E. patients fit into this category.

(b)   Being virtually unable to walk. Here the DSS is not terribly specific in terms of distance; however, anyone who is capable of walking unaided for more than a few hundred yards seems unlikely to qualify. Your walking ability does have to be *considerably* restricted.

(c)   The exertion required to walk constitutes either a danger to life, or could lead to a serious deterioration in health. Again, the interpretation is far from clear when it comes to M.E. Those patients who have very severe limitations in their exercise capabilities before becoming exhausted may well find that they fulfil this part of the criteria.

The new lower rate of mobility component will be payable to anyone who fails the above tests but who:

'. . . is able to walk but is so severely disabled physically or mentally that, disregarding any ability he may have to use routes which are familiar to him on his own, he cannot take advantage of the faculty out of doors without guidance or supervision from another person most of the time.'

Children under 16 must require more guidance or supervision

than another child of the same age.

In the past many people with M.E. have had their application for Mobility Allowance rejected, but with this new lower rate it may be worth making a new application. The only way to find out is to fill in a claim form and see what happens.

A major change in the way this new benefit is administered is the fact that most claims will be assessed by non-medically qualified civil servants at the DSS, and no longer by examining doctors. Whether this will be a change for the better remains to be seen.

What remains a major cause for concern is the advice being given to these officials on the subject of M.E. and the disability it causes. In drawing up the new guidelines, I was involved in discussions with senior DSS civil servants and doctors and, although some changes were made, the result is still very unsatisfactory. I have no doubt that many perfectly valid claims will now be rejected as a result. Below are reproduced the relevant sections on M.E. which are contained in the guidelines on Disability Living Allowance. These were issued to DSS adjudicating officers in 1992 despite opposition from all the main M.E. self-help support groups.

Care Considerations

- Some studies have shown an association with allergy to or intolerance of certain foods, food products and additives but other studies have not confirmed this.
- A great deal of help may be expected by, and is often given to, a sufferer from CFS or ME. Sufferers are sometimes advised to rest completely, but muscles which are not used deteriorate rapidly. There is, however, another school of thought which advocates graded exercises of muscles to assist the return to normal muscle function and power. In some studies of people affected by chronic fatigue syndrome objective tests of muscle power have shown it to be normal or near normal. A person affected by these syndromes may therefore be able to attend to bodily functions without the assistance of another but each case must be considered in the light of available evidence.

Mobility Considerations
- In some controlled clinical studies people with chronic fatigue syndromes have been shown to have adequate muscle power. They may, however, refrain from walking because they are fearful of the consequences.

If you do manage to successfully claim a DLA it's worth remembering that this benefit also acts as a passport to several other allowances and concessions. These include:
- Severe Disablement Allowance   (page 306)
- Orange Parking Badge   (page 283)
- British Rail Disabled Railcard   (page 285)
- Vehicle Tax Exemption   (page 284)
- Motability   (page 283)

Disability working allowance (DWA)

This second 'new' benefit was introduced in April 1992 and is designed to help disabled people who now feel capable of returning to work. It can be claimed by anyone who is:

- aged 16 or over
- working at least 16 hours per week as an employee or self-employed
- already claiming a qualifying benefit (e.g. Invalidity Benefit, Severe Disablement Allowance or Disability Living Allowance) in the eight weeks prior to making a DWA claim
- considered to be at a 'disadvantage in obtaining a job' because of a physical or mental disability
- able to pass the DWA means-test and has savings of less than £16,000.

If *all* the above conditions are met, a claim for DWA can be made as soon as you commence work. This has to be done on a complicated self-assessment form which is available from the DSS. Most claims are decided by an adjudication officer on the basis of this self-assessment, although a medical examination may be necessary. Once a DWA has been granted, it should continue for at least 26 weeks, possibly longer.

The amount of benefit which is payable is worked out

according to a rather complex system that is very similar to the way Family Credit is calculated. This is based on what is termed the 'threshold' level and depends on whether you are single, married or have dependent children. If your total weekly earnings are equal to or below this threshold limit, you should be entitled to the maximum amount of DWA. For those whose income is above the threshold, their DWA will be proportionately reduced.

As with the DLA, an appeal can be made to the Disability Appeal Tribunal if you disagree with an adjudicating officer's decision.

The Disability Alliance has made a number of criticisms about this new benefit, which in the long term could create disincentives to disabled people becoming 'independent' through taking paid employment. The strict criteria exclude disabled people who can only work less than 16 hours per week, and those who are not already receiving one of the qualifying benefits. Even the Social Services Advisory Committee has criticised the fact that this new benefit may well force disabled people into low paid work (because of the poverty trap element) instead of allowing them to realise their capacity. Lastly, there is the problem of reclaiming Invalidity Benefit or Severe Disablement Benefit if there is a deterioration of health. According to the rules this should be possible within two years of claiming DWA, but the fact that you have managed to work for 16 hours+ per week, for up to two years, may well be used by the adjudicating officer as a means of challenging your re-entitlement. So, do think very carefully about the DWA option; in pure financial terms it may be just as beneficial to opt for the therapeutic earnings rule in addition to your existing benefit. If you are uncertain about the relative advantages and disadvantages of claiming DWA, do talk it over with an experienced welfare rights officer before submitting a claim.

The invalid care allowance

This is for people of working age (16–60 for women, and 16–65 for men) who can't go out to work because they're having to look after someone at home who is severely disabled.

National insurance contributions are not required, but the payment is taxable. There are additions for dependent relatives, but it can be affected by other social security benefits. Claim on form DS700.

To qualify for ICA you must be spending thirty-five hours or more in 'caring'; any earnings above £30 per week may affect this benefit. You don't, however, have to be related to the person you're looking after.

If a claim for ICA is refused, you can appeal to the Social Security Appeals Tribunal.

Home responsibilities protection

If you're not eligible for Invalid Care Allowance, but still having to stay at home to look after a severely disabled person you may qualify for this. If you're claiming certain other social security benefits you may already be having your national insurance contributions credited by the DSS, and so protecting pension rights. If this isn't the case then you should check with the DSS if you ought to apply for HRP.

The *Disability Rights Handbook* also covers the benefit in detail.

Independent living fund

The Independent Living Fund is a charitable trust financed by central government. It was established in 1988 as part of the government's major reforms in social security payments. The fund is discretionary and there is only a limited amount of money available each year. However, for some severely disabled people with M.E. it could be of enormous benefit. Unfortunately, there has been very little in the way of publicity from the DSS, and I am not aware that anyone with M.E. has been awarded a grant from the Fund.

The aim of this fund is to help severely disabled people on low incomes to live independently in the community by providing some extra financial help towards the employment of domestic help or personal care. In theory the Fund is supposed to provide whatever extra money is necessary for such care, and payments of well over £100 per week can be awarded. It is particularly aimed at those who are less able or likely to organise their own care. A claim can be accepted from disabled people who live alone or with a carer/partner who cannot provide all the practical help that is required. Remember, though, the degree of disability has to be *severe*, and this means being able to satisfy the strict criteria relating to the Disability Living Allowance or the old Attendance Allowance. Anyone over the age of 16 can apply to the Fund and there is no upper age limit.

As far as income is concerned you or your partner must be receiving Income Support or can show that the cost of care is more than your current income. You should also have less than £8000 in savings.

To make a claim to the Fund fill in an application form (obtainable from your local social security office or by phoning the Benefit Enquiry Line on 0800 882200) and return it to the Fund managers. This should be followed a few weeks later by a thorough assessment in your own home by what is known as a 'voluntary visitor'. It will then take several weeks to process the application before a decision is made. If you don't hear anything more then contact the Fund directly. Payment for any claim that is accepted should be backdated to the application date.

If you feel that you might be eligible for this benefit do make a claim and see what happens. The address of the Fund is given in the reference section.

Income support

This is a benefit to help people aged 18 or over whose income is below a certain level. Some 16–17 year olds can get it, but only in special circumstances. The benefit is mainly designed for people who are able to obtain work, but the chronically sick, single parents and people over the age of 60 can also qualify.

Normally, you or your partner, if you have one, must not be working 24 hours or more a week. Income Support can be paid on top of other DSS benefits (including Unemployment Benefit) or earnings from part-time work, or if you have no money at all. Your right to Income Support doesn't depend on your NI contributions, it depends on how much money you have coming in each week. You can claim even if you have savings but not if you, or you and your partner together, have more than £8000. Savings between £3000 and £8000 will make a difference. Income Support may be taxable and you can also obtain help from the Social Fund.

If you are currently registered as unemployed because of M.E., ask for an Income Support claim form at the Unemployment Benefit Office. Anyone else should fill in the form in leaflet IS 1 from a Social Security office or local post office. Leaflet IS 20 (*A guide to Income Support*) gives further details.

Family credit

This is a tax-free benefit for working families with children. It is not a loan and does not have to be paid back. To obtain Family Credit you must be responsible for at least one child under 16 (or under 19 if in full-time education).

You or your partner must be working at least 24 hours a week to qualify. You can claim if you are employed or self-employed, a couple or a lone parent bringing up a child on your own. Your right to Family Credit does not depend on your National Insurance record.

The amount you receive depends on your income, your partner's income, how many children you have and their respective ages. You don't even have to be on a very low income or have a very large family to qualify.

You can also claim if you have savings, though not if you and your partner together have more than £8000. Savings between £3000 and £8000 will affect the amount you get. If your claim is accepted your family will be automatically entitled to NHS benefits.

Family Credit is claimed by post. You can obtain a claim pack FC1 (Family Credit) from a post office or local Social Security Office.

Housing benefit

If you are finding it hard to pay your full rent, you may be able to get some help from your local council, whether you are working or not. If you are a council tenant you can apply for a rent rebate. If you are a private tenant, you can claim for a rent allowance. You can still claim for Housing Benefit if you live in a hotel, hostel, guesthouse or similar accommodation.

Your right to Housing Benefit does not depend on your National Insurance contributions, and is tax free. The amount of help you can get depends on how much money you have coming in each week, the size of your family, your savings and how much rent you have to pay.

You can obtain a claim form from your council offices if you are not claiming Income Support. For those on Income Support a claim form should be automatically provided at the time. Return the form to your local Social Security office or your local council.

For further details see leaflet RR1 (*Housing Benefit – help with your rent*) from council offices and post offices.

Social fund

If you are faced with an exceptional expense which you find difficult to pay from your regular income, you may be able to obtain a payment from the Social Fund. Savings over £500 (or £1000 for those aged 60 or over) owned by you, or your partner together, are taken into account. There are several types of payment.

During a period of cold weather, you may qualify for a *Cold Weather Payment*. You qualify for this if you receive Income Support and you or your partner are over 60, or if someone you claim for is also disabled, or if you have a child under 5.

You may be able to obtain a *Community Care Grant* if you are receiving Income Support. These grants are given to help people lead independent lives in the community.

If you are on Income Support and need help to spread the cost of more expensive items, you may be entitled to a *Budgeting Loan*. These loans are interest free and repayable, normally from your weekly benefit.

Whether or not you are receiving Social Security benefits, you may need a *Crisis Loan* to help pay for living expenses or something you need urgently. These loans are also interest free and repayable. They are for people who have no other way of meeting their needs in an emergency or disaster.

For details about the Social Fund see leaflet SFL 2 (*How the Social Fund can help you*) and booklet SB16 (*A Guide to the Social Fund*). If you need to know more about any of the special benefits phone the DSS on their Freephone number on the BELL advice line.

Community charge benefit

If you are on a low income and find it hard to pay your full Community Charge you may be able to get help from your local council, whether you are working or not.

Most of the rules that apply to Housing Benefit also apply to Community Charge Benefit. If you are already claiming Income Support you should have filled in a claim form for Community Charge Benefit at the same time. If not, you should obtain leaflet CCB 1 (*Help with the Community Charge*) from your local post office, council office or Social Security office. When the new Council Tax comes into operation in April 1993 this benefit will obviously be replaced by something very similar.

N.B. Regulations regarding eligibility for the various social security benefits included in this chapter are constantly changing, and the capital limits are often linked to the rate of inflation. If you feel that you may be able to claim one of these benefits or wish to appeal against the DSS do check carefully that you have the most up-to-date information to hand.

PART 4:

APPENDICES

1. Useful Names
And Addresses

The M.E. Association

This is a particularly important source of practical advice, help and support. It is a self-help group, formed in 1976, which now has nearly 10,000 members. Dr Betty Dowsett, a consultant microbiologist with a long-standing interest in the illness is the Association's President. The Very Reverend Michael Mayne, Dean of Westminster, and Dr Charles Shepherd are Vice Presidents.

The Association is run by a central committee of volunteers, and organised into a large number of locally-based groups. These local groups are starting to cover most of the country, and exist in most large towns, or counties covering rural areas. As they become established they're starting to hold regular meetings throughout the year, and arranging guest speakers. There are also full-time paid employees at the office in Essex, who deal with an ever mounting number of queries and letters arriving each day (sometimes over 1,000 after a piece of television publicity) from patients, doctors, journalists — in fact anyone wanting to know more about M.E. The Association is actively involved with all aspects of the illness, and this includes:

- An education and information department which deals with day-to-day enquiries as well as the provision of literature for both doctors and patients. A full list is available on request.
- A welfare department which is able to give advice on DSS

benefits, employment and all the practical problems associated with disability.

- A 'listening ear' service run by volunteers which enables members to ring up and talk a problem over with someone who is not only understanding, but may also be able to offer some practical advice.
- The organisation of special groups for children/young people, and severely affected members.
- Sponsoring research via the Breakthrough Trust at various university departments into both the cause(s) and management of M.E. The M.E. Association is not opposed to complementary approaches to management, but believes that they should all come under the same close scrutiny and safety checks that apply to orthodox therapies.
- A scientific and medical advisory panel consisting of doctors working in the areas of virology, neurology, immunology, psychiatry, etc. These experts are available to advise on research grants and other medical matters as they arise.
- Close and regular contact with government departments and Members of Parliament on matters of concern, particularly benefits and government-sponsored research.
- Helping journalists from national newspapers, radio and television with background information in order to achieve a more positive coverage of the illness.

The Association also holds an Annual General Meeting in London each year, usually in April, at which research scientists are invited to discuss the latest medical findings.

Membership of the M.E. Association currently costs £12 per annum; this includes four issues each year of their journal called *Perspectives*. For further details send an SAE to:

M.E. Association
Stanhope House
High Street
Stanford-le-Hope
Essex SS17 0HA
Tel (0375) 642466
Fax (0375) 360256

The M.E. Association also have two regional offices in Northern Ireland and Scotland. Their addresses are on pages 342 and 343.

M.E. Action

M.E. Action is a national membership campaign offering help, information and other services to people with M.E. It was founded in 1987 by Sue Findlay, and now has Clare Francis, the well-known yachtswoman and author, as President.

It has campaigned to bring about the full recognition of M.E. as a genuine physical illness, and in this respect was actively involved in persuading Jimmy Hood MP to introduce a Bill in the House of Commons (see *Hansard*, 23 February 1988: pages 167–168) to draw attention to the multiple number of problems faced by people with M.E. The Bill received widespread all-party support, which was probably helped by the fact that there are several members in both houses ill with M.E.

M.E. Action accepts that both orthodox and some of the more controversial alternative approaches to management must be researched and assessed. They recently helped to fund a trial into the use of magnesium sulphate injections.

Members receive three copies per year of the journal *InterAction*. They also run a therapy helpline, postal library and, like the M.E. Association, produce various information leaflets.

M.E. Action welcomes enquiries from both patients and health professionals. For further details please send a large SAE to:

M.E. Action
PO Box 1302
Wells
Somerset BA5 2WE
Tel (0749) 670799

Westcare

This is a registered charity which provides information and services for people with M.E., their relatives, friends, doctors and other health care professionals. Westcare operates mainly in Bristol and the South West of England but nobody is excluded. Its clinic in Bristol offers consultations with a doctor who is familiar with M.E. and with professional counsellors.

Westcare works in co-operation with other M.E. charities and with the medical profession, particularly in the Bristol hospitals. Lectures and study days are provided and research projects are encouraged.

The charity is now hoping to develop further services such as facilities for respite care. Anyone who requires further information should contact Westcare at:

> 15 Queen Victoria Road
> Redland
> Bristol BS6 7PE
> Tel (0272) 738317

Overseas Organisations

Similar self-help support groups are also operating in various overseas countries:

America:

> The CFIDS Association
> PO Box 220398
> Charlotte
> NC 28222-0398
> Tel (1800 - toll free) 442 3437
> Fax 704/365-9755

Australian states:

Australian Capital Territory:

> ACT ME Society Inc
> PO Box 717
> Mawson
> ACT 2607
> Tel (06) 290 1984

New South Wales:

> ME/CFS Society of New South Wales Inc
> PO Box 449
> Crows Nest
> NSW 2065
> Tel (02) 439 6026

Queensland and Northern Territory:	ME Support Group PO Box 12 Oxenford Queensland 4210 Tel (075) 73 2772
South Australia:	ME/CFS Society Inc PO Box 383 Adelaide South Australia 5001 Tel (08) 49 1913
Victoria and Tasmania:	ME/CFSS Society of Victoria Inc 24 Livingstone Close Burwood Victoria 3125 Tel (03) 8888–798
Western Australia:	CFSS of Western Australia 92 Powell Street Joondanna Perth Western Australia 6060 Tel (09) 483 6667
Belgium:	AFZ M.E. Predikherenstraat 2 B–3000 Leuven Belgium
Canada:	M.E. Canada 246 Queen Street Suite 400 Ottawa Ontario Canada K1P 5E4 Tel (613) 563 1565 Fax (613) 567 0614

Denmark:	Danish ME/CFS Association co/ A Midsem Maglehøj 86 DK-3520 Farum Denmark
Holland:	M.E. Stichting Du Perronstraat 34 HS 1064 JT Amsterdam Holland
Italy:	C.F.S. Associazione Italiana Segreteria: Via Moimacco 20 33100 Udine Italy
New Zealand:	ANZMES PO Box 35 429 Browns Bay Auckland 10 New Zealand
Norway:	Norges M.E. Forening Eiksveien 96A 1345 Osteras Norway
South Africa:	M.E. Association of South Africa PO Box 461 Hillcrest 3650 South Africa

IFMEA (International Federation of M.E. Associations) is an organisation that collects and disseminates up-to-date medical information to patient-support groups on a worldwide basis. Groups who would like to join should contact:

Dr E Goudsmit
Director, IFMEA
23 Melbourne Road
Teddington
Middx TW11 9QX
UK

List of Useful Addresses A—Z

Please note that where an organisation uses the words 'British' or 'National' in its title the address will be listed under the name of the subject it is involved with. So, the British Allergy Foundation can be found under A — Allergy.

Also remember that when writing to any of these charities it would be appreciated if a large SAE is included as most of them are not well off financially.

Special addresses relevant to Northern Ireland, Scotland and Wales are listed separately at the end.

ACTION FOR VICTIMS OF MEDICAL ACCIDENTS (AVMA)
Bank Chambers
1 London Road
Forest Hill
London SE23 3TP
Tel (081) 291 2793
Advises patients who feel that something has gone wrong with their medical treatment and refers them to appropriate solicitors if legal action is possible

Acupuncture
MEDICALLY QUALIFIED ACUPUNCTURISTS
British Medical Acupuncture Society
Newton House, Newton Lane
Whitley
Warrington
Cheshire WA4 4JA
Tel (0925) 73727

NON-MEDICALLY QUALIFIED ACUPUNCTURISTS
British Acupuncture Association
34 Alderney Street
London SW1V 4EU
Tel (071) 834 1012
Produces a handbook with a directory of practitioners in the U.K. and abroad at £2.00 inc P&P

ADVISORY CENTRE FOR EDUCATION (ACE)
1b Aberdeen Studios
22-24 Highbury Grove
London N5
Tel (071) 354 8321
A telephone advice line is available from 2-5.00 p.m. daily

ALEXANDER TECHNIQUE, THE SOCIETY OF TEACHERS OF
10 London House
266 Fulham Road
London SW10 9EL
Tel (071) 351 0828

ALLERGY, THE BRITISH ALLERGY FOUNDATION
St Bartholomew's Hospital
West Smithfield
London EC1A 7BE
Tel (071) 600 6127

ALTERNATIVE MEDICINE
Institute for Complementary Medicine
21 Portland Place
London WC1N 3AF
Tel (071) 636 9543

AMARANT TRUST
14 Lord North Street
London SW1
Information and advice on menopausal problems, including the use of hormone replacement therapy (HRT)

BACK PAIN ASSOCIATION
31-33 Park Road
Teddington
Middlesex TW11 0AB
Tel (081) 977 5474
Encourages and funds research into the treatment and causes of back pain. Has 50 local groups and produces a regular magazine along with leaflets and cassettes on how to cope with back pain – send a large SAE

BRITISH MEDICAL ASSOCIATION
Tavistock Square
London WC1H 9JP
Tel (071) 387 4499

CAPITAL RADIO HELPLINE
Euston Tower
London NW1 3DR
Tel (071) 388 7575
A confidential off-air advice and information service for people
in London which is open from 9.30a.m.–5.30p.m. Monday –
Friday. Experienced counsellors will try to advise on any sort of
problem, or put you in touch with a relevant organisation

CARERS NATIONAL ASSOCIATION
29 Chilworth Mews
London W2 3RG
Tel (071) 724 7776
Offers information and support to people caring for relatives
and friends who, because of illness or disability, cannot manage
without help. Promotes information, recognition and services
for carers. 70 branches with 600 support groups nationally.
Membership is £3 per annum

CENTRE FOR ACCESSIBLE ENVIRONMENTS
35 Great Smith Street
London SW1P 3BJ
Tel (071) 222 7980
Information service and publisher on practical design of
buildings accessible to the disabled

CHILDREN IN HOSPITAL, NATIONAL ASSOCIATION
FOR THE WELFARE OF
Argyle House
29-31 Euston Road
London NW1 2SD
Tel (071) 833 2041

CHIROPRACTIC – BRITISH CHIROPRACTORS'
ASSOCIATION
5 First Avenue
Chelmsford
Essex CM1 1RX
Tel (0245) 35378

CIVIL LIBERTIES, NATIONAL COUNCIL FOR
(LIBERTY)
21 Tabard Street
London SE1 4LA
Tel (071) 403 3888

COLLEGE OF HEALTH
St Margaret's House
21 Old Ford Road
London E2 9PL
Tel (081) 983 1225
Aims to improve self-care and self-help groups through proper
use of NHS facilities and alternative therapies. Publishes a wide
range of useful leaflets. HEALTHLINE service has over 350
tapes which can be heard over the phone – Tel (081) 681 3311
from 4–8.00p.m. Monday to Friday. A full directory is
available by post. Also publishes the journal *Self-Health* which
covers both orthodox and alternative medicine

COMMUNITY HEALTH COUNCILS
There are 215 CHCs in England and Wales. You can find out
where your local CHC is from the local library, Citizens Advice
Bureau or under 'Community' in the phone book

COUNSELLING, BRITISH ASSOCIATION FOR
37a Sheep Street
Rugby
Warwickshire CV21 3BY
Tel (0788) 578328/9
A registered charity which has developed a code of ethics for
counsellors and operates an accreditation scheme for courses and
individuals. Provides a source of literature and runs an
information office

COUNCIL FOR INVOLUNTARY TRANQUILLISER ADDICTION
Cavendish House
Brighton Road, Waterloo,
Liverpool L22 5NG
Tel (051) 525 2777
Advice and support for people using tranquillisers on a long-term basis — and how to get off them. Also publishes leaflets and audio cassettes on the subject

CROSSROADS CARE ATTENDANT SCHEMES
10 Regent Place
Rugby
Warwickshire CV21 2PN
Tel (0788) 73653
Practical help for families with a member who is disabled

CYTOMEGALOVIRUS (CMV) SUPPORT GROUP
69 The Leasowes
Ford
Shrewsbury SY5 9LU
Tel (0743) 850055
Support group for people affected by cytomegalovirus infections

DEPARTMENT OF EDUCATION AND SCIENCE
Elizabeth House
York Road
London SE1 7PH
Tel (071)934 9000

DEPARTMENT OF SOCIAL SECURITY
The Adelphi
1-11 John Adam Street
London WC2N 6HT
Tel (071) 962 8000

DEPARTMENT OF SOCIAL SECURITY (LEAFLETS BY POST)
PO Box 21
Stanmore
Middlesex HA7 1AY

Freephone advice line on benefits for the disabled is available
from 9.00am. −4.30p.m. Monday to Friday (0800 882200)

DEPARTMENT OF TRANSPORT
Disability Unit
2 Marsham Street
London SW1P 3EB
Tel (071) 276 5256/7

DIAL UK (DISABLEMENT INFORMATION AND ADVICE LINES)
St Catherine's Hospital
Dickhill Road
Balby
Doncaster DN4 8QN
Tel (0302) 310123
Free confidential information and advice on a wide variety of
issues concerning disabled people. Over 80 branches throughout
the U.K.

DIAL Barnsley	0226 240273
DIAL Barrow	0229 33553
DIAL Basildon	0268 551900
DIAL Bedfordshire	0582 400461
DIAL Belfast	0232 370240
DIAL Berkshire (Reading)	0734 505900
DIAL Berkshire (Slough)	0753 75707
DIAL Bradford	0274 594173
DIAL Bucks Aylesbury	0296 433937
DIAL Bucks (High Wycombe)	0494 442601
DIAL Chester	0244 45655
DIAL Doncaster	0302 310359
DIAL Dorset	0202 677559
DIAL Falkirk	0324 611567
DIAL Great Yarmouth	0493 857603
DIAL Hampshire	0705 824853/829329
DIAL Herefordshire	0432 277770
DIAL Herts	0923 30514

DIAL Honiton	0404 41212
DIAL Isle of Wight	0983 522823
DIAL Kendal	0539 740508
DIAL Kent	0227 450001
DIAL NW Kent	0322 91362
DIAL Kilbride	03552 22955
DIAL Kirklees	0484 510511
DIAL Leeds	0532 795583
DIAL Leicestershire	0533 700666
DIAL Livingston	0506 414472
DIAL Llantrisant	0443 237937
DIAL Lowestoft	0502 511333
DIAL Mansfield	0623 25891
DIAL Merthyr Tydfil	0685 79769
DIAL Mid Suffolk Rethink	0449 672781
DIAL Mid Sussex	0444 416619
DIAL Northamptonshire (Corby Branch)	0536 204742
DIAL Northamptonshire (Daventry Branch)	0327 704223
DIAL Nuneaton & Bedworth	0203 349954
DIAL Oxford	0865 791818

DIAL Peterborough 0733 265551	**DIAL** Surrey 0883 844255
DIAL Rotherham 0709 373658	**DIAL** Swansea 0792 587642
DIAL Rugby 0788 68368	**DIAL** Tameside 061 320 8333
DIAL Salford & Bolton	**DIAL** Trafford 061 865 5021
061 799 2222	**DIAL** Wakefield 0924 379181
DIAL Selby & District	**DIAL** Waltham Forest
0757 210495	081-520 4111
DIAL Sheffield 0742 727996	**DIAL** Warrington 0925 816318
DIAL Solihull 021 770 0333	**DIAL** West Lancs 0695 51819
DIAL Somerset 0823 278067	**DIAL** Weston Super Mare
DIAL Stoke on Trent	0934 41926
0782 269744	**DIAL** Wigan 0942 215725
	DIAL Wiltshire 0225 760610
	DIAL Worcester City 0905 27790
	DIAL Wyre Forest 0562 68248

DISABILITY ALLIANCE
Universal House
88–94 Wentworth Street
London E1 7SA
Tel (071) 247 8776
Pressure group which campaigns on benefits for the disabled.
Publishes the *Disability Rights Handbook*, an invaluable guide
through the DSS benefit maze. Also carries out research into the
financial problems of disability

DISABLED DRIVERS' ASSOCIATION
Ashwellthorpe
Norfolk NR16 1EX
Tel (050 841) 449
Self-help association aiming for independence through mobility

DISABLED DRIVERS' MOTOR CLUB
Cottingham Way
Thrapston
Northamptonshire NN14 4PL
Tel (08012) 4724
Offers advice on mobility problems, conversions, insurance,
discounts, etc.

DISABLED LIVING FOUNDATION
380–384 Harrow Road
London W9 2HU
Tel (071) 289 6111

Information and advice on a large number of practical aids which are available for the disabled. Equipment centres open Monday — Friday, 9.00a.m.—5.00p.m. by appointment. Telephone/letter enquiry service is open from 9.30a.m. to 4.45p.m. Monday to Friday.

Local centres in:

Aberdeen	0224 685247	Leicester	0533 700747
Aylesbury	0296 84111	Liverpool	051 228 9221
Belfast	0232 669501	London	071 289 6111
Birmingham	021 643 0980	Macclesfield	0625 661740
Bodelwyddan	0745 583910	Manchester	061 832 3678
(North Wales)		Middlesborough	0642 850222
Braintree	0376 21068	Newcastle	091 284 0480
Caerphilly	0222 887325	Nottingham	0602 420391
Cardiff	0222 566281	Paisley	041 887 0597
Colchester	0206 853535	Portsmouth	0705 737174
Edinburgh	031 447 6271	Semington (Wilts)	0380 871007
Exeter	0392 59260	Southampton	0703 796631
Huddersfield	0484 518809	Stockport	061 419 4476
Hull	0482 28631	Swansea	0792 580161
Inverness	0463 234151	Swindon	0793 643966
Leeds	0532 793140	Welwyn Garden City	0707 324581

DISABLEMENT INCOME GROUP (DIG)
Millmead Business Centre
Millmead Road
London N17 9QU
Tel (081) 801 8013

Operates advisory service on DSS benefits. Several publications — list on request

DYSPHASIA, ACTION FOR DYSPHASIC ADULTS
Canterbury House
Royal Street
London SE1 7LN
Tel (071) 261 9572

Information and advice for people with speech problems (dysphasia)

EQUIPMENT FOR THE DISABLED
Mary Marlborough Lodge
Nuffield Orthopaedic Centre
Headington

Oxford OX3 7LD
Tel (0865) 750103
Publishes a series of useful illustrated booklets on various aspects
of disability (eg wheelchairs) each acting as a reference source

FAMILY WELFARE ASSOCIATION
501–505 Kingsland Road
London E8 4AU
Tel (071) 254 6251
Professional counselling service for families in distress. Ten local
branches in the U.K.

GENERAL MEDICAL COUNCIL
44 Hallam Street
London W1N 6AE
Tel (071) 580 7642

HEALING – CHURCHES COUNCIL FOR HEALTH AND
HEALING
St Marylebone Parish Church
Marylebone Road
London NW1 5LT
Tel (071) 486 9644
An interdenominational organisation which can answer
enquiries concerning religion and medicine, and provide details
on healing services

HEALING – NATIONAL FEDERATION OF SPIRITUAL
HEALING
Old Manor Farm Studio
Church Street
Sunbury on Thames
Middlesex

HEALTH SERVICE COMMISSIONERS

England:	Church House
	Great Smith Street
	London SW1P 3BW
	Tel (081) 212 7676
Scotland:	11 Melville Crescent
	Edinburgh EH3 7LU
	Tel (031) 225 7465

Wales: 4th Floor
                                      Pearl Assurance House
                                      Greyfriars Road
                                      Cardiff CF1 3AG
                                      Tel (0222) 394621

HEALTHWATCH
(formerly the CAMPAIGN AGAINST HEALTH FRAUD)
PO Box CAHF
London WC1N 3XX
Tel (081) 673 4401
Healthwatch campaigns and promotes good practice in the
assessment and testing of treatments, whether 'orthodox' or
'alternative'. Membership costs £12 per year

HERBALISTS – BRITISH HERBAL MEDICINE ASSOCIATION
Field House
Lye Hole Lane
Redhill
Avon RS18 7TB
Tel (0934) 862994
Runs an information service and a list of herbal practitioners

HOLISTIC MEDICAL ASSOCIATION, BRITISH
179 Gloucester Place
London NW1
Tel (071) 262 5299

Homeopathy
BRITISH HOMEOPATHIC ASSOCIATION
Basildon Court
27a Devonshire Street
London W1N 1RJ
Tel (071) 935 2163
Maintains a membership of individual practitioners in
homeopathy and provides an information service. It also has
an up-to-date reference library on homeopathic medicines
and publishes a bi-monthly journal called *Homeopathy*

HOMEOPATHIC HOSPITALS AND CLINICS

Found in: Bristol

Glasgow

Liverpool

London

Tunbridge Wells

For more information, send SAE to:

The Faculty of Homeopathy

The Royal London Homeopathic Hospital

60 Great Ormond Street

London WC1N 3HR

Tel (071) 837 9469

HOMEOPATHIC MEDICINES

Ainsworths Homeopathic Pharmacy

38 New Cavendish Street

London W1M 7LH

Tel (071) 935 5330

These can be prescribed on the NHS, but are not usually too expensive to purchase without a prescription

HYPNOSIS

The British Society of Medical and Dental Hypnosis

42 Links Road

Ashtead

Surrey KT21 2HJ

Tel (03722) 73522

Provides a list of medical and dental hypnotherapists to whom referrals can be made

INDEPENDENT LIVING FUND

PO Box 183

Nottingham NG8 3RD

Tel (0602) 290423/7

INSURANCE OMBUDSMAN BUREAU

31 Southampton Row

London WC1B 5HJ

Tel (071) 242 8613

INVALID CHILDREN'S AID NATIONWIDE
Allen Graham House
198 City Road
London EC1V 2PH
Tel (071) 608 2462
Help and advice for parents with problems associated with
disabled children — will advise on educational difficulties

LIFESKILLS
Bowman House
6 Billetfield
Taunton TA1 3NN
TEl (0823) 451771
Produce a variety of self-help audio cassette tapes

LONDON DIAL-A-RIDE AND TAXICAB (LONDON DART)
St Margarets
25 Leighton Road
London NW5 2DQ
Tel (071) 482 2325

MARRIAGE GUIDANCE COUNCIL (RELATE)
Herbert Gray College
Little Church Street
Rugby
Warwickshire CV21 3AP
Tel (0788) 573241
Local branches in your phone book or ask at the CAB

M.E. ASSOCIATION
See beginning of this chapter

M.E. ACTION
See beginning of this chapter

MEDIC-ALERT FOUNDATION
17 Bridge Wharf
156 Caledonian Road
London N1 9RD
Tel (071) 833 3034
Identification scheme for people suffering from hidden medical

problems. Produces bracelets/medallions with twenty-four hour telephone number of their office, which keeps details of your personal medical condition

MIGRAINE TRUST
45 Great Ormond Street
London WC1N 3HD
Tel (071) 278 2676
Information, advice and research into migraine headaches

MIND (National Association for Mental Health)
22 Harley Street
London W1N 2ED
Tel (071) 637 0741
Campaigning group on a range of issues to do with mental health. Publishes booklets and leaflets on a variety of issues concerned with psychiatric illness. Has a legal department which will help with any mental health problem which requires this sort of advice, e.g. discharge from a psychiatric hospital. Two hundred local groups – see the phone book

MOBILITY ADVICE AND VEHICLE INFORMATION SERVICES (MAVIS)
Department of Transport
Transport and Road Research Laboratory
Crowthorne
Berkshire RG11 6AU
Tel (0344) 779014

MOBILITY INFORMATION SERVICE
Unit 2a, Atcham Industrial Estate
Upton Magna
Shrewsbury SY4 4UG
Tel (0743) 761889

MOTABILITY
2nd Floor
Gate House
Westgate
The High
Harlow
Essex CM20 1HR
Tel (0279) 635666

Helps people in receipt of Mobility Allowance get the best value
for money including hire purchase of cars and wheelchairs, and a
car leasing scheme

NATIONAL TRUST
36 Queen Anne's Gate
London SW1H

NATUROPATHY – THE BRITISH NATUROPATHIC
AND OSTEOPATHIC ASSOCIATION
Frazer House
6 Netherall Gardens
London NW3 5RR
Tel (071) 435 8728
Members use the initials ND, DO or MBNOA after a four-year
training, but do not advertise

NYSTAGMUS ACTION GROUP
4 Grove Road
Epsom
Surrey KT17 4DF
Tel (0372) 741764
Promotes the understanding and knowledge of the eye condition
nystagmus. Membership £5 per year

OCCUPATIONAL PENSIONS ADVISORY SERVICE
11 Belgrave Road
London SW1V 1RB
Tel (071) 233 8080

OPEN UNIVERSITY
Derek Child
Adviser on Education of Students with Disabilities
Walton Hall
Milton Keynes MK7 6AA
Tel (0908) 653442
Home study and courses suitable for disabled students

OPPORTUNITIES FOR PEOPLE WITH DISABILITIES
1 Bank Buildings
Princes Street
London EC2R 8EU
Tel (071) 726 4963

Employment service for job seekers and employers. Eleven regional offices

OSTEOPATHY – THE GENERAL COUNCIL AND REGISTER OF OSTEOPATHS
1 Suffolk Street
London SW1Y 4HG
Tel (071) 839 2060
Keeps a list of professionally qualified osteopaths

OSTEOPOROSIS SOCIETY, NATIONAL
Barton Meade House
Radstock
Near Bath
Avon BA3 3YB
Tel (0761) 32472
Produce a series of booklets on all aspects of osteoporosis including prevention, diagnosis and management. Membership costs £5 per year

PAIN SOCIETY, THE
9 Bedford Square
London WC1B 3RA
Tel (071) 631 1650

PATIENTS ASSOCIATION
18 Victoria Park Square
Bethnal Green
London E2 9PF
Tel (081) 981 5676/5695
Advice and help to patients on any aspect of health care. Can help in resolving complaints against doctors and hospitals. Campaigns for better monitoring of drugs and their side-effects, and allowing more freedom of information in regard to medical records

PHOBIC ACTION
Greater London House
547/551 High Road
Leytonstone
London E11 4PR
Tel (081) 558 6012 (helpline)
(081) 558 3463 (office)

Charity that helps people with anxiety and phobic conditions.
Over 50 local groups. Membership £10 per year

PHYSIOTHERAPISTS
Mrs M. Briggs
50 Mannering Gardens
Westcliff-on-Sea
Essex SS0 0BQ
Produces a directory of chartered physiotherapists working in
private practice

PREMENSTRUAL SOCIETY, THE
PO Box 102
London SE1 7ES

PSYCHIATRISTS, ROYAL COLLEGE OF
17 Belgrave Square
London SW1X 8PG
Tel (071) 235 2351

RADAR (ROYAL ASSOCIAION FOR DISABILITY AND
REHABILITATION)
25 Mortimer Street
London W1N 8AB
Tel (071) 637 5400
Umbrella organisation giving advice on all matters related to
disability: access, holidays (publishes useful guides), housing,
mobility, welfare and employment. Large number of
publications and leaflets

RAYNAUD'S AND SCLERODERMA ASSOCIATION
TRUST
112 Crewe Road
Alsager
Cheshire ST7 2JA
Tel (0270) 872776
Information, newsletters and practical advice on Raynaud's
syndrome (cold hands and feet). Membership £4 per year

RED CROSS SOCIETY, BRITISH
9 Grosvenor Crescent
London SW1X 7EJ

Tel (071) 235 5454
Local branches are listed in the phone book

REHABILITATION ENGINEERING MOVEMENT ADVISORY PANELS (REMAP)

J.J. Wright, National Organiser
Hazeldene
Ightham
Sevenoaks
Kent TN15 9AD
Tel (0732) 883818
Makes or adapts aids for disabled people when these are not commercially available

RELATE – see MARRIAGE GUIDANCE COUNCIL

RELAXATION FOR LIVING

29 Burwood Park Road
Walton-on-Thames
Surrey KT12 5LH
Information on relaxation techniques, and courses; send a large SAE

SAMARITANS

17 Uxbridge Road
Slough
Berkshire LS1 1SN
Tel (0753) 32713/4
About 180 local branches (see phone book) giving a confidential service over the phone for anyone in despair

SOCIAL SECURITY APPEALS TRIBUNALS AND MEDICAL APPEAL TRIBUNALS

Office of the President of
Clements House
Gresham Street
London EC2V 7DN

SOCIAL SECURITY COMMISSIONERS

Harp House
83 Farringdon Street
London EC4A 4DH

SOCIETY FOR HORTICULTURAL THERAPY
Goulds Ground
Vallis Way
Frome
Somerset BA11 3DW
Tel (0373) 64782
Promotes gardening as a form of therapy for people with disabilities

SHOPMOBILITY SCHEMES

Basildon	0268 533644	Kingston upon Thames	
Bexleyheath	081-301 5237		081-547 1255
Bradford	0274 754076	Leicester	0533 526694
Braintree	0376 46535	Lincoln	0522 544983
Brierly Hill	0384 481141	Luton	0582 412636
Cambridge	0223 463370	Milton Keynes	0908 670866
Cardiff	0222 399355	Newport	0633 258212
Chesterfield	0246 209668	Northampton	0604 233714
Cwmbran	06333 62951	Nottingham	0602 584486
Dartford	0322 220915	Peterborough	0733 313133
Gateshead	091 460 5299	Plymouth	0752 600633
Glasgow	041 353 2594	Redditch	0527 69922
Gloucester	0452 396898	Sandwell	021 553 1943
Harlow	0279 446188	Southend on Sea	0702 339682
Hatfield	0707 262731	Sutton	081-770 0691
Hereford	0432 342166	Sutton Coldfield	021 355 1112
Huddersfield	0484 453000	Telford	0952 291370
Ipswich	0473 222225	Worcester	0905 28010
Keighley	0274 758225	Yeovil	0935 75914

Shopmobility schemes planned to open soon in Barking, Bristol, Chelmsford, Colchester, Crawley, Derby, Edinburgh, Glenrothes, Irvine, Leeds, Lichfield, Liverpool, Luton, Rotherham, Welwyn Garden City and Woking

SJØGREN'S SYNDROME ASSOCIATION, BRITISH
19 White Hart Wood
Sevenoaks
Kent TN13 1RR
Tel (0732) 453572
Nationwide support group for S.S. patients linking them to centres of medical research. Regular information on research and treatment. Membership £5 year

SPOD (ASSOCIATION TO AID SEXUAL AND
PERSONAL RELATIONSHIPS OF PEOPLE WITH A
DISABILITY)
286 Camden Road
London N7 0BJ
Tel (071) 607 8851/2
Information and advice on sexuality and disability. Can put
patients in touch with experienced sexual counsellors. Also
publishes leaflets and information

SPORTS ASSOCIATION FOR THE DISABLED, BRITISH
Maryglen Haig Suite
34 Osnaburgh Street
London NW1 3ND
Tel (071) 383 7277
Encouragement and advice on all forms of sporting activities for
the disabled

SWIMMING THERAPY, ASSOCIATION OF
4 Oak Street
Shrewsbury SY3 7RH
Tel (0743) 4393

TINNITUS ASSOCIATION, BRITISH
c/o Royal National Institute for the Deaf
105 Gower Streeet
London WC1E 6AH
Tel (071) 387 8033
Local groups offer counselling and information on tinnitus

VOLUNTEER BUREAUX, NATIONAL ASSOCIATION
OF
St Peters College
College Road
Saltley
Birmingham B8 3TG
There are now 370+ Volunteer Bureaux in the U.K. The
address of a local bureau can be found by enquiring to the above
address or looking in the phone book under 'V'

WESTCARE
See beginning of this chapter

Northern Ireland Addresses
M.E. ASSOCIATION
Northern Ireland Region
Bryson House
28 Bedford Street
Belfast BT2 7FE
Tel (0232) 439831

CARERS NATIONAL ASSOCIATION
Northern Ireland Regional Office
113 University Street
Belfast BT7 1HP
Tel (0232) 439843

CROSSROADS CARE ATTENDANT SCHEMES
Unit 8
Comber Road Industrial Estate
Newtownards BT23 4RX
Tel (0247) 815978

DISABILITY, NORTHERN IRELAND COUNCIL ON
2 Annadale Avenue
Belfast BT7 3JR
Tel (0232) 491011
Forum for over 130 organisations in Northern Ireland concerned
with all forms of disability. Offers an information and training
service, driving assessment and mobility information

LABOUR RELATIONS AGENCY
Windsor House
Bedford Street
Belfast BT2
Tel (0232) 321442
Useful and helpful agency for anyone experiencing problems
with employment, especially when they have no trade union to
help with advice

SOCIAL SECURITY APPEAL TRIBUNALS AND
MEDICAL APPEAL TRIBUNALS
Office of the President of
6th Floor

Cleaver House
3 Donegall Square North
Belfast BT1 5GA

SOCIAL SECURITY COMMISSIONERS
Office of the
5 Linenhall Street
Belfast BT2 8AA

Scotland
M.E. ASSOCIATION
11 Queens Crescent
Glasgow G4 9AS
Tel (041) 332 1651
Fax (041) 332 0175

CROSSROADS CARE ATTENDANT SCHEMES
24 George Street
Glasgow G2 1EG
Tel (041) 226 3793
46 area schemes now in operation

DEPARTMENT OF SOCIAL SECURITY
Central Office for Scotland
Argyle House
3 Lady Lawson St
Edinburgh EH3 0QL
Tel (031) 229 9191

DISABILITY SCOTLAND
5 Shandwick Place
Edinburgh EH2 4RG
Tel (031) 229 8632
Information on all aspects of disability

DISABLEMENT INCOME GROUP SCOTLAND
ECAS House
28–30 Howden Street
Edinburgh EH8 9HW
Tel (031) 667 0249

LAW SOCIETY OF SCOTLAND
26 Drumsheugh Gardens
Edinburgh EH3 7YR
Tel (031) 226 7411
Provides details of Scottish solicitors

RED CROSS SOCIETY, BRITISH, SCOTTISH BRANCH
204 Bath Street
Glasgow G2 4HL
Tel (041) 332 9591

SOCIAL SECURITY COMMISSIONERS OFFICE
23 Melville Street
Edinburgh EH3 7PW

Wales
DISABILITY HELPLINE WALES
3 Links Court
Links Business Park
St Mellons
Cardiff
Tel (0222) 798633
Information and advice on all aspects of disability

DSS REGIONAL OFFICE
Block 3
Government Buildings
Gabalfa
Cardiff CF4 4YJ

WALES COUNCIL FOR THE DISABLED
'Llyslfor'
Crescent Road
Caerphilly
Mid Glamorgan CF8 1XL
Tel (0222) 887325

2. Further Reading

How to obtain medical references

References from medical journals are from publications which shouldn't be too hard to find in a medical library. There's no 'embargo' on the general public obtaining this sort of information if they decide to do so. Many doctors are very opposed to patients reading scientific literature of this type, as they feel (with some justification) that patients get the wrong ideas and misinterpret symptoms and management advice. And, a few of them don't actually like the idea of their patients knowing more about a condition than they do!

If you want to get a photocopy of a reference, phone your local public library librarian, and ask if they'll do this for you — they're usually very obliging, even finding references which are quite obscure. You'll have to pay a small fee, but it shouldn't cost too much.

Unfortunately, if you go to a medical library and try to look up M.E. in one of the large medical textbooks, you still won't find very much of use, and sometimes nothing at all. I recently surveyed a large number of new editions of standard medical textbooks on infectious diseases and neurology. The results were dismaying. Even the latest edition of probably the most influential textbook on infectious diseases in the U.K. failed to even mention M.E. As a result I'm now in the process of tackling individual editors of these reference books to try and persuade them to include accurate accounts in their next editions. If your own doctor says he can't find anything about M.E. in his books, this is the reason why!

General Reviews

1   Behan P.O. *Chronic Fatigue Syndrome, What is it?*
(in press)

2   Behan P.O. 'Postviral neurological syndromes' (Editorial).
(*British Medical Journal*, 1983, 287, 853-854.)

3   Behan P.O. et al. 'The Postviral Fatigue Syndrome – an
analysis of the findings in 50 cases.' (*Journal of Infection*, 1985,
10, 211-222.)

4   Behan P.O. and Behan W.M.H. 'Postviral Fatigue
Syndrome.' (*CRC Critical Reviews in Neurobiology*, 1988, 4
(2), 157-178.)

5   Daugherty S.A. et al. 'Chronic Fatigue Syndrome in North
Nevada.' *Reviews of Infectious Diseases, 1991*, 13 (Supplement
1), 39-44.

6   David A. et al. 'Postviral Fatigue Syndrome – time for a
new approach.' (*British Medical Journal*, 1988, 296, 696-699.)

7   David A. et al. 'Chronic Fatigue Syndrome: signs of a new
approach.' (*British Journal of Hospital Medicine*, 1991, 45,
158-163.)

8   Dowsett E.G. et al. 'Myalgic encephalomyelitis – a
persistent enteroviral infection?' (*Postgraduate Medical Journal*,
1990, 66, 526-530.)

9   Lloyd A.R. et al.'What is myalgic encephalomyelitis?'
(*Lancet*, 1988, 1, 1286-1287.)

10 Shafran S. 'The Chronic Fatigue Syndrome.' (*The American
Journal of Medicine*, 1991, 90, 730-739.)

11 Shepherd C. 'Myalgic encephalomyelitis – is it a real
disease?' (*The Practitioner*, 1989, 223, 41-46.)

12 Shepherd C. and Wessely S. 'Head to Head: Myalgic
encephalomyelitis – a psychological disease?' (*Pulse*,
December 14th 1991, 56-58.)

13 Wessely S. 'Chronic Fatigue Syndrome' (Editorial). (*Journal
of Neurology, Neurosurgery and Psychiatry*, 1991, 54, 669-671.)

14 Wessely S. and Thomas P.K. 'The Chronic Fatigue
Syndrome – Myalgic Encephalomyelitis or Postviral
Fatigue.' (In C. Kennard [Ed.].) *Recent Advances in Clinical
Neurology*. No. 6. Edinburgh: Churchill-Livingstone. 1990,
85-132.)

15 Wessely S. 'Old wine in new bottles: neurasthenia and

"M.E."' (*Psychological Medicine*, 1990, 20, 35-53.)

Brain and nervous system

16 Behan P.O. 'Postviral neurological syndromes' (Editorial). (*British Medical Journal*, 1983, 287, 853.)

17 Buchwald D. et al. 'A Chronic Illness Characterized by Fatigue, Neurologic and Immunologic Disorders, and Active Human Herpesvirus Type 6 Infection.' (*Annals of Internal Medicine*, 1992, 116, 103-113.)

18 Leon-Soto Mayor L. *Epidemic diencephalomyelitis. A possible cause of neuropsychiatric, cardiovascular and endocrine disorders.* (First edition. *Pageant Press*, New York, 1969.)

19 O'Connell R.A. et al. 'The role of SPECT brain scan imaging in assessing psychopathology in the medically ill.' (*General Hospital Psychiatry*, 1991, 13, 305-312.)

20 Johnson R.T. *Viral infections of the Nervous System*. (Raven Press, New York, 1982, Chapter 8: 'Para infectious Neurological syndromes'.)

21 Prasher Deepak et al. 'Sensory and cognitive event-related potentials in myalgic encephalomyelitis.' (*Journal of Neurology, Neurosurgery and Psychiatry*, 1990, 53, 245-253.)

22 Rosenstock L. et al, and the Pesticide Health Effects Study Group. 'Chronic central nervous system effects of acute organophosphate pesticide intoxication.' (*The Lancet*, 1991, 338, 223-227.)

Children and adolescents

23 *Ean's Story*, Interaction (M.E. Action), 1989, 3, 52-54.

24 *Guidelines for parents of children with M.E.* (available from the M.E. Association.)

25 Lask B. and Dillon M.J. 'Postviral Fatigue Syndrome.' (*Archives of Disease in Childhood*, 1990, 65, 1198.)

26 Lask B. 'What does M.E. mean to me?: the psychiatrist's viewpoint.' (*Maternal and Child Health*, 1991, 6-8.)

27 Smith M.S. et al. 'Chronic fatigue in adolescents'. (*Paediatrics*, 1991, 88, 2, 195-202.)

28 Wachsmuth J.R. and Macmillan H.L. 'Effective treatment for an adolescent with Chronic Fatigue Syndrome'. (*Clinical Paediatrics*, 1991, 30, 8, 488-490.)

29 Wilson P.M.J. et al. 'Features of Coxsackie B Virus (CBV)

infection in children with prolonged physical and psychological morbidity.' (*Journal of Psychosomatic Research*, 1989, 33, 1, 29–36.)

Clinical features and personal accounts

30 Behan P.O. *Diagnostic and Clinical Guidelines for Doctors, 1990* (available from the M.E. Association).

31 Behan P.O. and Barhem A.M.O. 'Clinical spectrum of Postviral Fatigue Syndrome.' (*British Medical Bulletin*, 1991, 47, 4, 793–808.)

32 Cotteril J.A. 'The Devil's Grip.' (*The Lancet*, 1973, 1, 1308–1309.)

33 Dille J.R. 'Chronic Fatigue Syndrome.' (*Aviation, Space and Environmental Medicine*, 1991, 62, 1008–9.)

34 English T.L. 'Skeptical of Skeptics.' (*Journal of the American Medical Association*, 1991, 265, 964.)

35 Hartnell L. 'Postviral Fatigue Syndrome: a Canker in my Brain.' (*The Lancet*, 1987, 1, 910.)

36 Harvey W.T. 'A flight surgeon's personal view of an emerging illness.' (*Aviation, Space and Environmental Medicine*, 1989, 60, 1199–1201.)

37 Holmes G.P. et al. 'Chronic Fatigue Syndrome – a working case definition.' (*Annals of Internal Medicine*, 1988, 108, 387–389.)

38 Hurst N.P. et al. 'Coxsackie B infection and arthritis.' (*British Medical Journal*, 1983, 286, 605.)

39 Moldovsky H. 'Nonrestorative sleep and symptoms after febrile illness in patients with fibrositis and Chronic Fatigue Syndromes.' (*Journal of Rheumatology*, 1989, Supplement 19, 16, 150–153.)

Differential Diagnosis

40 Gardner W. 'Hyperventilation disorders.' (*Journal of the Royal Society of Medicine*, 1990, 83, 755–756.)

41 Goldenberg D.L. 'Fibromyalgia, Chronic Fatigue Syndrome and Myofascial Pain Syndrome.' (*Current Opinion in Rheumatology*, 1991, 3, 247–258.)

42 Pilgrim J.A. et al. 'Low blood pressure, low mood?' (*British Medical Journal*, 1992, 304, 75–78.)

43 Rosen S.D. et al. 'Is Chronic Fatigue Syndrome

synonymous with effort syndrome?' (*Journal of the Royal Society of Medicine*, 1990, 83, 761–764.)

44 Wysenbeck et al. 'Primary fibromyalgia and the Chronic Fatigue Syndrome.' (*Rheumatology International*, 1991, 10, 227–229.)

Endocrinology (hormone imbalance)

45 Bakheit A.M.O. et al. *Abnormal arginine-vasopressin secretion and water metabolism in patients with Postviral Fatigue Syndrome.* (*British Medical Bulletin*, 1991, 47, 803–4.)

46 Bakheit A.M.O. et al. *Possible upregulation of hypothalamic 5-HT receptors in patients with the Postviral Fatigue Syndrome.* (*British Medical Journal*, 1992, 304, 1010–1012.)

47 Demitrack M.A. et al. 'Impaired activation of the hypothalamic – pituitary – adrenal axis in patients with Chronic Fatigue Syndrome.' (*Journal of Clinical Endocrinology and Metabolism*, 1991, 73, 1224–1234.)

48 Denman A.M. 'Sex hormones, autoimmune diseases and immune responses' (Editorial). (*British Medical Journal*, 1991, 303, 2–3.)

Epidemiology

49 David A. et al. 'Tired, weak or in need of a rest: fatigue among general practice attenders.' (*British Medical Journal*, 1990, 301, 1199–1202.)

50 Ho-Yen DO et al. 'General Practitioners' experience of the Chronic Fatigue Syndrome.' (*British Journal of General Practice*, 1991, 41, 324–326.)

51 Lloyd A.R. et al. 'Prevalence of Chronic Fatigue Syndrome in an Australian population.' (*Medical Journal of Australia*, 1990, 153, 522–528.)

Heart Involvement

52 Banatvala J.E. *Coxsackie B Viral Infections in Cardiac Disease in Clinical Virology*. (Waterson A.P. Ed., 1983, Churchill-Livingston.)

53 Bowles N.E. et al. 'Detection of Coxsackie B virus specific RNA sequences in myocardial biopsy samples from patients with myocarditis and dilated cardiomyopathy.' (*The Lancet*, 1986, 1, 1120–1122.)

54 Grist N.R. and Bell E.J. 'A six year study of Coxsackie B infections in heart disease.' (*Journal of Hygiene*, Cambridge, 1974, 73, 165-172.)

55 Grist N.R. 'Myalgic encephalomyelitis: postviral fatigue and the heart.' (*British Medical Journal*, 1989, 11th November, 1219.)

56 Lerner A.M. and Wilson F.M. 'Virus myocardiopathy.' (*Prog. Med. Virol.*, 1973, 15, 63-91.)

57 Montague T. et al. 'Cardiac function at rest and with exercise in the Chronic Fatigue Syndrome.' (*Chest*, 1989, 95, 779-784.)

58 Muir P. et al. 'Chronic relapsing pericarditis and dilated cardiomyopathy: serological evidence of persistent enterovirus infection.' (*The Lancet*, 1989, 1, 804-807.)

59 Reyes M.P. et al. in Bendinelli M. and Friedmann H. (Eds) 'Myocarditis, clinical and experimental correlates' *Coxsackie viruses – a general update*. (Plenum Press, New York and London, 1988, 253-270.)

60 Tilzey A.Z. et al. 'Persistent Coxsackie B virus IgM response in patients with recurrent pericarditis.' (*The Lancet*, 1986, 1, 1491-1492.)

Historical

61 Acheson E.D. 'The clinical syndrome variously called benign myalgic encephalomyelitis, Iceland disease and epidemic neuromyasthenia.' (*American Journal of Medicine*, 1959, 26, 569-695.)

62 Barnes D. 'Mystery disease at Lake Tahoe challenges virologists and clinicians.' (*Science*, 1986, 234, 541.)

63 Beard G. 'Neurasthenia, or nervous exhaustion.' (*Boston Medical and Surgical Journal*, 1869, 3, 217-220.)

64 Fegan K.G. et al. 'Myalgic Encephalomyelitis and report of an epidemic.' (*Journal of the Royal College of Practitioners*, 1983, 33, 335-337.)

65 Field E.J. 'Darwin's illness.' (*The Lancet*, 1990, 336, 826.)

66 Gillam A.G. 'Epidemiological study of an epidemic diagnosed as poliomyelitis occurring amongst the personnel of the Los Angeles County General Hospital during the summer of 1934.' (*Public Health Bulletin No. 240,* April 1938,

U.S. Public Health Service, Washington DC, Government Printing Office.)

67 Henderson D.A. and Shelokov A. 'Epidemic neuromyasthenia: clinical syndrome?' (*New England Journal of Medicine*, 1959, 260, 757–764.)

68 Keighley B.D. et al. 'Sporadic myalgic encephalomyelitis in a rural practice.' (*Journal of the Royal College of General Practitioners*, 1983, 33, 339–341)

69 Leading Article. 'New clinical entity?' (*The Lancet*, 1956, 1, 789.)

70 Maros K.A. 'Portrait of a plague.' (*Medical Journal of Australia*, 1991, 155, 132.)

71 McEvedy C.P. and Beard A.W. 'Royal Free Epidemic of 1955 – a reconsideration.' (*British Medical Journal*, 1970, 1, 7–11.)

72 'Medical Staff of the Royal Free Hospital. An outbreak of encephalomyelitis in the Royal Free Hospital group, London, in 1955.' (*British Medical Journal*, 1957, 2, 895–904.)

73 Poore M. et al. 'An unexplained illness in West Otago.' (*New Zealand Medical Journal*, 1984, 97, 351.)

74 Ramsay A.M. 'Epidemic neuromyasthenia (1955–1978).' (*Postgraduate Medical Journal*, 1978, 54, 718.)

75 Richmond C. 'Myalgic encephalomyelitis, Princess Aurora, and the Wandering Womb.' (*British Medical Journal*, 1989, 298, 1295–1296.)

76 Sigurdsson B. et al. 'A disease epidemic in Iceland simulating poliomyelitis.' (*American Journal of Hygiene*, 1950, 52, 222–238.)

77 Sigurdsson B. et al. 'Response to poliomyelitis vaccination.' (*The Lancet*, 1958, 1, 370.)

78 Wallis A.L. *An investigation into an unusual disease seen in epidemic and sporadic forms in General Practice in Cumberland in 1955 and subsequent years.* (M.D. Thesis Edinburgh University (1957).)

Immunology

79 Bendinelli M. et al. *Interactions with the Immune System.* Chapter 6, 81–102.

Huber S.A. *The role of immune mechanisms in pathogenesis in*

Coxsackie viruses (a general update). (Chapter 7, 103-116, Bendinelli M. and Friedmann H. Eds. Plenum Press, New York and London, 1988.)

80 Caligiuri M. et al. 'Phenotypic and functional deficiencies of natural killer cells in patients with Chronic Fatigue Syndrome.' (*Journal of Immunology*, 1987, 139, 3306-3313.)

81 Chao C.C. 'Serum neopterin and interleukin-6 levels in Chronic Fatigue Syndrome.' (*Journal of Infectious Diseases*, 1990, 162, 1412-1413.)

82 Cheyne P.R. et al. 'Interleukin-2 and the Chronic Fatigue Syndrome.' (*Annals of Internal Medicine*, 1989, 110, 4, 321.)

83 Eby N.L. et al. 'Natural Killer Cell Activity in the Chronic Fatigue-Immune Dysfunction Syndrome.' (In *Natural Killer Cells and Host Defence*, Ed. E.W. Ades and C. Lopez. Basle: Karger, 1989, 141-145.)

84 Gupta S. et al. 'A comprehensive immunological analysis in Chronic Fatigue Syndrome.' (*Scandinavian Journal of Immunology*, 1991, 33, 319-327.)

85 Hobbs J. R. et al. 'CD8 deficiency in patients with muscle fatigue following suspected enteroviral infections (myalgia encephalitica).' (*Protides of the Biological Fluids*, 1989, 36, 391-398.)

86 Ho-Yen D.O. et al. 'Myalgic encephalomyelitis and alpha interferon.' (Letter to *The Lancet*, 1988, 1, 125)

87 Klimas N.G. et al. 'Immunologic abnormalities in Chronic Fatigue Syndrome.' (*Journal of Clinical Microbiology*, 1990, 28, 1403-1410.)

88 Lever et al. 'Interferon production in Postviral Fatigue Syndrome.' (Letter to *The Lancet*, 1988, 2, 101.)

89 Landay A. et al. 'Chronic Fatigue Syndrome: clinical condition associated with immune activation.' (*The Lancet*, 1991, 338, 707-711.)

90 Lloyd A. et al. 'Interferon and myalgic encephalomyelitis' (Letter to *The Lancet*, 1988, 1, 471.)

91 Lloyd A.R. et al. 'Immunological abnormalities in the Chronic Fatigue Syndrome.' (*Medical Journal of Australia*, 1989, 151, 122-124.)

92 Lloyd A., Hickie I. and Wakefield D. 'Immunological abnormalities in the Chronic Fatigue Syndrome.' (*Medical*

Journal of Australia, 1990, 152, 51–2.)

93 Lloyd A.R. et al. 'Cytokine levels in serum and cerebrospinal fluid in patients with Chronic Fatigue Syndrome and control subjects.' (*Journal of Infectious Diseases*, 1991, 164, 5, 1023–1024.)

94 McDonald E.M. et al. 'Interferons as mediators of psychiatric morbidity.' (*The Lancet*, 1987, ii, 1175–1177.)

95 Morrison L.J.A. et al. 'Changes in natural killer cell phenotype in patients with Postviral Fatigue Syndrome.' (*Clinical and Experimental Immunology*, 1991, 83, 441–446.)

96 Wakefield D. et al. 'Immunoglobulin subclass abnormalities in patients with Chronic Fatigue Syndrome.' (*Paediatric Infectious Diseases Journal*, 1990, 9, S50–S53.)

97 Wemm K.M. et al. 'The effects of a laboratory stressor on natural killer cell function in Chronic Fatigue Syndrome patients.' (*Psychosomatics*, 1991, 32, 470–471.)

Muscle

98 Arnold D.L. et al. 'Excessive intracellular acidosis of skeletal muscle on exercise in a patient with a Postviral Exhaustion/Fatigue Syndrome.' (*The Lancet*, 1984, i, 1367–1369.)

99 Astrom E. et al. 'Effects of viral and mycoplasma infections on ultrastructure and enzyme activities in human skeletal muscle.' (*Acta Pathol. Microbiol. Scand. 84*, 113.)

100 Behan W.M.H. et al. 'Mitochondrial abnormalities in the Postviral Fatigue Syndrome.' (*Acta Neuropathologica*, 1991, 83, 61–65.)

101 Byrne E. et al. 'Chronic Fatigue and Myalgia Syndrome: mitochondrial and glycolytic studies in skeletal muscle.' (*Journal of Neurology, Neurosurgery and Psychiatry*, 1987, 50, 743–746.)

102 Jamal G.A. and Hansen S. 'Electrophysiological studies in the Postviral Syndrome.' (*Journal of Neurology, Neurosurgery and Psychiatry*, 1985, 48, 691–694.)

103 Jamal G.A. and Hansen S. 'Postviral Fatigue Syndrome: Evidence for underlying organic disturbance in the muscle fibre.' (*European Neurology*, 1989, 29, 273–276.)

104 Jamal G.A. and Miller R.G. 'Neurophysiology of the Postviral Fatigue Syndrome.' (*British Medical Bulletin*, 1991, 47, No. 4, 809–825.)

105 Lloyd A. et al. 'Muscle strength, endurance and recovery in the Post-infectious Fatigue Syndrome.' (*Journal of Neurology, Neurosurgery and Psychiatry*. 1988, 51, 1316–22.)

106 Lloyd A.R. 'Muscle and brain: Chronic Fatigue Syndrome.' (*Medical Journal of Australia*, 1990, 153, 530–534.)

107 Lloyd A.R. et al. 'Muscle performance, voluntary activation, twitch properties and perceived effort in normal subjects and patients with Chronic Fatigue Syndrome.' (*Brain*, 1991, 114, 85–89.)

108 Pacy P.J. et al. 'Post-absorptive whole body leucine kinetics and quadriceps muscle protein synthetic rate (MPSR) in the Postviral Syndrome.' (*Clinical Science*, 1988, 75, 36–37.)

109 Shumate J.B. 'Myodenylate deaminase deficiency.' (*Seminars in Neurology*, 1983, 3, 242.)

110 Stokes M.J. et al. 'Normal muscle strength and fatiguability in patients with effort syndromes.' (*British Medical Journal*, 1988, 297, 1014–1017.)

111 Teahon K. et al. 'Clinical studies of the Postviral Fatigue Syndrome (PVFS) with special reference to skeletal muscle function.' (*Clinical Science*, 1988, 75, 45.)

112 Yonge R.P. 'Magnetic resonance muscle studies; implications for psychiatry.' (*Journal of the Royal Society of Medicine*, 1988, 81, 322–326.)

Pregnancy and neonatal infection

113 Anonymous – Leading Article. 'Avoiding the dangers of enteroviruses to infants.' (*The Lancet*, 1986, 1, 194–195.)

114 Blattner R.S. et al. 'Role of viruses in the aetiology of congenital malformations.' (*Progress in Medical Virology* 15 (Melnick J.L. Ed) Karger, Basle, 1973, 1–41.)

115 Brady W.K. and Purdon A. 'Intrauterine fetal demise associated with enterovirus infection.' (*Southern Medical Journal*, 1986, 79, 770–772.)

116 Gear J.H.S. and Measroch Y. 'Coxsackie virus infections of the Newborn.' (*Progress in Medical Virology* 15 (Melnick J.L. Ed) Karger, Basle, 1973, 42–62.)

Psychiatry

117 Butler S. et al. 'Cognitive behaviour therapy in the Chronic Fatigue Syndrome.' (*Journal of Neurology, Neurosurgery and*

Psychiatry, 1991, 54, 153–158.)

118 Goudsmit E.M. and Gadd R. 'All in the mind? The psychologicalisation of illness.' (*The Psychologist*, 1991, 4, 449–453.)

119 Hickie I. et al. 'The psychiatric status of patients with the Chronic Fatigue Syndrome.' (*British Journal of Psychiatry*, 1990, 156, 534–540.)

120 Hickie I. et al. 'Chronic Fatigue Syndrome.' (*British Journal of Psychiatry*, 1990, 157, 447–460.)

121 Kendell R. 'Chronic fatigue, viruses, and depression.' (*The Lancet*, 1991, 337, 160–163. Follow-up letters on pages 564, Shepherd, Simpson and Cathébras et al, and 992 Hickie et al.)

122 Lane T.J. et al. 'Depression and somatization in the Chronic Fatigue Syndrome.' (*American Journal of Medicine*, 1991, 91, 4, 335–344.)

123 Lynch S. et al. 'Antidepressant therapy in the Chronic Fatigue Syndrome.' (*British Journal of General Practice*, 1991, 41, 339–342.)

124 Manu P. et al. 'Somatization disorder in patients with chronic fatigue.' (*Psychosomatics*, 1989, 30, 4, 388–395.)

125 Ray C. 'Chronic Fatigue Syndrome and depression: conceptual and methodological ambiguities' (Editorial). (*Psychological Medicine*, 1991, 21, 1–9.)

126 Sharpe M. 'Psychiatric management of Postviral Fatigue Syndrome.' (*British Medical Bulletin*, 1991, 47, 4, 989–1005.)

127 Wessely S. 'Old Wine in New Bottles: neurasthenia and "M.E." ' (*Psychological Medicine*, 1990, 20, 35–53.)

128 Wessely S. and Powell R. 'Fatigue Syndromes: a comparison of chronic "postviral" fatigue with neuromuscular and affective disorders.' (*Journal of Neurology, Neurosurgery, and Psychiatry*, 1989, 52, 940–948.)

129 Wessely S. 'Myalgic encephalomyelitis — a warning: discussion paper.' (*Journal of the Royal Society of Medicine*, 1989, 82, 215–217.)

130 Winbow, A. 'Myalgic Encephalomyelitis presenting as a psychiatric illness.' (*British Journal of Clinical and Social Psychology*, 1986, 4, 30–31.)

131 Wood G.C. et al. 'A comparative psychiatric assessment of

patients with Chronic Fatigue Syndrome and muscle disease.' (*Psychological Medicine*, 1991, 21, 619–628.)

Research: miscellaneous

132 Bowles N.E. et al. 'Dermatomyositis, Polymyositis and Coxsackie B virus infection.' (*The Lancet*, 1987, 1, 1004–1007.)

133 Demitrack M.A. and Greden J.F. 'Chronic Fatigue Syndrome: The Need for an Integrative Approach.' (*Biological Psychiatry* (Editorial). 1991, 30, 747–752.)

134 McKinlay M.A. et al. 'Use of WIN 51711 to prevent Echo virus type I induced paralysis in suckling mice.' (*Journal of Infectious Diseases*, 1986, 154, 678–681.)

135 Middleton D. et al. 'No Association of HLA Class II antigens in Chronic Fatigue Syndrome.' (*Disease Markers*, 1991, 9, 47–49.)

136 Oldstone M.B.A. 'Viral alteration of cell function.' (*Scientific American*, 1989, 261, 34–40.)

137 Oldstone M.B.A. 'Viral persistence and disease, cytopathology in the absence of cytolysis.' (*British Medical Bulletin*, 1991, 47, 4. 838–851.)

138 Riley M.S. et al. 'Aerobic work capacity in patients with Chronic Fatigue Syndrome.' (*British Medical Journal*, 1990, 301, 953–956.)

139 Roberts A. 'Loss of form in young athletes due to viral infection.' (*British Medical Journal*, 1985, 290, 357–358.)

140 Sharpe M.C. et al. 'A report — Chronic Fatigue Syndrome: Guidelines for research.' (*Journal of the Royal Society of Medicine*, 1991, 84, 118–121.)

141 Simpson L. 'Nondiscocytic erythrocytes in Myalgic Encephalomyelitis.' (*New Zealand Medical Journal*, 1989, 22 March, 126–127.)

142 Simpson L.O. 'Are M.E. and Chronic Fatigue Syndrome the same disease?' (*New Zealand Medical Journal*, 1990, 103, 305.)

143 Southern P. and Oldstone M.A. 'Medical consequences of Persistent Viral Infection.' (*New England Journal of Medicine*, 1986, 314, 359.)

Treatment

144 Anon. 'Fluoxetine (Prozac), suicide and aggression.' (*Drug and Therapeutics Bulletin*, 1992, 30, 5-6.)

145 Collignon P. 'Immunoglobin treatment for Chronic Fatigue Syndrome.' (*American Journal of Medicine*, 1991, 94, 4, 443.) See also reply by Lloyd A. et al. pages 443-3.

146 Cotton P. 'Treatment with Ampligen' (news item). (*Journal American Medical Association*, 1991, 226, 2667-2668.)

147 Gantz N.M. and Holmes G.P. 'Treatment of patients with Chronic Fatigue Syndrome.' (*Drugs*, 1989, 36, 6: 855-862.)

148 Ho-Yen DO. 'Patient management of Postviral Fatigue Syndrome.' (*Journal of the British Journal of General Practice*, 1990, 40, 37-39.)

149 Kaslow J.E. et al. 'Liver extract — folic acid — cyanocobalamin vs placebo for Chronic Fatigue Syndrome.' (*Archives of Internal Medicine*, 1989, 149, 2501-2503.)

150 Lane R.J.M. et al. 'A double-blind, placebo-controlled, crossover study of verapamil in exertional muscle pain.' (*Muscle and Nerve*, 1986, 9, 635-641.)

151 Lloyd A. et al. 'A double-blind, placebo-controlled trial of intravenous immunoglobulin therapy in patients with Chronic Fatigue Syndrome.' (*American Journal of Medicine*, 1990, 89, 561-568.)

152 Peel M. 'Rehabilitation in Postviral Syndrome.' (*Journal of the Society of Occupational Medicine*, 1988, 38, 44-45.)

153 Peterson R.K. et al. 'A controlled trial of intravenous immunoglobulin G in Chronic Fatigue Syndrome.' (*American Journal of Medicine*, 1990, 89, 554-560.)

154 Rozenberg G.A. et al. 'Amantadine, fatigue and multiple sclerosis.' (*Arch Neurology*, 1988, 45, 1104-1106.)

155 Shepherd C. 'Helping M.E. patients help themselves.' (*Mims Magazine*, 1990, 1st July, 39-41.)

156 Shepherd C. 'Relieving Postviral Fatigue.' (*Pulse*, 1991, October 5th, page 69.)

157 Straus S.E. et al. 'Acyclovir treatment of Chronic Fatigue Syndrome. Lack of efficacy in a placebo-controlled trial.' (*New England Journal of Medicine*, 1988, 26, 1692-1698.)

158 Walton J. 'Diffuse exercise-induced muscle pain of undetermined cause relieved by verapamil.' (*The Lancet*, 1981, 1, 993.)

159 Webster. 'Intravenous immunoglobulins' (Editorial). (*British Medical Journal*, 1991, 303, 375–376.) Letter 716 (Shepherd).

Treatment: alternative approaches

160 Baldwin C.A. et al.'What pharmacists should know about ginseng'. (*The Pharmaceutical Journal*, 8 November 1986, 583–586.)

161 Behan P.O. and Behan W.M.H. 'Essential fatty acids in the treatment of Postviral Fatigue Syndrome.' In D.F. Horrobin (Ed.) *Omega-6 Essential Fatty Acids. Pathophysiology and Roles in Clinical Medicine.* (NY: Wiley-Liss, 1990, 275–282.)

162 Behan P.O., Behan W.M.H. and Horrobin D. 'Effect of high doses of essential fatty acids on the Postviral Syndrome.' (*Acta Neurologica Scandinavica*, 1990, 82, 209–216.)

163 Brush M. 'Is Pyridoxine safe?' (*Mims Magazine*, 15.8.86, 31–32.)

164 Campbell D. and Townson N. 'Pretty Poison (Germanium).' (*New Statesman and Society*, 8 September 1989, 10–12.)

165 Campbell D. and Townson N. 'Let them eat shit (probiotics).' (*New Statesman and Society*, 8 June 1989, 10–12.)

166 Cohen M. 'Chinese Medicine in the treatment of chronic immunodeficiency: diagnosis and treatment.' (*American Journal of Acupuncture*, 1990, 18, 111–112.)

167 Cox I.M. et al. 'Red Blood Cell magnesium and Chronic Fatigue Syndrome.' (*The Lancet*, 1991, 337, 757–760.) See also letters on pages 1094–1095 (Wessely, Young and Trimble, Richmond, Shepherd), 1295 (Cox et al, Davies, Walden), 338: 66 (Ganz), 641 (Deulofeu).

168 Dalton K. 'Toxicity of Vitamins (B6).' (*British Medical Journal*, 1986, 292, 903.)

169 Dismukes W.E. et al. 'A randomized, double-blind trial of Nystatin therapy for the candidiasis hypersensitivity syndrome.' (*New England Journal of Medicine*, 1990, 323, 1717–1723. Editorial in the same issue on pages 1766–1767, and follow-up letters on pages 1592–1594.)

170 Evans C.D.H. and Lacey J.H. 'Toxicity of Vitamins:

complications of a health movement.' (*British Medical Journal*, 1986, 292, 509-510.)

171 Fisher P. et al. 'Effect of homoeopathic treatment on fibrositis (primary fibromyalgia).' (*British Medical Journal*, 1989, 299, 365-366.)

172 Hunter J.O. 'Food allergy — or enterometabolic disorder?' (*The Lancet*, 1991, 338, 495-496.)

173 Jenkins M. 'Thoughts on the management of M.E.' (*British Journal of Homoeopathy*, 1989, 78, 6-14.)

174 Katelaris, C.H. et al. 'Vega testing in the diagnosis of allergic conditions.' (*Medical Journal of Australia*, 1991, 155, 113-114.)

175 Lewis J.G. 'Adverse Reactions to Vitamins.' (*Adverse Drug Reaction Bulletin*, 82, 296-299.)

176 Matsusaka T. et al. 'Germanium-induced nephropathy: report of two cases and review of the literature.' (*Clinical Nephrology*, 1988, 30, 341-345.)

177 MacGregor F.B. et al. 'Hepatotoxicity of herbal remedies (Valerian).' (*British Medical Journal*, 1989, 299, 1156-1157.)

178 Renfro L. et al. 'Yeast connection among 100 patients with chronic fatigue.' (*American Journal of Medicine*, 1989, 86, 165-168.)

179 Shepherd C. *Alternative Approaches to M.E.* Available from the M.E. Association.

180 Straus S.E. et al. 'Allergy and the Chronic Fatigue Syndrome.' (*Journal of Allergy and Clinical Immunology*, 1988, 82, 791-795.)

Virology: enteroviruses

181 Archard L.C. et al. 'Postviral Fatigue Syndrome: persistence of enteroviral RNA in muscle and elevated creatine kinase.' (*Journal of the Royal Society of Medicine*, 1988, 81, 326-329.)

182 Bell E.J. 'Coxsackie B viruses and myalgic encephalomyelitis.' (*Journal of the Royal Society of Medicine*, 1988, 81, 329-331.)

183 Bendinelli M. and Friedmann H. *Coxsackie Viruses — A General Update.* (Plenum Press, New York and London 1988.) The most authoritative reference book on Coxsackie infections.

184 Calder B.D. et al. 'Coxsackie B Viruses and the Postviral Syndrome — a prospective study in General Practice.' (*Journal of the Royal College of General Practitioners*, 1987, 37, 11–14.)

185 Cunningham L. et al. 'Persistence of enteroviral RNA in Chronic Fatigue Syndrome is associated with the abnormal production of equal amounts of positive and negative strands of enteroviral RNA.' (*Journal of General Virology*, 1990, 71, 1399–1402.)

186 Dowsett E.G. 'Human enterovirus infections.' (*Journal of Hospital Infection*, 1988, 11, 103–115.)

187 Gow J.W. et al. 'Enteroviral sequences detected by polymerase chain reaction in muscles of patients with Postviral Fatigue Syndrome.' (*British Medical Journal*, 1991, 302, 692–696.)

188 Halpin D. and Wessely S. 'VP-1 Antigen in Chronic Postviral Fatigue Syndrome.' (*The Lancet*, 1989, May 6th, 1028–1029.)

189 Loria R.M. 'Host conditions affecting the course of Coxsackie virus infections' in Bendinelli and Friedmann Eds. *Coxsackie viruses — A general update*. (Plenum Press, New York and London, 1988, 135–157.)

190 Lynch S. and Seth R. 'Postviral Fatigue Syndrome and the VP-1 antigen.' (*The Lancet*, November 11th, 1989, 1160–1161.)

191 Matteucci D. et al. 'Group B Coxsackie viruses readily establish persistent infections in human lymphoid cell lines.' (*Journal of Virology*, 1985, 56, 651–654.)

192 Melnick J.L. 'Enteroviruses' in *Textbook of Virology by Fields*. (Raven Press, New York, 1985, 739–794.)

193 Miller N.A. et al. 'Antibody to Coxsackie B virus in diagnosing Postviral Fatigue Syndrome.' (*British Medical Journal*, 1991, 302, 140–143.)

194 Yousef G.K. et al. 'Chronic enteroviral infection in patients with Postviral Fatigue Syndrome (the VP1 test).' (*The Lancet*, 1988, 1, 146–150.)

Virology: Epstein–Barr, HHV6 and retroviruses
195 Archard L. et al. 'Detection of Epstein–Barr virus DNA in

muscle from patients with Postviral Fatigue Syndrome.'
(*Journal of Experimental Clinical Cancer Research*, 1988, 7,
142.)

196 Buchwald D. et al. 'Frequency of "chronic active Epstein-
Barr Infection" in a General Medical Practice.' (*Journal of
The American Medical Association*, 1987, 257, 2303-2307.)

197 De Freitas et al. 'Retroviral sequences related to human
T-lymphotrophic virus type 11 in patients with Chronic
Fatigue Immune Dysfunction Syndrome.' (*Proceedings of the
National Academy of Sciences* (USA), 1991, 81, 2922-2926.)

198 Gold D. et al. 'Chronic fatigue: a prospective clinical and
virological study.' (*Journal of the American Medical
Association*, 1990, 264, 1, 48-53.)

199 Hamblin T.J. et al. 'Immunological reasons for ill-health
after infectious mononucleosis.' (*British Medical Journal*,
1983, 287, 85-88.)

200 Holmes G.P. et al. 'A cluster of patients with a chronic
mononucleosis-like syndrome. Is Epstein-Barr Virus the
Cause?' (*Journal of The American Medical Association*, 1987,
259, 2297-2302.)

201 Hotchin N.A. et al. 'Active Epstein-Barr virus infection in
Postviral Fatigue Syndrome.' (*Journal of Infection*, 1989, 18,
143-150.)

202 Jones J. 'Serological and immunological responses in
Chronic Fatigue Syndrome with emphasis on Epstein-Barr
virus.' (*Reviews of infectious diseases*, 1991, 13 (Supp), 26-31.)

203 Josephs S.F. et al. 'HHV-6 reactivation in Chronic Fatigue
Syndrome.' (*The Lancet*, 1991, 337, 1346-1347.)

204 Straus S.F. 'EB or not EB — that is the question!' (*Journal of
the American Medical Association*, 1987, 259, 2335-2336.)

Research into myalgic encephalomyelitis

This is a list of the most useful books, magazine articles and
research papers which have been published in the medical
journals.

Books

British Medical Bulletin, 1991, 47, 4 — 'Postviral Fatigue Syndrome' edited by P.O. Behan, D. Goldberg and J.F. Mowbray

with an introduction by Sir Donald Acheson. Detailed coverage of molecular biology, clinical aspects, history and psychiatry. Available from Churchill Livingstone, 1–3 Baxter's Place, Edinburgh EH1 3AF. Price £29.95 (U.K.), $56 (Canada/USA) and £35 overseas.

CFIDS: A Disease of a Thousand Names by Dr David Bell. (M. D. Pollard Publications U.S.A., 1991). A comprehensive account of recent American research and approaches to management by a paediatrician who has looked after a large number of children with M.E. Obtainable by post from CFIDS (see Useful Addresses) in America.

Post-Viral Fatigue Syndrome, edited by Dr Rachel Jenkins and Professor James Mowbray (Wiley, Chichester, 1991.) An expensive (£60) and comprehensive medical textbook which includes contributions from a variety of specialists and researchers. Available from the publishers direct: John Wiley and Sons Ltd, Baffins Lane, Chichester, West Sussex, PO19 1UD, U.K.

A Year Lost and Found by the Very Reverend Michael Mayne, Dean of Westminster. A personal account of living with the illness by the M.E. Association's Vice President. Available from Darton, Longman and Todd Ltd, 89 Lillie Road, London SW6 1UD.

Myalgic Encephalomyelitis and Postviral Fatigue States — The Saga of Royal Free Disease by Dr Melvin Ramsay. This book gives an excellent historical account of the numerous outbreaks of the illness that have occurred throughout the world since 1934. Published by Gower Medical Ltd, London, 1988.

Magazine articles

'Raggedy Ann Town' by William Boly (*In Health* July/August 1987). An excellent review that pieces together the CFIDS puzzle in America, the Lake Tahoe outbreak, and the subsequent involvement of medical and political figures in the ensuing debate.

'Chronic Fatigue Syndrome: A Modern Medical Mystery', by Geoffrey Cowley and others (*Newsweek*, 12 November 1990). An in-depth study of the latest research findings from America along with several patient profiles.

Reprints of both are available from CFIDS in America (see Useful Addresses).

'On the Track of an Elusive Disease' by Joseph Palca (*Science*, 1991, vol. 254, pages 1726-1728), takes a critical look at the American research into retroviruses and spumaviruses as possible causes of M.E.

Other Useful Books and Pamphlets

General

The Health Directory compiled by Fiona Macdonald with help from the Patients Association and the College of Health. An invaluable book that lists about 1,000 organisations which have been set up to help patients and their families with common (and not so common) health problems. Available from bookshops, price £6.95, or from Plymbridge Distributors Ltd, Estover Road, Plymouth PL6 7PZ, price £7.82.

Patients' Rights is a helpful free leaflet published by the National Consumers Council and the Association of Community Health Councils for England and Wales. It explains how to use the NHS without compromising your personal rights and responsibilities. Topics covered include how to find a general practitioner, referral to hospital, obtaining a second opinion, being informed about your medical records, confidentiality and complaints against doctors and hospitals. The leaflet is printed in nine ethnic languages as well. Available from your local Community Health Council (see the phone book) or by writing to the Association of Community Health Councils, 30 Drayton Park, London N5 1PB.

Allergies

Allergy: the facts by R Davies and S Ollier (Oxford University Press, 1989), £4.95. This is a sound book for lay readers on a topical and controversial subject. I would recommend it to patients with allergies who wish to find out more.

The Complete Guide to Food Allergy and Intolerance by Dr Jonathan Brostoff and Linda Gamlin (Bloomsbury, 1989, £4.99). Explains why certain foods can cause problems for some people and how to identify and eliminate the culprits. Also covers many of the unorthodox approaches to allergy investigation and treatment.

The British Allergy Foundation (see Useful Addresses) is a national charity whose aims are to increase the understanding of allergy, to help patients overcome its effects and to fund various research projects. They publish a series of useful leaflets on eczema, hay fever, rhinitis, urticaria, etc.

Alternative approaches
The Readers Digest Family Guide to Alternative Medicine (£24.95) is a comprehensive but rather uncritical guide to most aspects of alternative medicine.

Anxiety, panic attacks and tranquillisers
Understanding Anxiety is available by post from MIND Mail Order, 4th Floor, 24–32 Stephenson Way, London NW1 2HD, price 25p.

Understanding Stress is published by the Consumers Association, and is available from them direct at Which? Books, Castlemead, Gascoyne Way, Hertford X, SG14 1LH, price £8.95.

Self-help for your Nerves by Clare Weeks (Angus and Robertson, 1981).

Phobias and Obsessions by Joy Melville (Unwin Press, 1979).

Agoraphobia — Simple Effective Treatment by Clare Weeks (Angus and Robertson, 1990).

Coming off Tranquillisers and Sleeping Pills by Shirley Trickett (Thorsons, 1986). A step-by-step guide to withdrawal from tranquillisers which takes into account the wide variety of withdrawal symptoms and ways of coping with them.

Candida albicans
The Yeast Connection by Dr William Crook MD (Random House, 1988). Describes the alternative view on the yeast allergy syndrome and its treatment.

Carers
Caring at Home by Nancy Kohner (National Extension College, Cambridge, £2.50). Essential reading for any carer, and packed with useful information. Available by post from the King's Fund Centre, 126 Albert Street, London NW1 7NF. Tel (071) 267 6111.

Help at Hand from the Association of Carers (see Useful Addresses), price £1.

Depression
Understanding Depression is available by post from MIND Mail Order (for address see *Anxiety*), price 25p.
Coping with depression by Ivy Blackburn (Chambers).
Depression, The Way Out of Your Prison by Dorothy Rowe (Routledge, 1983).

DSS Benefits
Disability Rights Handbook is published by the Disability Alliance (see Useful Addresses), £4.50 post free. This is the most comprehensive publication available on all the different DSS benefit entitlements. It also covers appeal procedures in detail and is thoroughly updated every April.

Also from the Disability Alliance:
Guide to Benefits for Children with Disabilities and their Families.
Guide to the Disability Living Allowance and Disability Working Allowance.
Severe Disablement Allowance — hard to claim, impossible to live on.

Disability: practical problems
The A—Z of Disability is a directory of information, services, organisations and manufacturers by Pat Saunders (Marlborough: Crowood Press, 1989, £8.95). The author, who is severely disabled, provides a lively and entertaining read as he gives his experiences of coping and helping others to cope with disability.

Everyday Aids and Appliances includes articles from the British *Medical Journal* edited by G P Mulley. Published by the British Medical Association (see Useful Addresses) 1989, £6.95. Sixteen different chapters dealing with practical aids for all manner of disability.

More Everyday Aids and Appliances acts as a companion volume to the first book, and concentrates on aids which enable people to manage at home despite impaired mobility, those that improve mobility both at home and outside, and appliances that compensate for damage to the eyes, teeth, hair, etc. Published by the *British Medical Journal*, London, 1991, £8.95.

The Department of Transport publishes an excellent guide called *Door to Door* giving information on all kinds of mobility problems. Available from libraries and the HMSO, or by writing to the Department of Transport (Door to Door Guide), Freepost, Victoria Road, South Ruislip, Middlesex HA4 0NZ.

Drug information

The best source for reliable information on common drugs is your local pharmacist. Most large hospitals also have a drug information officer in their pharmacy department. They are usually extremely helpful, especially with more unusual queries, but are not always happy about responding to requests from members of the general public.

The British National Formulary is concise and revised every six months. It gives a fairly comprehensive guide to costs, side-effects, drug interactions and comparisons of drugs used for treating specific conditions. Published by the British Medical Association and the Royal Pharmaceutical Society of Great Britain.

Martindale: The Extra Pharmacopoeia is the best book for anyone seeking detailed information on drugs. It is particularly useful for information on adverse effects, precautions and interactions, with numerous references to relevant medical papers and brief summaries of original articles describing clinical use. Martindale is very expensive to buy, but it may be available in some large libraries or at the local hospital. Your local pharmacist may even have a copy if you ask nicely! Published by The Pharmaceutical Press, London.

Herbal medicines

The Drug and Therapeutics Bulletin (15 December 1986) is a publication for doctors: it carried an excellent review of both the benefits and possible side-effects from herbal medicines.

Information on individual herbs can be found in:

British Herbal Pharmacopoeia, published in three volumes by the British Herbal Medicine Association, London, a scientific committee of herbalists, pharmacologists, pharmacists and doctors. It's very comprehensive.

The Encyclopedia of Herbs and Herbalism by M. Stuart (Orbis, 1979) gives medicinal uses of 400-plus herbs.

Mary Grieve's *A Modern Herbal* (Penguin, 1977) combines ancient and traditional folklore on the subject, as well as botanical descriptions, medicinal usage and dosage.

Homeopathy
Introduction to Homeopathic Medicine by H. Boyd (Beaconsfield, 1981).

Relaxation
Breath of Life — Undoing Muscular Tension is a tape produced by the British Holistic Medical Association (see Useful Addresses), which some patients have found helpful.

Cassette tapes to help with relaxation can also be obtained from Relaxation for Living and Lifeskills (see Useful Addresses).

Addendum: further references

Dowsett E.G. and Welsby P.D. 'Conversation Piece.' (*Postgraduate Medical Journal*, 1992, 68, 63–65.)

Ehud U. et al. 'Hypothesis: cytokines may be activated to cause depressive illness and chronic fatigue syndrome.' (*European Archives of Psychiatry and Clinical Neuroscience*, Spring 1992.)

Ho-Yen D.O. et al. 'Natural Killer Cells and the Post-Viral Fatigue Syndrome.' (*Scandinavian Journal of Infectious Diseases*, 1991, 23, 711–716.)

Lloyd A. et al. 'Cell-mediated immunity in patients with chronic fatigue syndrome, healthy control subjects and patients with major depression.' (*Clinical and Experimental Immunology*, 1992, 87, 76–79.)

Riccio M. et al. 'Neuropsychological and psychiatric abnormalities in myalgic encephalomyelitis: A preliminary report.' (*British Journal of Clinical Psychology*, 1992, 31, 111–120.

Wood C. et al. 'Fluctuations in perceived energy and mood among patients with chronic fatigue syndrome.' (*Journal of the Royal Society of Medicine*, 1992, 85, 195–198.)

Wessely S. 'The measurement of fatigue and chronic fatigue syndrome.' (*Journal of the Royal Society of Medicine*, 1992, 85, 189–90.)

INDEX

A Full List of Cedar Books

While every effort is made to keep prices low, it is sometimes necessary to increase prices at short notice. Mandarin Paperbacks reserves the right to show new retail prices on covers which may differ from those previously advertised in the text or elsewhere.

The prices shown below were correct at the time of going to press.

☐ 7493 0794 3	**Finding Love, Keeping Love**	Judith Sills	£4.99
☐ 7493 0526 6	**Coming Back**	Ann Kaiser Sterns	£5.99
☐ 7493 0936 9	**The Courage to Grieve**	Judith Tatelbaum	£5.99
☐ 7493 0718 8	**Seeds of Greatness**	Denis Waitley	£4.99
☐ 7493 1210 6	**Divorce Hangover**	Anne Walther	£5.99
☐ 7493 1049 9	**Irritable Bowel Syndrome**	Geoff Watts	£5.99

All these books are available at your bookshop or newsagent, or can be ordered direct from the publisher. Just tick the titles you want and fill in the form below.

Mandarin Paperbacks, Cash Sales Department, PO Box 11, Falmouth, Cornwall TR10 9EN.

Please send cheque or postal order, no currency, for purchase price quoted and allow the following for postage and packing:

UK including BFPO   £1.00 for the first book, 50p for the second and 30p for each additional book ordered to a maximum charge of £3.00.

Overseas including Eire   £2 for the first book, £1.00 for the second and 50p for each additional book thereafter.

NAME (Block letters) ....

ADDRESS...

....

☐ I enclose my remittance for ....

☐ I wish to pay by Access/Visa Card Number ☐☐☐☐☐☐☐☐☐☐☐☐☐☐☐☐

Expiry Date ☐☐☐☐